PREVENTION'S GIANT BOOK OF HEALTH FACTS

The Ultimate Reference for Personal Health

By the Editors of *Prevention* Magazine Health Books

Introduction by Mark Bricklin, Editor, *Prevention* Magazine

Edited by John Feltman

 Rodale Press, Emmaus, Pennsylvania

If you have any questions or comments concerning this book, please
write:
    Rodale Press
    Book Readers' Service
    33 East Minor Street
    Emmaus, PA 18098

Library of Congress Cataloging-in-Publication Data

Prevention's giant book of health facts : the ultimate reference for
    personal health / by the editors of Prevention magazine health
    books ; introduction by Mark Bricklin ; edited by John Feltman.
        p.   cm.
    Includes index.
    ISBN 0-87857-909-5   hardcover
    1. Medicine, Popular—Handbooks, manuals, etc.   I. Feltman,
John.   II. Prevention (Emmaus, Pa.)   III. Title: Giant book of
health facts.
RC81.P857   1990
613—dc20   90-45939
                                                            CIP

Distributed in the book trade by St. Martin's Press

    6 8 10 9 7   hardcover

Contributors

Editor: John Feltman

Contributing Writers: Lance Jacobs
William LeGro
Judith Lin
Claudia Allen
Ellen Michaud
Don Wade
Russell Wild

Book Designer: Denise Mirabello

Associate Designer: Greg Imhoff

Technical Artist: Lisa Carpenter

Intern: Stacia Hickman

Illustrators: Byrne Advertising
Jack Crane
Leslie Flis
Greg Imhoff
Stewart Jackson
Narda Lebo
Karen Mettejat
Patti Rutman
Robert Zimmerman

Research Chief: Ann Gossy

Research Planning Editor: Holly Clemson

Research/Fact-Checking Staff: Anne Castaldo
Anna Crawford
Christine Dreisbach
Jan Eickmeier
Staci Hadeed
Karen Lombardi
Paris Mihely-Muchanic
Linda Miller
Cynthia Nickerson
Sandra Salera-Lloyd

Production Editor: Jane Sherman

Copy Editor: Mary Green

Office Staff: Roberta Mulliner
Eve Buchay
Karen Earl-Braymer

Senior Managing Editor, Prevention *Magazine Health Books:* Debora Tkac

Executive Editor, Prevention *Magazine Health Books:* Carol Keough

Vice President and Editor in Chief, Prevention *Magazine Health Books:* William Gottlieb

Group Vice President, Health: Mark Bricklin

CONTENTS

INTRODUCTION

Nothing is growing faster than health knowledge these days. Except maybe health confusion.

You know, for instance, that if your blood pressure is 120 over 80, it's well within the normal range. And you know that's good because high blood pressure puts you at greater risk for stroke and heart disease. But . . . what if your pressure is 158/85? Is that still normal? And what about your 16-year-old son's blood pressure? What's normal for a teenager?

A friend asked me that question a while ago, and I didn't know the answer.

"Wouldn't it be good," he said, "if there was a book that had very specific information like that about all kinds of health questions?"

An excellent suggestion, I thought. And since my friend was Robert Teufel, president of Rodale Press, we wasted little time in making that suggestion a reality.

In these pages, you'll be able to find exact answers to a host of health questions that most people are . . . well, *confused* about. We *should* know the answers, but don't. And confusion is a poor starting point for building good health habits, or knowing when and where to find the right medical answer to your problem.

Do you know, for instance, the very best exercises for strengthening a low back that's been giving you grief? In my experience, not even people with a long history of back problems know the answer to that one. But . . . it's right here in this book.

Can you get AIDS in a public restroom? Rest easy, that answer is here, too.

Are those aches and pains just a nuisance, or are they announcing arthritis? The answer's important, because early treatment can make a world of difference if you *do* have arthritis. While only a doctor can make the diagnosis, this book will give you the clues to watch out for.

How safe are coronary bypasses? What about balloon angioplasty?

Just what constitutes a "safe" cholesterol level? Is 220 really dangerous? And what does the HDL level on my cholesterol report mean? Is a "60" high or low?

What should I eat to lower my cholesterol if it's really high? I've heard this and that, but what are the *facts*?

Is the Midwest the worst place to retire to if you have allergies? And is that new home going to be smack in the middle of a "tornado alley"? Where should you live (or not live) if you have a near-phobia of lightning?

Those answers, too, are now here at your fingertips.

So are an amazing wealth of other answers, ranging from the super practical to the simply amazing.

How do I choose the best antacid?

How can I avoid the osteoporosis that gave Aunt Marian a broken hip?

How should I handle a lost filling until the dentist can see me?

What causes gallstones? Is surgery the only answer?

How dangerous is it for my son to play high school football?

A friend just gave me some herbal medicines that are supposed to boost my immune system. Do they really work? Are they *safe*?

What does that odd writing on my prescription label mean? Why can't they write it in plain English?

I get flu nearly every year. But a nurse told me I'm too young to get flu shots. Is she right?

I'm taking a vacation to New Zealand. Is traveler's diarrhea a serious risk there?

I drink very little milk. How can I get enough vitamin D in my diet to avoid bone problems?

Are the ads on TV for diet pills true? Is there any danger they don't tell you about?

Can someone give me the facts, please, about all the different kinds of contact lenses?

I've been taking beta-blockers for years. But what exactly are they doing for me, and how?

Prevention's Giant Book of Health Facts is here to guide you through all these tricky questions and more. We think you will find it a fascinating "read" and a valued reference work as well.

Mark Bricklin, Editor
Prevention Magazine

1

ACCIDENTS

Just when you least expect it, there's an accident. Yet car crashes, drownings, falls, fires, poisonings, and other mishaps occur with such numbing regularity that they can hardly be considered unexpected. Your chances of being involved in a fatal accident within a one-year period are about half that of Americans who lived a couple of generations ago, but that doesn't mean you can stop looking both ways when you cross the street. Chances are still about 1 in 2,600 that you will die as the result of an accident, and that's no small risk.

More than 73 million accidental injuries occur in the United States every year. And the consequences are serious. In 1987, for example, almost 9 million people were disabled and 94,000 others died as a result of accidents. Every hour, 11 Americans die from accidents and another 1,000 are injured. Americans lose more working years through accidents than from all forms of cancer and heart disease combined. The price paid for these mishaps, from doctor bills to property damage, is astronomical. In 1987, for instance, accidents cost $133.2 billion, an amount equal to almost half the U.S. defense budget.

Most disabling accidents occur in the home. But most accidental deaths occur out on the streets, where cars, motorcycles, trucks, and other vehicles swerve into trees, run red lights, and otherwise do life-threatening damage. And just in case you think you're safe once you leave the dangerous confines of your home and arrive in one piece at work, take note: Americans suffered nearly 2 million disabling injuries and 11,000 deaths on the job in 1987.

Your own chances of having an accident depend on a wide variety of factors. Your age, your sex, your job, your personality—these things and more figure into the equation. What's certain is that two out of every three Americans suffer some sort of accidental injury each year. So be careful out there.

1

Who Dies in Accidents

Your statistical risk of being fatally injured in an accident changes as you age. The danger is especially great between the ages of 15 and 24. Then it declines, but only for awhile. Once you reach 75, you have three times the risk you had at a younger age.

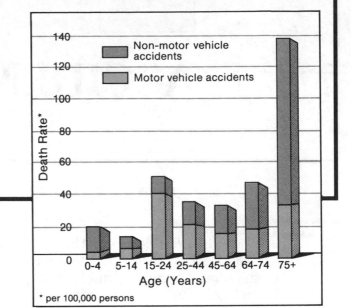

* per 100,000 persons

Number of accidents each year related to amusement park rides and attractions: 6,484.

Number of accidents each year related to bunk beds: 33,629.

Leading Causes of Death

Among people aged 75 and older, falls are the leading cause of accidental death, in part because of the high incidence of life-threatening hip fractures. Motor vehicles are the single most common cause of accidental death in every other age group.

Age	No. 1 Cause of Accidental Death	No. 2 Cause of Accidental Death
0–4	Motor vehicles	Fires and burns
5–14	Motor vehicles	Drowning
15–24	Motor vehicles	Drowning
25–44	Motor vehicles	Poisoning by solids or liquids
45–64	Motor vehicles	Falls
65–74	Motor vehicles	Falls
75+	Falls	Motor vehicles

Choking on food or another object is the second leading cause of accidental death (after falls) for persons aged 90 and over.

Men Are at Greater Risk

A man is more likely than a woman to be involved in a fatal accident. In one recent year, 93,457 accidental deaths occurred. Men accounted for 64,160 of them, or 69 percent. The chart shows a breakdown according to type of accident.

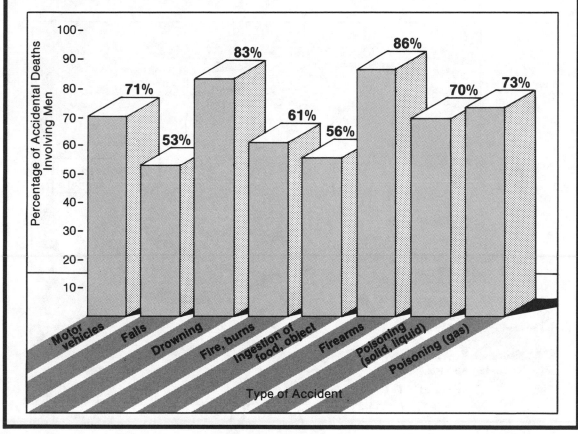

Percentage of Accidental Deaths Involving Men

- Motor vehicles: 71%
- Falls: 53%
- Drowning: 83%
- Fire, burns: 61%
- Ingestion of food, object: 56%
- Firearms: 86%
- Poisoning (solid, liquid): 70%
- Poisoning (gas): 73%

Type of Accident

Some studies suggest that left-handers have more accidents than right-handers. In reviewing records of 2,300 deceased major-league baseball players, researchers at the University of British Columbia found that lefties had more serious accidents and died earlier than right-handers. And a study of university students showed that 44 percent of left-handers, compared to 36 percent of right-handers, suffered accidents that required medical attention.

Where It Hurts

Of the more than 73 million accidental injuries that occur in the United States every year, open wounds and lacerations are the most common (nearly 18 million). Bruises, fractures, and sprains also occur frequently.

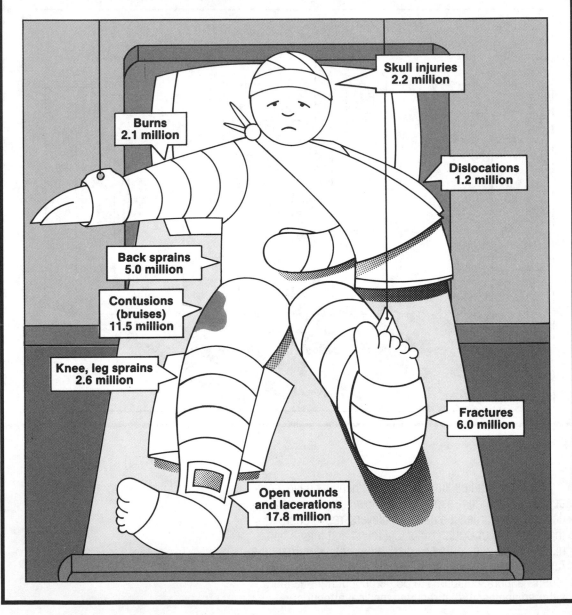

Every 4 Seconds . . .

In the time it takes for the second hand on your watch to tick four times, someone will suffer an accidental injury in the United States. Every 6 minutes, one of those accidents will be fatal.

Type of Accident	One Injury Every . . .	One Death Every . . .
All accidents	4 seconds	6 minutes
Home	10 seconds	26 minutes
Motor vehicle	18 seconds	11 minutes
Work	18 seconds	47 minutes

People who talk on cellular telephones in their cars may be "an accident waiting to happen," says the Insurance Information Institute. Riskier yet, the stress of receiving emotional news — whether good or bad — over a car phone could be all a driver needs to go over the (center) line.

A ring on your finger can lead to severe injury, reports a University of Wisconsin Medical School surgeon, if you accidentally catch it on something during a fall or get it too near a moving piece of equipment. Such an accident might even result in amputation.

The Most Dangerous Months

Summer is the peak season for fatal accidents in the United States. While January and February start the year slowly, with accidental deaths running below the overall average of 7,830 per month, things start hopping come spring. Fatal accidents reach their peak in August, then decline toward the year's close.

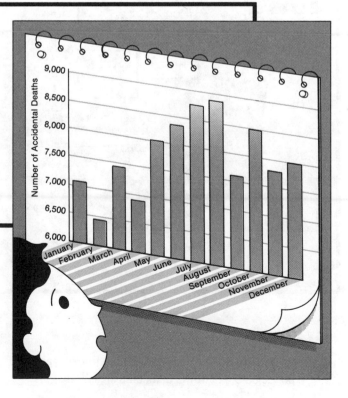

The first reported motor vehicle death in the United States occurred in New York City on September 14, 1899.

Trampoline accidents bounced almost 14,000 people into the hospital in 1988.

The Most Dangerous States

So you like living on the edge? Pack your things and move to Alaska, if you're not already there. More people die in accidents in that state than in any of the lower 49. But you needn't go north to satisfy a desire to live dangerously. New Mexico, Nevada, Mississippi, and South Carolina are also near the top of the high-risk list. Those of us who prefer to live on the safe side would do well to reside in New Jersey, New York, Ohio, or Hawaii.

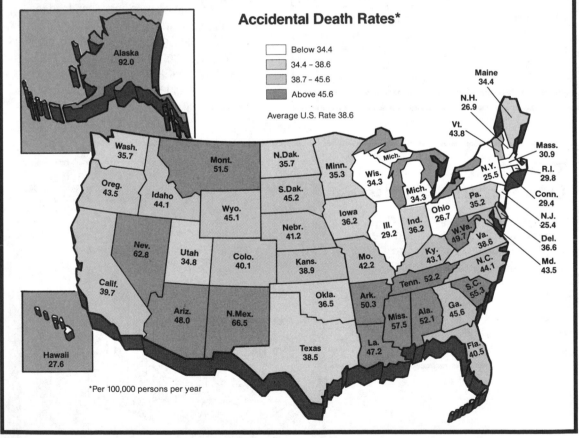

Accidental Death Rates*

Below 34.4
34.4 – 38.6
38.7 – 45.6
Above 45.6

Average U.S. Rate 38.6

Alaska 92.0

Maine 34.4
N.H. 26.9
Vt. 43.8
Mass. 30.9
N.Y. 25.5
R.I. 29.8
Conn. 29.4
N.J. 25.4
Del. 36.6
Md. 43.5

Wash. 35.7
Mont. 51.5
N.Dak. 35.7
Minn. 35.3
Mich.
Wis. 34.3
Mich. 34.3
Pa. 35.2

Oreg. 43.5
Idaho 44.1
Wyo. 45.1
S.Dak. 45.2
Iowa 36.2
Ohio 26.7
W.Va. 49.7
Va. 38.6

Nev. 62.8
Utah 34.8
Colo. 40.1
Nebr. 41.2
Ill. 29.2
Ind. 36.2
Ky. 43.1
N.C. 44.1

Calif. 39.7
Kans. 38.9
Mo. 42.2
Tenn. 52.2
S.C. 55.3

Ariz. 48.0
N.Mex. 66.5
Okla. 36.5
Ark. 50.3
Miss. 57.5
Ala. 52.1
Ga. 45.6

Hawaii 27.6
Texas 38.5
La. 47.2
Fla. 40.5

*Per 100,000 persons per year

About 3,600 ambulances, 3,700 fire trucks, and 20,600 police cars had traffic accidents in 1985.

Peril Is Greatest for Motorcyclists

An accident on a motorcycle, motor scooter, or motor bike is about 17 times more likely to be fatal than one involving a car or other vehicle that affords greater protection. Motorcycle accidents also lead to a higher proportion of injuries, both minor and severe. More than 4,000 people riding motorcycles were killed and another 460,000 injured in motorcycle accidents in 1987.

A sobering fact: A drunk driver is 25 times more likely to have a traffic accident than a person who doesn't drink and drive. More than half of fatal traffic accidents — 22,000 fatalities in 1987 — may have involved alcohol. Alcohol was also implicated in about 320,000 injuries and 1.6 million accidents that caused property damage. The estimated annual cost of alcohol-related motor vehicle accidents is $13 billion.

High Risks on the Highway

If you're going to have any sort of accident, chances are high that it will involve a passenger car. Most accidents in the United States involve some kind of motor vehicle — 33 million in 1987. Of these, more than three-fourths, or about 26 million, involve passenger cars.

Type of Vehicle	Accidents per Year
Passenger cars	25,900,000 (78.5%)
Trucks	6,000,000 (18.2%)
Motorcycles	360,000 (1.1%)
Commercial buses	140,000 (0.4%)
Taxicabs	100,000 (0.3%)
School buses	50,000 (0.1%)
Motor scooters, motorbikes	20,000 (0.1%)
Other	430,000 (1.3%)

Seventy-eight percent of adults reported in a 1988 survey that they never drive after drinking. But don't stop driving defensively: A small but nevertheless dangerous 3 percent of adults said that they drive after they drink *all the time*.

More people die in motor vehicle accidents at night than during the day. Driving at night in rural areas holds the highest risk for motor vehicle fatalities.

Is THAT A FACT?

People thrown clear from a vehicle in an accident have a lower risk of injury than those remaining inside.

Not true. There is a higher risk of serious injury or death for passengers who are ejected during an accident. A British study shows that 32 percent of ejected passengers suffered serious injury or died, compared with 6 percent of those who remained in the vehicle.

Best and Worst Drivers

That wild 17-year-old down the block may be a maniac behind the wheel, and indeed drivers under age 20 do have the highest accident rate. But drivers aged 20 to 24 and 75 or over, not teenagers, have the highest rate of fatal traffic accidents. Drivers in the 55-to-64 category have the lowest fatal accident rate.

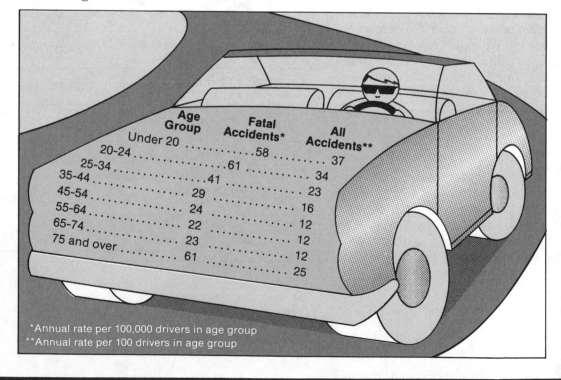

Age Group	Fatal Accidents*	All Accidents**
Under 20	58	37
20-24	61	34
25-34	41	23
35-44	29	16
45-54	24	12
55-64	22	12
65-74	23	12
75 and over	61	25

*Annual rate per 100,000 drivers in age group
**Annual rate per 100 drivers in age group

How Not to Drive

People may simply blame foul weather, poor road conditions, and other factors for their accidents, but traffic authorities say improper driving techniques account for nearly 70 percent of accidents.

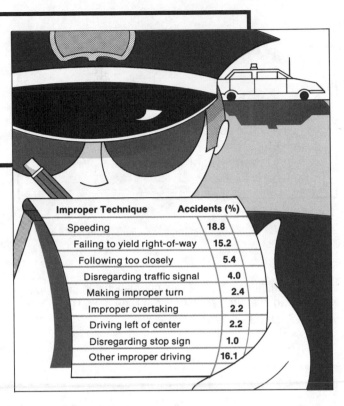

Improper Technique	Accidents (%)
Speeding	18.8
Failing to yield right-of-way	15.2
Following too closely	5.4
Disregarding traffic signal	4.0
Making improper turn	2.4
Improper overtaking	2.2
Driving left of center	2.2
Disregarding stop sign	1.0
Other improper driving	16.1

Drivers in 72 percent of fatal traffic accidents were less than 25 miles from home at the time the accident occurred.

Is THAT A FACT?

Drunk drivers are more likely to escape injury in a car accident because intoxication makes them more "flexible."

Not true. Actually, alcohol intoxication substantially *increases* your chances of injury in a traffic accident, say researchers from the University of North Carolina who reviewed the results of more than a million car crashes. Alcohol has a weakening effect on bones, which can make them more likely to break during an accident. Even more dangerous, alcohol slows blood clotting, making it more likely that you could bleed to death after a severe injury.

High-Risk Holidays

It's just as newscasters say: The holidays really are more dangerous for driving. Traffic deaths during five holiday periods sampled were 6 percent higher than during similar non-holiday periods at the same time of year.

Holiday	Total Deaths	Daily Deaths
Memorial Day (3 days)	550	183.3
Fourth of July (3 days)	550	183.3
Labor Day (4 days)	600	150.0
Christmas Day (4 days)	490	122.5
New Year's Day (4 days)	470	117.5

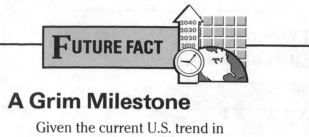

A Grim Milestone

Given the current U.S. trend in motor vehicle deaths, the 3-millionth highway fatality will probably occur in the early 1990s.

Reaching for a soft drink has been the death of some, the cause of severe injuries for others. At least 15 serious accidents have involved people trying to rock a can of soda from a machine that toppled onto them. Injuries included fractures of the toes, ankles, legs, pelvis, and skull, as well as dislocated knees and torn ligaments. Several victims were crushed to death. Soda machines can weigh up to a half-ton when fully loaded.

The highest accident rate per million vehicle-miles in the world is estimated to occur in Nigeria and other East African countries.

Accidents at Home

All may look quiet on the home front, but accidents abound. Americans sustained more than 22 million accidental falls, burns, poisonings, and other injuries at home in 1986. That means that about 1 person in 11 sustained an injury that required medical attention or restricted their activity for a half-day or more. Three million of those injuries were disabling, and 20,500 of them resulted in death.

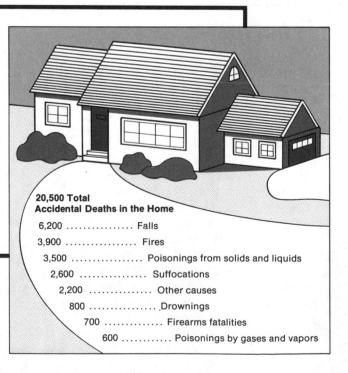

**20,500 Total
Accidental Deaths in the Home**

6,200 .... Falls
3,900 .... Fires
3,500 .... Poisonings from solids and liquids
2,600 .... Suffocations
2,200 .... Other causes
800 .... Drownings
700 .... Firearms fatalities
600 .... Poisonings by gases and vapors

Is Nothing Safe?

Accidents can happen in the weirdest ways. Sometimes, like a scene from a horror film, seemingly innocent objects turn on us, cutting or jabbing, crushing or gagging. The table lists some of the seemingly innocuous objects that landed Americans in the emergency room in 1988.

Item	Injuries	Item	Injuries
Jewelry	40,417	Combs or hairbrushes	3,308
Paper money or coins	29,418	Towels or washcloths	3,130
Light bulbs	8,730	Candles or candlesticks	2,908
Tie and belt racks	8,531	Window shades or venetian blinds	2,875
Pet supplies	7,998		
Toothpicks, hors d'oeuvres picks	7,668	Ironing boards or covers	2,513
		Musical instruments	2,482
Paper products	6,698	Umbrellas	1,960
Luggage	5,964	Hairspray	1,815
Laundry baskets	5,143	Drinking fountains	1,810
Decorative yard equipment	4,756	Clocks	1,755
Mixing bowls or canisters	3,492	Drinking straws	1,669
Baby bottles or nipples	3,403	Deodorant	1,236

Fired Up on the Fourth

Fireworks set off an explosive surge of accidental injuries every year, especially when everybody gets into the act around the Fourth of July. In 1988, more than 10,000 Americans suffered injuries requiring medical care when their fun with fireworks backfired.

Children and young adults get blasted more than anyone else: Three-fourths of fireworks victims are between the ages of 5 and 24. Burns, skin abrasions, fractured bones, and cuts are all common results of fireworks gone awry. Losing all or part of a finger is not uncommon.

Eye injuries are frightfully frequent, with 40 percent of all victims suffering permanent visual damage. Bottle rockets, firecrackers, cherry bombs, M-80s, salutes, roman candles—these are the culprits behind most eye injuries. But even allegedly "safe" fireworks can do serious damage. Sparklers, for instance, burn at more than 1800°F. Precious metals can melt at that temperature. So, not surprisingly, can a person's precious eye.

The Dangers of Child's Play

Playtime can be perilous. Just ask any of the 113,000 children—and grownups behaving like children?—whose toys landed them in emergency rooms during 1988. Balloons that burst, toy guns that miss their target, wagons that wipe out—these and other mishaps with toys can bring an abrupt end to anyone's fun.

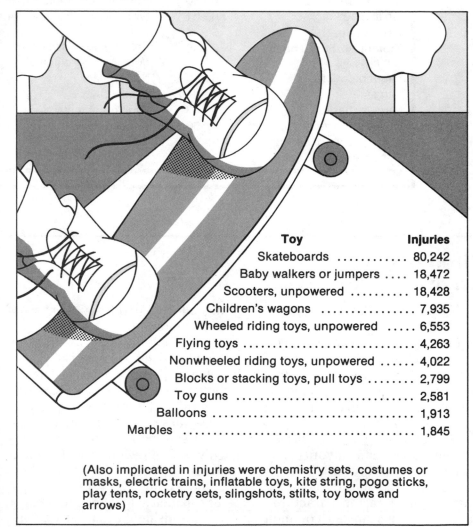

Toy	Injuries
Skateboards	80,242
Baby walkers or jumpers	18,472
Scooters, unpowered	18,428
Children's wagons	7,935
Wheeled riding toys, unpowered	6,553
Flying toys	4,263
Nonwheeled riding toys, unpowered	4,022
Blocks or stacking toys, pull toys	2,799
Toy guns	2,581
Balloons	1,913
Marbles	1,845

(Also implicated in injuries were chemistry sets, costumes or masks, electric trains, inflatable toys, kite string, pogo sticks, play tents, rocketry sets, slingshots, stilts, toy bows and arrows)

Rating the Workplace

Historically, the manufacturing industry has posed a greater risk to worker safety than most other industries, according to the U.S. Department of Labor. Working for a company that manufactures wood and lumber products, for instance, is an unlucky 13 times as risky as working for a bank.

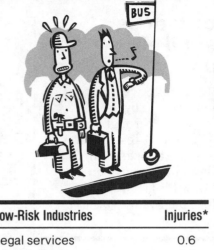

High-Risk Industries	Injuries*
Manufacturers of wood and lumber products	18.6
Manufacturers of food and related products	16.2
Manufacturers of furniture and fixtures	14.9
Construction industry	14.5
Air transportation industry	14.0
Water transportation	12.8
Production of paper products	12.4
Trucking and warehousing	12.3
Agricultural production	12.0
Forestry	11.4

*per 100 full-time workers

Low-Risk Industries	Injuries*
Legal services	0.6
Insurance agencies	1.0
Banks	1.4
Movie theaters	2.8
Apparel stores	3.2
Education	3.3
Real estate	4.6
Social services	5.7
Museums, botanical gardens, and zoos	5.9
Auto repair, services, and garages	6.5

*per 100 full-time workers

When Alertness Goes Off Duty

Most accidents attributed to human error take place inside one of two "zones of vulnerability," say researchers. Occurring between 2:00 A.M. and 7:00 A.M. and again from 2:00 P.M. to 5:00 P.M., these are periods of the day when brain functions are at their lowest, diminishing your capacity to concentrate. The researchers note, for example, that the accidental meltdown of radioactive fuel rods at Three Mile Island occurred between 4:00 A.M. and 6:00 A.M., when workers failed to recognize the need for corrective action.

Sleep deprivation can also affect your accident-preventing alertness. Investigators of the space shuttle *Challenger* explosion said that the human error and poor judgment leading up to the event could be linked to sleep loss during shift work. Some key managers in the launch had less than 2 hours' sleep preceding the tragedy.

When Tornadoes Are Most Likely to Strike

Nearly 600 people were accidentally injured or killed by the 746 tornadoes that swept through the United States in 1986. Texas had 132 tornadoes, more than any other state. But Oklahoma is considered stormier yet, having the greatest number of tornadoes *per square mile* of any state.

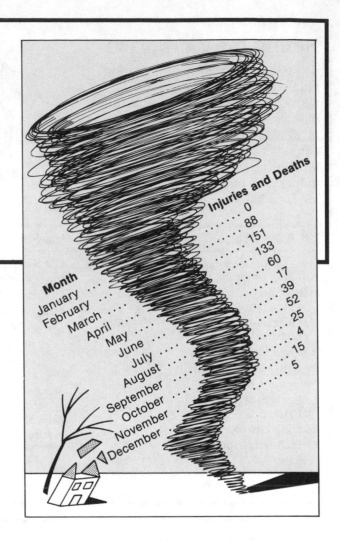

Month	Injuries and Deaths
January	0
February	88
March	151
April	133
May	60
June	17
July	39
August	52
September	25
October	4
November	15
December	5

Accidents in the Arts

All those action-packed movies and television shows that we can't seem to get enough of can be a real pain for the folks responsible for all the excitement: the stunt crew. Whether they're being gunned down in the Old West or blown up in an old warehouse, whether they're falling off the Sears Tower or screeching around hairpin turns at 150 miles an hour, stunt people risk their lives every workday. During a recent five-year period, 4,998 members of the Screen Actors Guild were injured while making movies and television shows. Their fatality rate is actually higher than that of people who work in law enforcement or the construction industry, says the Center for Safety in the Arts. At the top of the risk list are helicopter scenes, car chases, fires, falls, explosions, being shot at with "blank" ammunition, and handling animals.

All-terrain vehicles (ATVs), mopeds, and minibikes were responsible for more than 138,589 injuries in 1987. During one three-year period, ATVs alone caused more than 100 deaths and 100,000 injuries, about half of them to children under the age of 16, and 22 percent to children ages 5 through 12.

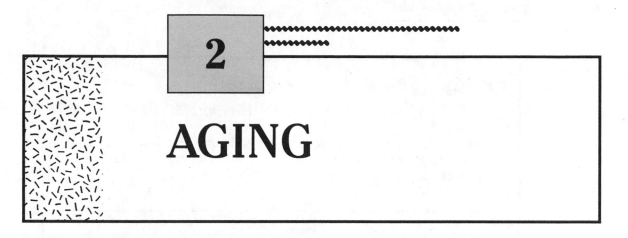

2

AGING

Today, one out of every five Americans is 55 or older—more of them women than men—and their ranks are growing. In fact, in the past two decades, the older population has grown more than twice as fast as the rest of the population.

People may be living longer for a variety of reasons—a reduction in smoking, improvements in diet and exercise habits, better control of blood pressure, declines in infectious diseases, and a decreased incidence of heart attacks. And the trend should continue: A baby born in 1900 could expect to live an average of 47.3 years; a 1985 baby can expect to live 74.7 years.

Although older people are more prone to illness than the young, aging and disease are not synonymous. Still, physiological changes that accompany aging can heighten a person's susceptibility to disease. An illness or accident which hardly affects a young person may be of much greater consequence to an elderly person.

More than four out of five persons 65 and over have at least one chronic health condition, and multiple conditions are commonplace.

Contrary to popular belief, only about 5 percent of the elderly live in nursing homes at any given time. And older people generally view their health positively. Nevertheless, 25 percent of all elderly persons suffer some degree of physical limitation in their ability to prepare meals, bathe, or otherwise personally care for themselves.

The elderly are the heaviest users of health services in the United States, accounting for 30 percent of all hospital discharges. One-third of the country's personal health-care expenditures involve the elderly, even though they constitute only 12 percent of the population. As the aging population grows, U.S. government expenditures on medical care during the next 40 years are expected to increase at one of the most rapid rates in the developed world. In 1965, federal budget expenditures for health and pension programs totaled about 25 percent of the budget. By 2040, these expenditures will equal about 60 percent.

An Aging Nation

America's elderly comprise a rapidly increasing proportion of the population. In 1900, just 4 percent of the U.S. population was 65 and older. By 2050, when people born in 1985 turn 65, nearly one in four Americans will be that age or older, and more than 5 percent of the population will be over 85.

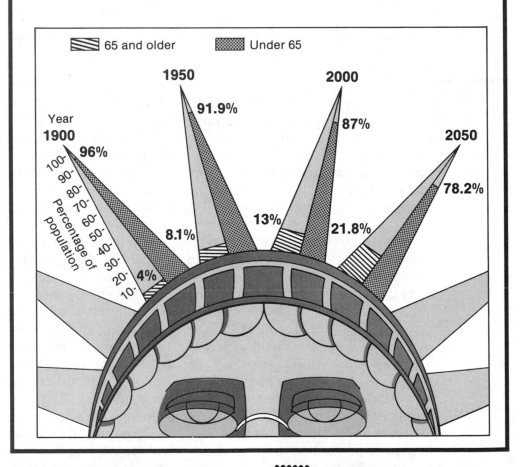

In 1900, the average woman could look forward to 19 years of caring for a child and 9 years of caring for a parent. Today, she will spend 17 years caring for a child and 18 years assisting an elderly parent.

There were more than 25,000 centenarians—people 100 years old—in the United States in 1985. By 1990, that figure is expected to double.

Men: Outnumbered and Outlived

Older women greatly outnumber older men in most nations. The average life expectancy for a person born today in the United States is 74.7 years. But American women outlive men by an average of seven to eight years, a gender-based difference in life expectancy that is one of the most extreme in the world.

This imbalance becomes even more pronounced with advancing age. Over the age of 85, there are three American women for every two American men.

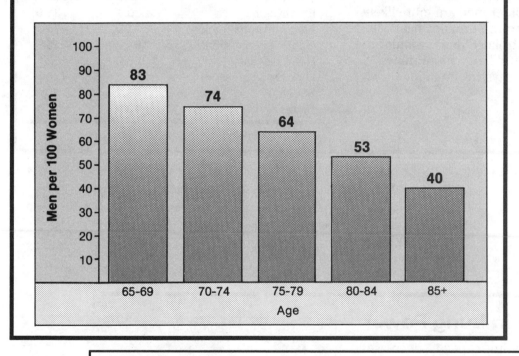

Why Women Live Longer

Women age better than men do. According to the National Institute on Aging, women are more likely than men to eat carefully and to avoid excess alcohol. The gap between men's and women's life spans may also have something to do with their lifestyles after retirement, theorizes the director of Britain's Royal College of Physicians Research Unit. Men, he says, tend to adopt an unhealthy lifestyle after retirement, eating too much, drinking, smoking, and being less active mentally and physically, whereas women continue cooking, cleaning, shopping, and following other routines that may actually help them live longer. Male and female animals other than humans appear to live to about the same age, probably because male animals have no retirement age, he notes.

The Ailments That Come with Age

There's a difference between the sexes when it comes to the kinds of old-age health problems they encounter. Older men are more likely to suffer from coronary heart disease and stroke. Elderly women are more likely to have chronic illnesses that cause physical limitations, such as arthritis.

Condition	Rate of Occurrence*	
	Men 65 and Older	Women 65 and Older
Arthritis	361.5	550.5
Cataracts	104.3	205.7
Emphysema	80.1	21.9
Frequent constipation	31.9	75.4
Hearing impairment	364.2	245.9
Heart disease	328.0	288.1
High blood pressure	351.4	458.4
Stroke	76.7	50.3
Ulcers	43.9	27.1

*per 1,000 persons

Want to live to 100? Your chances of doing so are highest if you reside in one of these ten states: Hawaii, Minnesota, South Dakota, Iowa, Nebraska, North Dakota, Kansas, Florida, Idaho, or Arizona.

Lapse in Lung Power

Breathing capacity decreases with age. According to a study summarized here, the total volume of oxygen inhaled with each breath declines. The oxygen intake of a person over the age of 80 is only half that of someone under 30.

Average number of days per year that health problems restricted activities or led to bed confinement among people over 65: 23.

Average number of days per year that health problems restricted activities or led to bed confinement among people 45 to 64: 34.

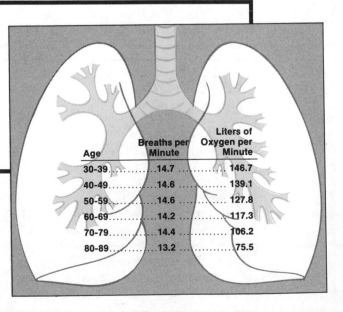

Age	Breaths per Minute	Liters of Oxygen per Minute
30-39	14.7	146.7
40-49	14.6	139.1
50-59	14.6	127.8
60-69	14.2	117.3
70-79	14.4	106.2
80-89	13.2	75.5

How We Age: A Blow-by-Blow Account

No two people age in the same ways or at the same rate. One's chronological age is not a very good index of performance capabilities, an extensive study of older people showed. Some 80-year-olds may be in better physical condition than those much younger. Even within a single individual, the organs do not age at the same rate. For example, a 50-year-old man may have the skin of a 40-year-old and the liver of a 60-year-old. Some general patterns emerge, however, when observing changes in different body systems through the passing years.

Skin

Skin changes over the years are a natural process, though the extent to which a person "shows his age" is partially determined by heredity. Sun damage also plays a large part in the skin's loss of youthfulness. Using sunscreens throughout your life may give skin a chance to repair itself.

Aging skin grows flabby as the long-term effects of gravity take their toll, pulling tissues downward. Wrinkles emerge as the dermis, the deep layer of the skin, loses moisture and elasticity. This causes the epidermis, or top skin layer, to become loose and form creases and folds.

Age 20: Wrinkles may start to appear horizontally across the forehead.

Late 20s or early 30s: Wrinkles may form between the eyebrows, especially among people who frown frequently.

Age 40: "Crow's feet" start to form along the sides of the eyes.

Age 50: Tiny wrinkles begin at the corners of the mouth. Among smokers, these can start to form in the forties.

Late 50s: The spine of the nose may begin to atrophy, causing the tip of the nose to descend.

Age 60: Wrinkles begin to encircle the lips. In addition, as we age, bags form beneath the eyes, forehead tissues sag, eyebrows descend, and the upper eyelids may seem to droop. Some people accumulate fat and develop a double chin. Age spots result if pigment gathers in patches. Elderly skin has more spots, warts, and moles.

Itching is more common as aging skin loses oils and dries out. The elderly also have a diminished sweat response.

Hair

By age 50: Half the population will have gray hair. Graying results as the production of coloring pigment slows in the hair follicles. This is largely determined by genetics and is irreversible.

Among men, baldness is a common problem. The condition, regulated by male sex hormones, usually begins with a receding hairline and a balding spot at the back of the head. The two eventually converge, leaving the entire top of the head bald or with a few strands of vellus hair, the thin, sparse hair produced by aging hair follicles.

As women age, there is a general thinning of head hair. But many older women experience an increase in hair elsewhere: An estimated 40

(continued)

How We Age: A Blow-by-Blow Account — *Continued*

percent of women over the age of 80 are likely to be troubled by excessive facial hair.

Vision

With age, the lenses of the eyes become less elastic, and the muscles that flex or flatten them to change focus gradually lose their tone. The result is presbyopia, a term that literally means "elderly vision."

By age 40: Many people will need reading glasses.

By age 65: Virtually every person will suffer some loss in the ability to focus, to resolve images, to discern colors, and to adapt to light. More than half of all cases of visual impairment are among people 65 or older.

By age 80: A person needs three times more light than at age 20 to achieve the same visual clarity.

Between ages 65 and 74: As many as two-thirds of the elderly will have cataracts or some other form of clouding of the normally transparent lens. An estimated 3 out of every 100 people over 65 will suffer from glaucoma. And blindness may result from age-related macular degeneration, a disease that affects the part of the retina responsible for clear vision.

Hearing

Starting at age 55: Age-related hearing loss, or presbycusis, begins to occur in many people. One-fourth of those between ages 65 and 74 will have hearing impairment, as will 39 percent of those 75 and older. But only 2 percent of those 55 and over are legally deaf.

This progressive hearing degeneration includes loss of nerve cells in the auditory pathways. Hearing loss initially occurs at high frequencies. You may still be able to hear speech but may have difficulty distinguishing words or tolerating loud sounds. The incidence of tinnitus, or ringing in the ear, also increases with age.

Taste

Between ages 50 and 60: Taste sensitivity and the flow of saliva do not change dramatically with age in healthy, nonmedicated men and women. There is, however, a gradual decrease in the number of taste buds on the tongue. As many as two-thirds of them may atrophy.

Muscles

Between ages 20 and 30: Muscle strength is at its maximum.

At about age 40: Lean body mass begins to gradually shrink. Decreasing muscle mass is slowly replaced by fat. So a person who maintains a consistent weight may actually be putting on fat.

A steady decline in muscle tone, strength, and stamina also starts at around 40. This occurs despite physical exercise, although it is more marked in sedentary people. Older persons are more likely to experience strains, pulls, and cramping after exercise. But a well-conditioned 65-year-old may still possess far better muscle tone than a 25-year-old who doesn't exercise.

By age 65: Muscle strength drops by as much as 80 percent.

By age 80: About half of one's muscle mass has been lost.

Bones

By age 40: Both men and women begin to lose bone mineral because of decreased ability to absorb calcium. Bone mass actually reaches its peak at about age 35. Severe loss of bone density, called osteoporosis, may produce bones that are so weak and porous that they spontaneously break.

Hip fractures start to rise in frequency in the early forties and thereafter double every six years.

The elderly are at increased risk for developing osteomalacia, a decrease in bone density resulting from vitamin D deficiency, often because of an inadequate diet, lack of sunlight exposure, or problems with vitamin absorption.

The incidence of back problems increases as vertebrae in the spine weaken and disks degenerate, shrink, and sometimes collapse.

Brain

An older brain can function just as well as a younger one. Although the brain shrinks with age, losing millions of nerve cells, the remaining cells sprout more dendrites, the projections that foster communication between brain cells.

Apparent memory losses among the elderly may be due to a poor attention span, poor motivation, anxiety, or the increased time it takes to "search" one's memory for a piece of information. Intellectually active individuals retain healthy mental abilities, regardless of age.

After age 65: One in ten people will develop symptoms of dementia, a serious condition characterized by poor memory, confusion, and an inability to perform simple math.

Alzheimer's disease, with its profound confusion and disorientation, affects people mostly over the age of 80.

Heart

The heart of a disease-free older person pumps about as well as that of a younger adult, although changes do occur. The aging heart shrinks, while surrounding fat increases. It beats at a slower rate and responds less quickly to increasing workloads, but it pumps more blood per heartbeat than a younger heart does.

Between ages 30 and 70: Systolic blood pressure (when the heart is contracting) gradually rises by 20 to 30 percent. There is also a slight rise in diastolic pressure (when the heart is relaxed).

Over age 40: Heart disease becomes the number-one cause of death in men. Women develop heart disease 10 to 20 years later than men do.

Kidneys

Older people's kidneys gradually lose filtering cells, decreasing the ability to filter blood and excrete waste materials. The elderly also face greater risk of dehydration because their kidneys are less able to conserve water. This inability may also cause an increasing need to get up at night to urinate.

(continued)

How We Age: A Blow-by-Blow Account —
Continued

Urogenital System

The incidence of urinary incontinence, the inability to control the passing of urine, increases with age. A common form in women is stress incontinence, which occurs during mild physical exertion such as lifting, coughing, or sneezing.

Over age 50: As many as 80 percent of men experience enlargement of the prostate, a gland at the base of the bladder that produces fluid needed to transport and nourish sperm. While the problem doesn't generally affect sexual capacity or enjoyment, it causes more frequent or difficult urination.

After age 65: The incidence of bladder cancer increases. Bladder cancer is three times more common in men than women, and is more common among cigarette smokers, male or female.

Older women become more prone to nonmalignant bladder disorders, due to hormonal changes after menopause which impair resistance to infection.

Sexuality

Sexual activity can continue well into later years, although changes do occur in the sex organs.

Between ages 45 and 55: Most women will experience menopause. A small number will reach menopause in their early thirties, while others will have normal menstrual cycles into their sixties. During menopause, hormone levels decrease, the ovaries become smaller, and the mucus-producing lining of the vagina grows thinner. During sex, an older woman may take longer to become aroused and to lubricate, but these changes needn't interfere with pleasure. Women can remain as sexually responsive in later life as they ever were, although they are sterile after menopause.

The decline of sexual functioning in men is very gradual, beginning just after the peak of sexual prowess around age 20 and culminating by age 60 or 70. The sperm counts of older men are about the same as those of younger men, but the proportion of immature sperm increases with age. Other changes include a decrease in the size of the testes, a delayed and less firm erection, less seminal fluid, and a briefer orgasm followed by longer recovery period (the time that passes before it's possible to have another erection and orgasm). Men are able to reproduce until very late in life.

Immune System

After age 40: Infection-fighting lymphocytes have a decreased ability to kill tumor cells. Neutrophils, which fight acute infection, also grow less efficient with age. These changes may influence susceptibility to cancer and infectious diseases.

Systematic Slowdown

Basal metabolism—the energy-generating level of your body at rest—declines with age. At its high point during infancy, it drops suddenly in childhood. After the age of 20, it undergoes a steadier decline. As a result, the older you get, the fewer calories you require for energy. In fact, an 80-year-old requires about 300 fewer calories per day to fuel the body at rest than a 30-year-old does.

Is That A Fact?

Older people take longer to stop bleeding when they get a cut.

Actually, men and women over 50 exhibited a 1-minute *decrease* in bleeding time for every additional 20 years in age, according to one study. Even the very elderly, those over 85, have systems that can effectively stem bleeding and repair extensive wounds.

Limitations of the Aged

Disease and dysfunction in older people often lead to limitations in the types of activities they are able to perform by themselves. The chart shows some of the most common limitations among 26 million people aged 65 and older who were living outside of nursing homes or other institutions in 1984.

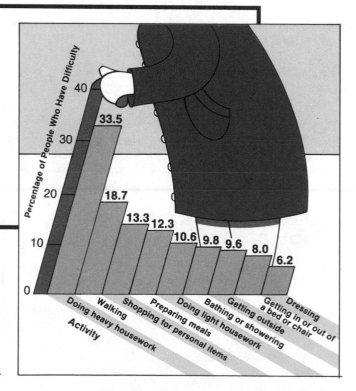

Percentage of People Who Have Difficulty

40

33.5

30

20

18.7

13.3 12.3

10.6 9.8 9.6 8.0

10

6.2

0

Activity — Doing heavy housework — Walking — Shopping — Preparing meals — Doing light housework — Bathing or showering — Getting outside — Getting in or out of a bed or chair — Dressing

 The oldest man in the world was reported to be Shigechiyo Izumi of Japan, who was 120 when he died in 1986. The oldest American was Mrs. Fannie Thomas, who was nearly 114 when she died in 1981.

Where People Fall

Falls are a leading cause of injury and death among the elderly. More than half of all such injuries take place in and around the home. Experts say many could be prevented with better lighting, skid-resistant mats or rugs, well-placed railings and grips, and other commonsense measures. Here's a breakdown of where falls are most likely to occur.

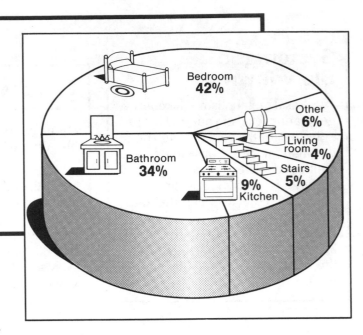

Bedroom **42%**

Other **6%**

Living room **4%**

Bathroom **34%**

Stairs **5%**

9% Kitchen

Money may be a partial antidote for aging. About 25.6 percent of older people with incomes over $35,000 said they considered their health excellent as compared with others their age. Only about 11 percent of those with incomes less than $10,000 were able to say the same.

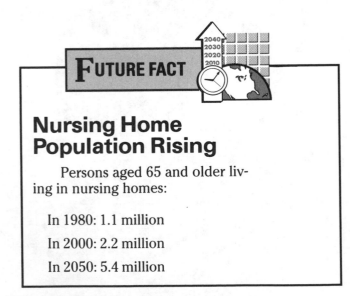

FUTURE FACT

2040
2030
2020
2010

Nursing Home Population Rising

Persons aged 65 and older living in nursing homes:

In 1980: 1.1 million

In 2000: 2.2 million

In 2050: 5.4 million

Signs of a Mature Personality

Personality traits may vary with age. Certain features such as rebelliousness toward authority and impulsiveness appear to decline with age. A personality test administered to people in different age groups showed that compared with those aged 25 to 40, people over 47 were more outgoing, conscientious, adventurous, tender-minded, imaginative, shrewd, guilt-prone, and liberal-thinking, and they were less bright, stable, assertive, happy-go-lucky, suspicious, independent, and tense.

Who Takes Care of the Elderly?

More than 2 million people provide unpaid assistance to elderly people living outside of nursing homes or institutions. Almost three-fourths of the caregivers live with the persons receiving the care.

eople born to parents of advanced age may be at higher risk of developing Alzheimer's disease later in life, say Japanese researchers. They found that a high proportion of people with the disease had been born to older parents whose age, they theorize, may cause chromosomal abnormality.

Daughters 29%

Wives 23%

Other males 7%

Other females 20%

Sons 8%

13% Husbands

Eat Light, Live Longer

A lighter diet may help prolong life. Studies have shown that laboratory animals whose caloric intake was restricted to 10 to 50 percent of what they normally ate lived as much as 50 percent longer than those on nonrestricted diets. And the longer animals' diets were restricted, the longer they lived.

Food restriction delays age-related physiological deterioration and retards kidney and heart disease, researchers postulate. Eating a lighter diet appeared to be effective in extending animals' lives whether or not the change in diet started early or later in life.

Overmedication among the elderly could be responsible for 10 to 20 percent of cases of mental confusion resembling Alzheimer's. Medications taken for high blood pressure, arthritis, cardiovascular problems, and diabetes are common culprits.

Use It or Lose It

Exercise may help delay the effects of aging, including lower aerobic capacity and reduced muscle mass. One study showed that men between ages 35 and 74 who exercised regularly had a lower risk of dying than their sedentary counterparts. These men could expect to live an hour or two longer for every hour they exercised.

The Ten Best Strategies for Living Longer

Many of us have the potential to live longer simply by developing habits that help prevent life-threatening problems. The most important steps:

1. Don't smoke. Cigarettes shorten life by causing heart disease, emphysema, cancer, and other diseases.

2. Eat a balanced diet and maintain a desirable weight. This increases overall well-being and the health of cells.

3. Exercise regularly. Fitness increases resistance to disease.

4. Drink alcohol only in moderation. Heavy alcohol intake has been linked to numerous disorders, from malnutrition to stroke.

5. Have regular medical checkups. Also, see a doctor as soon as you've detected a problem, and follow his advice.

6. Get enough sleep, whether it's at night or includes a nap during the day.

7. Avoid overexposure to sun and cold. Older persons are more vulnerable to excesses of heat and cold because the aging body doesn't handle temperature variations as efficiently as it once did.

8. Practice good safety habits at home. Falls and fires take the lives of many older people.

9. Stay involved with family and friends. Depression is a major problem of the elderly, often brought on by loneliness.

10. Maintain a positive outlook on life. Your attitude is extremely important in determining the quality and duration of life. Satisfaction and pleasure seem to contribute to good health and long life just as surely as any pill or medication does.

Men tend to wrinkle about ten years later than women—partly because their skin is thicker and oilier and partly because the scraping of the razor during a daily shave promotes rejuvenation of the skin's lower layers.

Is THAT A FACT?

Older people daydream about the past more than young people.

Not true. A study of 1,100 men and women aged 17 to 92 showed no correlation between age and the past, present, or future settings of their daydreams. Young people were just as likely to daydream about days past as the elderly were.

Slower to React

Your ability to react to stimuli decreases with age. In one study, a group of people aged 60 to 70 were tested against a group aged 17 to 38. The subjects were individually tested on several "bits" of stimulus: Electric lights were flashed on and off in varying combinations. In both the old and the young group, reaction time slowed when stimulus complexity increased. Older subjects showed slower reaction time overall.

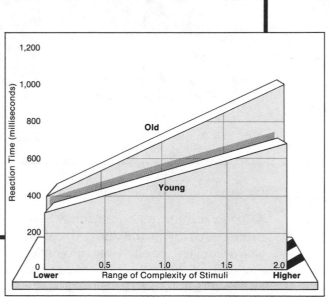

Marriage and a satisfying sex life may contribute to a longer life. Married people have lower mortality rates than those who are divorced, widowed, or never married, one study has shown.

Liking your job and continuing to work may lengthen your life. Work satisfaction was one of the strongest predictors of longevity among men over the age of 60, probably because of its effects on exercise, mental health, and social support, says a researcher at Duke University. Among women in this age group, involvement in churches, clubs, and volunteer organizations was a stronger predictor of a long life than work. As more women enter the work force, the researcher says, work will probably become more important for them, as well.

FUTURE FACT

Alzheimer's Will Increase Drastically

Alzheimer's disease, possibly America's greatest future health problem, currently accounts for more than 60 percent of all admissions to nursing homes. As the population ages, the number of Alzheimer's victims is projected to increase as much as eightfold by the year 2050. More than half of them will be aged 85 or older.

3

AIDS

Acquired immune deficiency syndrome—AIDS—is the most dreaded worldwide disease epidemic since influenza killed 20 million people at the end of World War I. AIDS has already killed more Americans than the Vietnam War—more than 72,000 through January 1990.

AIDS is caused by the human immunodeficiency virus (HIV). Up to 1.5 million Americans are infected with this virus; more than 100,000 actually have AIDS. Like any virus, HIV doesn't discriminate: It doesn't care whether you're male or female, young or old, black or white, straight or gay, on drugs or off them. It's spread by sex and blood. The percentage of heterosexual AIDS cases nearly doubled between 1986 and 1989, and the 1989 rate of heterosexual HIV infection was the same as the early 1980s rate of homosexual infection.

The AIDS virus is new as viruses go; the earliest infection is believed to have occurred in Africa in the 1950s. The first American case may have occurred as early as 1968. But HIV became epidemic only in 1980. Why?

The virus may have changed genetically. People may have changed their sexual practices. They may have increased the number of their sexual partners.

HIV attacks white blood cells, the body's defense against bacterial, fungal, and viral infections, leaving the body vulnerable to illnesses that normally don't kill but in AIDS patients can be deadly. HIV also attacks brain cells, digestive system cells, and skin cells.

The body doesn't give up without a fight. It produces antibodies to the AIDS virus. The primary diagnostic test for infection detects the presence of HIV antibodies in the blood. Antibodies can keep the virus under control for a period of time. No one knows why some people get AIDS six months after HIV infection and others can go as long as 15 years. One ominous finding is that infection can be as old as 4 or more years without producing the telltale antibodies—a "silent infection."

Many leading scientists think that if other infections could be controlled, a person might live with AIDS for a long period of time.

3 Ways You Can Get AIDS, and 15 Ways You Can't

It isn't easy to get AIDS. Experts say you have to do one of three things:

1. Have sex with a person infected with the human immunodeficiency virus (the most common way AIDS is transmitted). Protect yourself by avoiding sex partners who are at high risk (homosexual and bisexual men, intravenous drug users, prostitutes), by practicing monogamy, and by using condoms and spermicides.

2. Receive infected tissue or blood into your body—via either an organ transplant, a blood transfusion, or a contaminated needle. If you've received a transplant or tranfusion since April 1985, when blood screening for HIV was begun, your risk is very low.

3. Be born to a mother infected with HIV.

There are many ways you *cannot* get AIDS. Here are 15. Study after study has failed to turn up any AIDS cases developing from these contacts, even when family members and friends shared such contacts with loved ones who had AIDS.

1. Sharing an elevator with people who have AIDS. The virus isn't spread through the air.

2. Sharing food or drink with a person who has AIDS. The virus is rarely found in saliva in the first place, and in the second place, saliva inactivates the virus.

3. Shaking hands with someone with AIDS. There's no HIV in sweat or on the skin.

4. Being sneezed on or coughed on by someone with AIDS. The virus has never been found in phlegm or nasal mucus.

5. Using a toilet seat previously occupied by a person with AIDS. The virus is not a hardy one; it dies immediately in open air. There's so little HIV in urine or feces that experts think it can't be transmitted this way.

6. Swimming in a pool or sitting in a hot tub with someone who has AIDS. HIV can't survive in water. And again, there's no HIV in sweat or on skin, and too little in urine to cause infection.

7. Kissing an infected person on the lips or cheek. There's no known case of saliva transmitting the virus. Caution: Saliva has been found to contain the virus in rare instances, so French kissing is probably not a good idea.

8. Eating food prepared by a chef who has AIDS. Forget the chef's saliva, sweat, and skin. But what if he cuts himself and bleeds on your

(continued)

3 Ways
You Can Get AIDS,
and 15 Ways
You Can't—*Continued*

food? Fear not: Your digestive system would make short work of any AIDS virus that got that far.

9. Donating blood. A twist of the getting-AIDS-by-tranfusion risk. Needles used for blood donation in America are used only once. There's no risk whatsoever. Unsterilized needles used for acupuncture, tattooing, or ear piercing could spread the virus, but sterilization kills the virus.

10. Being bitten by mosquitoes. There's no evidence the AIDS virus can live in insects. This mosquito myth arose from the high incidence of AIDS in Belle Glade, Florida. Research found that the residents were getting AIDS from sex and intravenous drug use.

11. Being immunized against hepatitis-B (with the hepatitis-B vaccine) or hepatitis-A (with gamma globulin). Gamma globulin and one form of the hepatitis-B vaccine are derived from blood. But the process of making the vaccine and gamma globulin inactivates HIV and all other viruses.

12. Being infected by pets, or by animals that have AIDS-like diseases. The viruses that cause feline leukemia and certain immunodeficiency diseases in horses and goats can't grow in humans. HIV can grow in chimpanzees, gibbons, and rabbits, while a similar virus can infect macaques, green monkeys, and baboons. So if you injected yourself with their blood, you could get infected. Otherwise, the odds are negligible.

13. Working or going to school with someone who has AIDS. What if an infected child bleeds, and the blood enters another child's open wound? Experience with health workers accidentally exposed this way shows infection is highly unlikely. Even when health workers accidentally stick themselves with infected needles, infection rarely results—one study showed a risk of 1 in 286 instances. There's no evidence from anywhere in the world that has traced a case of AIDS to the kind of casual contact experienced at work or school.

14. Visiting an infected person's home. You can't get AIDS from living in the same house as an infected person, much less visiting there.

15. Having sex with someone who isn't infected. That should be obvious. (Even with someone who *is* infected, the virus isn't easily transmitted in one or a few exposures.)

AIDS across the Nation

Where are AIDS cases most concentrated in the United States, its territories, and possessions? The top table shows the ten areas with the highest AIDS rates from November 1988 through October 1989 (with the number of new cases in the period).

Among the top ten, the rate declined from the same period in the previous year only in New York, Puerto Rico, New Jersey, and the Virgin Islands. Florida's rate soared by more than a third and Georgia's by nearly 72 percent.

The bottom table shows the ten areas with the lowest AIDS rates.

Only in Vermont did the rate drop from the previous year. Idaho's rate more than doubled, while West Virginia's jumped 210 percent.

State or Region	Rate*	New Cases
1. District of Columbia	83.7	519
2. New York	36.0	6,474
3. Puerto Rico	35.4	1,172
4. New Jersey	29.1	2,251
5. Florida	27.8	3,486
6. Virgin Islands	24.3	28
7. California	22.5	6,438
8. Georgia	18.7	1,202
9. Nevada	16.2	167
10. Maryland	15.1	687

*per 100,000 persons

State or Region	Rate*	New Cases
1. U.S. Pacific Islands	0.7	1
2. South Dakota	0.8	6
3. North Dakota	0.9	6
4. Guam	1.5	2
5. Montana	2.0	17
6. Iowa	2.1	59
6. Idaho	2.1	22
7. Vermont	2.5	14
8. West Virginia	2.8	53
9. Alaska	3.1	19

*per 100,000 persons

When Ignorance Is Not Bliss

In 1987, a survey of doctors' knowledge of AIDS was conducted in the Washington, D.C., area. The results were alarming, to say the least. Of the primary-care physicians surveyed, more than half couldn't name the two major diagnostic tests for HIV infection—the ELISA and the Western Blot. Even worse, 12 percent didn't even know that HIV causes AIDS.

Seventy-five percent of the doctors preferred not to ask their patients about their sex lives, hoping the patients would bring up the subject themselves. Twenty percent of the doctors thought that heterosexual family members should not share bathrooms with their gay brethren. And a third didn't specifically recommend that their patients use condoms when having sex with an HIV-infected man.

AIDS Rates around the World

The United States has the highest number of AIDS cases in the world, but your chance of meeting someone with AIDS is three to four times higher in Bermuda or the Bahamas. The African nation of the Congo, however, may have the highest AIDS rate of all: 57 cases per 100,000 population in 1987 (the most recent year for which figures were available).

On the map, the first number shown is each country's 1987 incidence rate; the second is the rate for 1988. Note that the U.S. rate rose about 10 percent in one year, while Argentina's—although still only a fraction of America's—tripled, and Ghana's grew sevenfold. Nations of South and East Asia and the Islamic world have almost no AIDS cases. Tiny countries like Monaco may have rel-

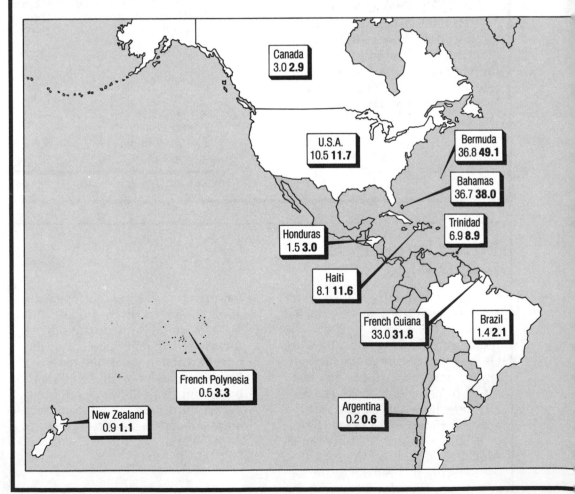

Canada
3.0 **2.9**

U.S.A.
10.5 **11.7**

Bermuda
36.8 **49.1**

Bahamas
36.7 **38.0**

Honduras
1.5 **3.0**

Trinidad
6.9 **8.9**

Haiti
8.1 **11.6**

French Guiana
33.0 **31.8**

Brazil
1.4 **2.1**

French Polynesia
0.5 **3.3**

Argentina
0.2 **0.6**

New Zealand
0.9 **1.1**

〰〰〰
AIDS is beginning to spread to smaller cities. In 1984, U.S. metropolitan areas with less than 500,000 people had 12 percent of the nation's AIDS cases. In 1989, they had 19 percent.

〰〰〰
HIV infection was the fifteenth leading cause of death in the United States in 1987 — the first year HIV statistics were included.

atively high rates but a low number of cases — Monaco has had four cases since AIDS reporting began.

And even these figures don't tell the whole story because of incomplete reporting and underreporting, especially in the Third World. The official tally as of October 1989 stood at 182,000 cases worldwide; the estimated cumulative number of cases is 600,000.

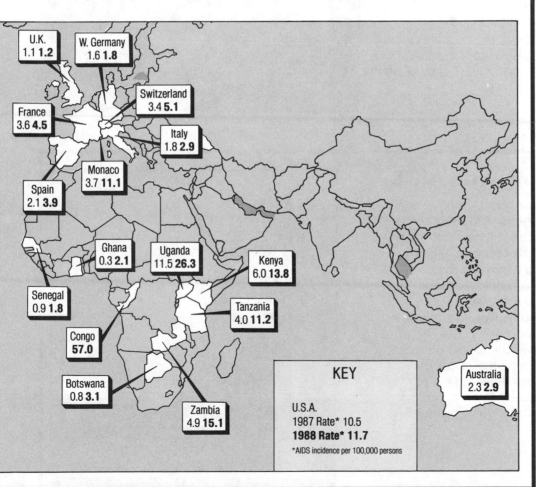

U.K.
1.1 **1.2**

W. Germany
1.6 **1.8**

Switzerland
3.4 **5.1**

France
3.6 **4.5**

Italy
1.8 **2.9**

Monaco
3.7 **11.1**

Spain
2.1 **3.9**

Ghana
0.3 **2.1**

Uganda
11.5 **26.3**

Kenya
6.0 **13.8**

Senegal
0.9 **1.8**

Tanzania
4.0 **11.2**

Congo
57.0

Botswana
0.8 **3.1**

Zambia
4.9 **15.1**

Australia
2.3 **2.9**

KEY

U.S.A.
1987 Rate* 10.5
1988 Rate* 11.7
*AIDS incidence per 100,000 persons

The AIDS Iceberg

The long latent period of AIDS virus infection—averaging close to ten years—means a lot of infected people don't have symptoms, while many with symptoms don't yet have full-blown AIDS. The huge mass of HIV-infected people were infected during the 1980s, and most will not reach the tip of the iceberg until sometime in the 1990s.

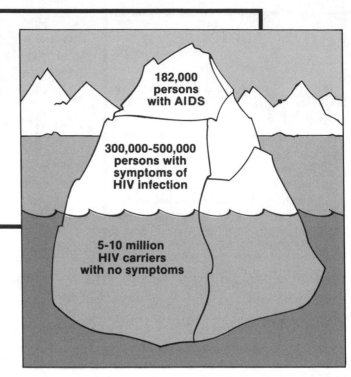

More has been learned about the AIDS virus in a shorter time than about any other microbe in history.

Surviving with AIDS

For some reason, a few people with AIDS manage to live substantially longer than others. As this chart shows, about 3.4 percent of gay men with AIDS in a San Francisco study survived into their sixth year with the usually fatal disease. No one could say these people would continue to survive, and no one could say why they were still alive. Some researchers believe the long-term survivors may have been dealt a good genetic hand that enables their immune systems to fight the virus more effectively.

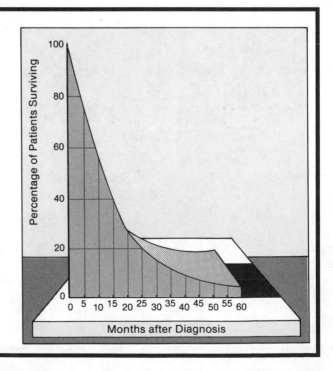

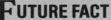
AIDS Incidence Rising in New Decade

Worldwide, the number of people with AIDS is rising sharply, says the World Health Organization (WHO). The cumulative figure was projected to double between 1989 and 1991 to more than 1 million. But the rest of the 1990s will see the most dramatic rise, as many of the millions of people infected during the 1980s develop the disease. In fact, nine times more adults are expected to get AIDS during the 1990s than did so in the previous decade. WHO estimates that one-third of these potential cases could be prevented through education and behavior changes.

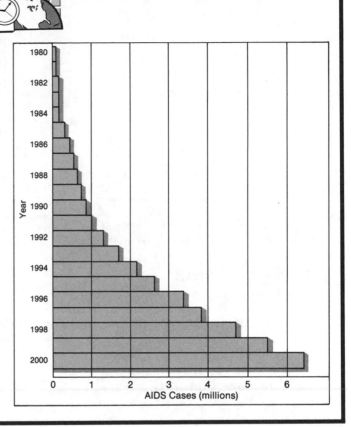

AIDS Index

Risk of HIV infection from blood transfusion: 1 in 250,000 units.

Estimated lifetime cost of treating an AIDS patient: $60,000.

Estimated cost of treating all AIDS patients in 1988: $2.6 billion.

Estimated cost of treating all AIDS patients in 1992: $7.5 billion.

In 1988, percentage of Americans who thought AIDS is likely to become epidemic in the general population: 69.

Percentage who said they were worried about getting AIDS: 38.

Percentage who said they took steps to avoid catching AIDS: 49.

Percentage of English-speakers who said they hadn't received AIDS information: 11.5.

Percentage of Spanish-speakers who said they hadn't: 46.6.

Hispanics in America need more intensive education about AIDS delivered in their own language, says a Johns Hopkins University study. Researchers found Hispanics have less access to AIDS information because of language barriers and inadequate reading skills.

WARNING SIGNALS

The Symptoms of Infection

When a person is infected by any virus, he or she usually develops antibodies to fight the virus. This call to arms of the body's defenses is called seroconversion. It is often accompanied by symptoms, the first signs of infection.

When the infection is caused by HIV, certain symptoms are likely to be reported—such as fever, sore throat, and lethargy—but these symptoms are also found with many less-serious illnesses. But HIV seroconversion is twice as likely to produce symptoms, and it's clearly marked by swollen lymph nodes, rash, depression, loss of appetite, weight loss, and eye pain—symptoms very similar to those of mononucleosis.

The illness that goes along with HIV seroconversion also usually lasts longer than seroconversion from other viral infections, and patients are more likely to need hospitalization. And also unlike most other viral infections, white blood cell counts drop significantly in HIV seroconversion. Seroconversion, however, is *not* AIDS—it's the body's reaction to the initial infection.

Symptom	Percentage of People Reporting
Fever	76.9
Lethargy	66.7
Malaise	66.7
Sore throat	56.4
Loss of appetite	56.4
Muscle pain	56.4
Headache	48.7
Joint pain	48.7
Weight loss	46.2
Swollen lymph nodes	43.5
Pain behind the eye	38.5
Dehydration	30.8
Nausea	30.8
Depression	28.2
Diarrhea	28.2
Irritability	28.2
Rash on the torso	23.1
Dry cough	23.1
Abdominal pain	15.4
Runny nose	15.4
Dark urine	15.4

~~~**D**espite the fact that many prison inmates report intravenous drug use and homosexual activity, less than 8 percent tested positive for HIV in a Johns Hopkins University study.

What's Your Risk of HIV Infection?

People at highest risk for HIV infection include homosexual and bisexual men, intravenous drug users, and hemophiliacs. Others with high risk are prostitutes, heterosexuals from countries where HIV infection is prevalent, and people who received multiple blood transfusions between 1983 and 1985 in areas where HIV infection is common. High-risk behavior includes sexual intercourse or needle sharing with a member of a high-risk group. This table attempts to quantify a person's risk, depending on risk category and number of sexual encounters.

Risk Category of Partner	Estimated Risk of Infection	
	1 Sexual Encounter	500 Sexual Encounters
HIV blood status unknown		
Not in any high-risk group		
Using condoms	1 in 50,000,000	1 in 110,000
Not using condoms	1 in 5,000,000	1 in 16,000
High-risk group		
Using condoms	1 in 100,000 to 1 in 10,000	1 in 210 to 1 in 21
Not using condoms	1 in 10,000 to 1 in 1,000	1 in 32 to 1 in 3
HIV blood test negative		
No history of high-risk behavior		
Using condoms	1 in 5,000,000,000	1 in 11,000,000
Not using condoms	1 in 500,000,000	1 in 1,600,000
Continuing high-risk behavior		
Using condoms	1 in 500,000	1 in 1,100
Not using condoms	1 in 50,000	1 in 160
HIV blood test positive		
Using condoms	1 in 5,000	1 in 11
Not using condoms	1 in 500	2 in 3

~~~**O**ne "worst-case" scenario says that more than 14 million Americans will be infected with HIV, and more than 2.7 million will have died of AIDS, by 2002.

4

ALCOHOL

Drinking alcohol is one of our culture's longest-standing traditions. Americans drink the equivalent of 500 million gallons of pure alcohol a year. That's a little over 2½ gallons per person. Why so much alcohol?

People drink because they like the taste (although most first-time drinkers would agree it's an acquired taste), because alcohol warms their tummies, and because of the myths that equate drinking with sophistication and maturity. But mostly people drink to be sociable. A few stiff drinks can relax the inhibitions of even the most bashful wallflower.

But drinking has a dark side that begins—but far from ends—with a pounding head the morning after that we call a hangover. Continued use (and abuse) of alcohol has been linked to cirrhosis of the liver, stroke, cancer, high blood pressure, diabetes, gout, insomnia, impotence, and various digestive problems.

There are social costs to drinking as well. At least half of all highway fatalities, suicides, murders, drownings, and on-the-job accidents are related to alcohol consumption. Public intoxication accounts for 40 percent of all arrests.

That figure of 2½ gallons of alcohol per person is a bit misleading. No one drinks pure alcohol. Instead, dozens of more palatable ways of consuming the substance have been invented, including mixing it with everything from orange juice to coffee and cream.

The most popular drink overall is beer, which Americans down to the tune of 5.7 *billion* gallons per year (or 23 gallons per person). Next comes wine, of which Americans sip nearly 500 million gallons each year (or 2 gallons per person). These are followed by spirits: Americans down gin, vodka, bourbon, and the like containing about 150 million gallons of pure ethanol yearly.

Alcohol consumption in the United States fluctuates from year to year, but the general trend has been downward for the past decade. By the end of the 1980s, total consumption was the lowest in three decades.

Most Drinks Pack the Same Punch

Generally, whether it's a mug of beer, a glass of wine, or a shot of whiskey, the amount of alcohol in any standard drink is about the same. That's because, although there is a much smaller percentage of alcohol in a mug of beer than in a glass of bourbon, for example, the mug of beer is usually much larger. As shown here, the alcohol content of a 12-ounce glass of beer equals that in one average glass of wine. That glass of wine equals one average glass of sherry, port, or other "fortified" wine, which in turn equals one average shot of hard stuff.

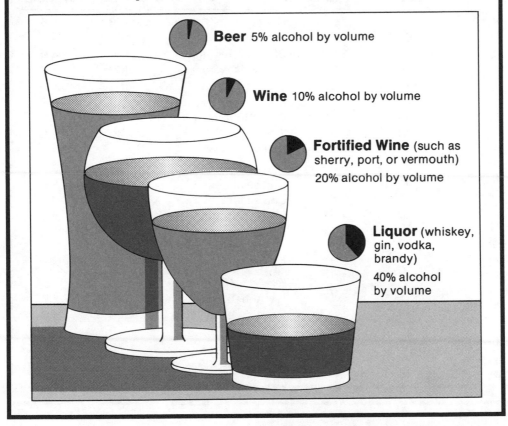

Beer 5% alcohol by volume

Wine 10% alcohol by volume

Fortified Wine (such as sherry, port, or vermouth) 20% alcohol by volume

Liquor (whiskey, gin, vodka, brandy) 40% alcohol by volume

While driving and drinking is known to be a bad combination, studies show that driving with a hangover may also diminish driving ability by as much as 20 percent—even though all alcohol has long since disappeared from the blood.

Beer: The Kick and the Calories

Some beers have more alcohol —and more calories—than others. As a rule of (tipped) thumb, the "light" or reduced-calorie beers tend to have less alcohol than regular beers. That's because two-thirds of the calories in beer comes from the alcohol content.

	Calories (per 12 oz.)	Percentage of Alcohol by Volume		Calories (per 12 oz.)	Percentage of Alcohol by Volume
Regular Beer			Olympia	153	4.6
Anchor Steam	154	4.7	Pabst Blue Ribbon	152	4.9
Augsberger	175	5.5	St. Pauli Girl (light)	150	4.9
Beck's	150	4.7	St. Pauli Girl (dark)	150	4.8
Blatz	144	4.6	Schlitz	151	4.9
Budweiser	144	4.7	Schmidt's	147	4.7
Busch Bavarian	156	4.9	Stroh Bohemian	149	4.7
Coors	140	4.6	Tuborg	140	4.8
Dos Equis	145	4.5	**Light Beer**		
Guinness Stout	192	5.8	Amstel Light	95	3.7
Hamm's	136	4.4	Budweiser Light	108	3.5
Heileman's Old Style	144	4.9	Coors Light	102	4.1
Heineken	152	5.0	Michelob Light	135	4.2
Kirin	149	5.0	Miller Lite	99	4.3
Kronenbourg	170	5.2	Schlitz Light	97	4.2
Labatt's	147	5.0	Stroh Light	115	4.1
Löwenbräu	157	4.9	**Low-Alcohol Beer**		
Michelob	162	5.0	LA, Anheuser-Busch	110	1.7
Miller	149	4.7	Break Special Lager	115	1.8
Molson	154	5.1	Pace	85	1.7
Newcastle Brown Ale	144	4.6	Blatz L.A.	73	1.8
O'Keefe Ale	135	5.0	Black Label L.A.	73	1.8
Old Milwaukee	145	4.6			

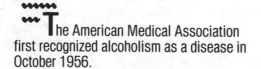

The American Medical Association first recognized alcoholism as a disease in October 1956.

What to Expect from That Next Drink

If you're going to a party tonight and planning to drink, here is how you can expect your mind and body to react, according to the American Medical Association. The chart is intended to guide a person who weighs 154 pounds—if you weigh less, adjust intake accordingly. (It is assumed that all the drinks are consumed during a single drinking session of a few hours.)

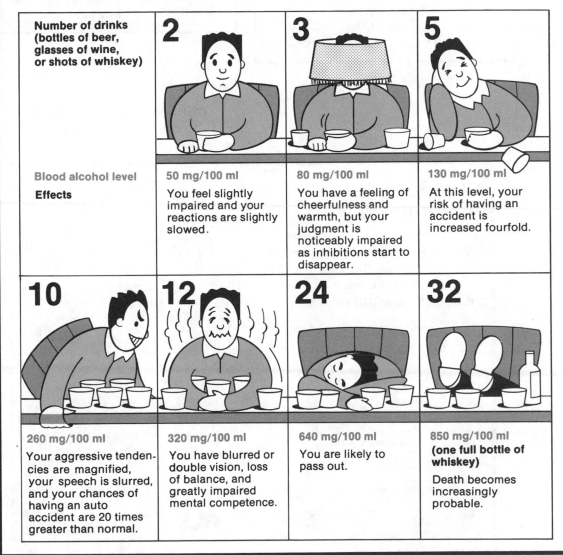

Number of drinks (bottles of beer, glasses of wine, or shots of whiskey)	**2**	**3**	**5**
Blood alcohol level / **Effects**	50 mg/100 ml — You feel slightly impaired and your reactions are slightly slowed.	80 mg/100 ml — You have a feeling of cheerfulness and warmth, but your judgment is noticeably impaired as inhibitions start to disappear.	130 mg/100 ml — At this level, your risk of having an accident is increased fourfold.
	10	**12**	**24**	**32**
	260 mg/100 ml — Your aggressive tendencies are magnified, your speech is slurred, and your chances of having an auto accident are 20 times greater than normal.	320 mg/100 ml — You have blurred or double vision, loss of balance, and greatly impaired mental competence.	640 mg/100 ml — You are likely to pass out.	850 mg/100 ml (one full bottle of whiskey) — Death becomes increasingly probable.

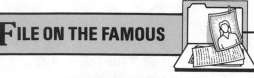

FILE ON THE FAMOUS

Writers on the Rocks

Great writers of the past who have fallen victim to serious problems with alcohol include Sinclair Lewis, Edgar Allan Poe, Eugene O'Neill, Jack London, O. Henry, Dylan Thomas, and F. Scott Fitzgerald.

IS THAT A FACT?

Alcoholism is often inherited.

True. Most scientists now feel that alcoholism is in part a hereditary disorder, although they are uncertain about the degree to which it is hereditary and the degree to which it is a learned behavior.

Alcoholics have a death rate 2.5 times higher than nonalcoholics.

Worldwide Alcohol Use

The nations that rank tops in beer, wine, and liquor consumption are shown here. Figures for the United States and Canada have been included for comparison.

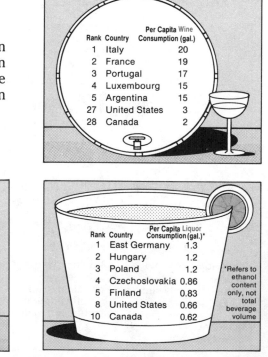

Rank	Country	Per Capita Wine Consumption (gal.)
1	Italy	20
2	France	19
3	Portugal	17
4	Luxembourg	15
5	Argentina	15
27	United States	3
28	Canada	2

Rank	Country	Per Capita Beer Consumption (gal.)
1	West Germany	39
2	East Germany	37
3	Czechoslovakia	34
4	Denmark	32
5	Belgium	31
13	United States	23
15	Canada	26

Rank	Country	Per Capita Liquor Consumption (gal.)*
1	East Germany	1.3
2	Hungary	1.2
3	Poland	1.2
4	Czechoslovakia	0.86
5	Finland	0.83
8	United States	0.66
10	Canada	0.62

*Refers to ethanol content only, not total beverage volume

Where Americans Drink the Most . . . and Least

People in Nevada consume more alcohol per capita than in any other place in the United States, but Washington, D.C., is close behind.

Utah and Arkansas residents drink the least. Here, state by state, is a look at how much Americans drink.

State	Per Capita Alcohol Consumption (gal.)	State	Per Capita Alcohol Consumption (gal.)
1. Nevada	5.07	24. Minnesota	2.56
2. Washington, D.C.	4.77	25. New York	2.55
3. New Hampshire	4.52	26. Oregon	2.54
4. Alaska	3.52	27. Virginia	2.53
5. Vermont	3.18	28. South Carolina	2.50
6. Wisconsin	3.16	29. Georgia	2.44
7. Arizona	3.15	30. Louisiana	2.43
8. Delaware	3.13	31. North Dakota	2.40
9. California	3.12	32. Missouri	2.37
10. Florida	2.97	33. Idaho	2.33
10. Massachusetts	2.97	34. Nebraska	2.28
11. Hawaii	2.89	35. South Dakota	2.24
12. Colorado	2.88	36. Pennsylvania	2.23
13. Rhode Island	2.87	37. Ohio	2.18
14. Connecticut	2.80	38. North Carolina	2.16
15. New Jersey	2.78	39. Indiana	2.15
16. Maryland	2.76	40. Iowa	2.05
17. Montana	2.74	40. Mississippi	2.05
18. New Mexico	2.70	41. Tennessee	1.96
19. Illinois	2.68	42. Alabama	1.91
20. Washington	2.66	43. Kansas	1.89
21. Wyoming	2.64	44. Kentucky	1.85
22. Texas	2.63	45. West Virginia	1.84
U.S. average	**2.63**	46. Oklahoma	1.81
23. Michigan	2.57	47. Arkansas	1.64
24. Maine	2.56	48. Utah	1.58

It's estimated that 10 percent of the U.S. population drink about half of all the alcohol consumed.

How Alcohol Harms Society

Drinking too much not only harms individuals but society as a whole. Here is how alcohol abuse is related to many of our nation's most pressing problems. The numbers represent the percentage of all cases that are related to alcohol.

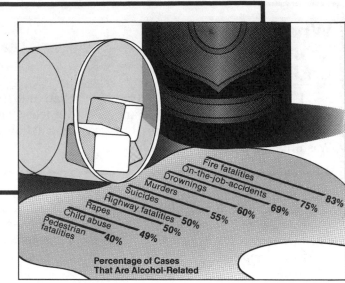

Fire fatalities
On-the-job-accidents
Drownings
Murders 83%
Suicides 75%
Highway fatalities 69%
Rapes 60%
Child abuse 55%
Pedestrian 50%
fatalities 50%
49%
40%

Percentage of Cases That Are Alcohol-Related

~~~~~**F**at-rich foods like peanut butter and cheese slow the absorption of alcohol.

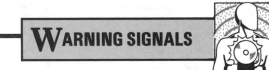

WARNING SIGNALS

Are You an Alcoholic?

If you've asked yourself that question, this itself may be reason to consider the possibility that you are suffering from alcoholism. According to Peter Nathan, Ph.D., director of the Center of Alcohol Studies at Rutgers University, these are some signs that indicate you have a condition that warrants attention.

▼ You drink to intoxication four or more days a week.

▼ You've been in trouble lately. This may mean trouble with the law (for drunken driving or spouse abuse), with your boss (for coming in late or doing shoddy work), or with a teacher (for low grades).

▼ You continue to drink, even though you are aware that it is affecting your body in negative ways. You may be having problems with your heart or liver.

▼ You continue to drink after having made one or more unsuccessful attempts to stop.

▼ You spend a great deal of time either drinking or in activities connected to drinking, such as nursing a hangover.

▼ On days when you try not to drink, you experience signs of withdrawal, like nausea, restlessness, and irritability.

5

ALLERGIES AND ASTHMA

The world can seem like an unfriendly place to the 44 million Americans who suffer from allergies and asthma. They put on a ring and they itch. They eat a certain food and they choke. They take a deep breath of a fresh spring breeze and start to sneeze their heads off.

What causes this misery? For those with allergies, it's usually a hypersensitive immune system. Instead of recognizing a grain of pollen or a bite of egg for the innocent that it is, the immune system perceives the innocent as an invader and calls out the immune system's cellular defending forces to destroy it.

Unfortunately, the chemicals used to signal this aggressive response—histamines, prostaglandins, and leukotrienes—are also the ones that cause allergy symptoms. If they're released in the gastrointestinal tract, as they would be in the case of a food allergy, the result can be vomiting or diarrhea. If they're released in the nose, eyes, and sinuses of someone who has hay fever, the result can be sneezing, a runny nose, and itchy eyes. Or if they're released in the skin, the result can be swelling and redness. Maybe even hives.

If these chemicals find their way to the lungs, they can cause airway swelling and the overproduction of mucus which will, in those who have inherited a tendency toward a "twitchy" airway, trigger an asthma attack. There are other triggers of asthma—exercise and infections are two—but for between 50 and 90 percent of those who have asthma, allergy is the cause.

How are asthma and allergies handled? Some people simply try to avoid the things that trigger their condition—pollen, dust, a particular food or fabric, whatever. Others try immunotherapy—a series of gradually more potent injections of a particular allergen—that may eventually desensitize them to the offending substance. Still others turn to a variety of drugs designed to counteract symptoms.

Who's Allergic to What?

In a joint survey of 1,000 Americans commissioned by the American Academy of Allergy and Immunology, the American College of Allergists, and the American Association for Clinical Immunology and Allergy, 37 percent of the people surveyed said they had allergies.

Forty-two percent of the women said they had allergies, compared with 32 percent of the men. And while women were more likely to suffer from allergies to food and medication, men were slightly more likely to suffer from hay fever and insect stings. Here's a breakdown of the results.

Type of Allergy	Percentage of All Allergy Victims*	Percentage of Allergic Women*	Percentage of Allergic Men*
Hay fever (pollen, grass, trees, weeds)	58	57	59
Medication	19	21	15
Dust	18	16	17
Food	16	19	12
Asthma	4	4	3
Insect sting	4	3	4
Other	24	6	6

*Since some people have more than one allergy, totals may exceed 100 percent.

An Allergy to Being Female

Some women are allergic to their own hormones. Preliminary studies of four women indicate that the release of progesterone after ovulation can apparently cause hives, vomiting, diarrhea, bloating, low blood pressure, flushing, and a life-threatening episode of airway constriction and shock—called anaphylaxis—in some women.

If you're allergic to shellfish, exposure to even the steam from a boiling or frying crustacean could leave you gasping for air.

If the December holidays make you sneeze, check your Christmas tree. It may be shedding mold—or dust, if it's artificial—along with needles and tinsel. Or maybe a male mountain cedar tree is pollinating in your living room.

An Insect Sting Can Be Fatal

Every year 50 to 100 people in the United States die from an allergic reaction to an insect sting. Yellow jackets are the most common attackers, although honeybees are more prevalent offenders in the western United States, and wasps are more common in the south-central United States.

What kind of a reaction can a susceptible person expect if stung? Here's a list of symptoms reported by 245 people. Because the more serious symptoms are potentially life-threatening, prompt medical attention is important.

Symptom	Percent reporting
Skin only	14
Hives and swelling	78
Dizziness; low blood pressure	61
Difficulty breathing; wheezing	53
Throat tightness; hoarseness	40
Loss of consciousness	33

Born to Sneeze

French scientists have discovered a link between when you're born and when you sneeze.

A study of 1,301 people indicates that those with grass pollen allergies are most likely to be born from January to May, while people with mold allergies are least likely to be born in April, May, and December.

The researchers found no association, however, between month of birth and a sensitivity to tree or weed pollen.

Is That A Fact?

Allergy shots don't usually work.

That's no longer true. Allergy shots—a series of increasingly more potent injections of whatever it is you're allergic to—used to be somewhat unpredictable because the extracts they contained weren't standardized. Today, however, that's no longer a problem, and the shots are between 75 and 90 percent effective in eliminating allergies.

Regional Sneezes

An amazing variety of allergy-triggering trees, weeds, grasses, and molds grow and thrive across the United States—each with its own favorite location and optimal season. Here's a breakdown of what blooms where and when.

Southwest. Cedar, ash, oak, and poplar trees start pollinating in February. Mulberry and olive trees pollinate from March through May. Bermuda grass, Kentucky bluegrass, and Johnsongrass spread their seed from May through September, although the season lasts from April through October around Phoenix, and never ends in southern Texas and the Gulf states. Pigweed and salt brush are an allergy problem in New Mexico from June through September, although they both cause problems in southern Texas until November. Russian thistle and ragweed bloom in Oklahoma during August and September, while amaranth pollen can distribute sneezes from May through November.

Far West. Along the West Coast, trees pollinate from January through May in the north and February through May in the south. Oak, poplar, and sycamore are particularly active, while olive trees kick up a fuss around Fresno and Los Angeles. Bermuda grass, Kentucky bluegrass, and ryegrass are waving their blades from May through July in many areas. Bromegrass, ryegrass, and Kentucky bluegrass will tickle your nose from April through December around San Francisco. Plantain and goosefoot are common throughout the region. Sagebrush is common around Reno and Los Angeles, while dock and plantain are plentiful around Seattle and Portland from May through September. Russian thistle blooms in southern California from July through October and at least a dusting of ragweed seems to be everywhere.

The Rockies. Box elder, birch, and poplar trees bloom from mid-March through May, while sagebrush, Russian thistle, and false ragweed pollinate from August through mid-October. Kentucky bluegrass, orchard grass, and redtop shed their seed

Dutch scientists found evidence of an allergy to various spices in 9 out of 12 blood samples they were checking for suspected food allergies. The allergy-provoking spices? Coriander, curry, mace, celery seed, and white pepper.

When the nose encounters an allergen, it sneezes. And, in a way, so does the heart. Its rate doubles, its beats are 43 percent stronger, and—just like the nose—it produces a flood of histamine.

from May through August. There's no ragweed season here!

The Plains states. Oak, box elder, alder, ash, birch, and sycamore blossom from March through October. Kentucky bluegrass perks up in May and lasts until July. Russian thistle and amaranth bloom in July around Kansas. Russian thistle and hemp pollinate from July through early September in Nebraska, while sagebrush causes sneezes from mid-August through September in the Dakotas. There's heavy ragweed in August and September throughout the region.

Midwest. Oak, poplar, walnut, box elder, and ash trees pollinate from March through May. Kentucky bluegrass, timothy, orchard grass, and redtop bloom from May through mid-July. The ragweed season in August and September is four times heavier than in other areas of the United States.

New England. Birch, oak, sycamore, willow, hickory, and maple trees blossom from mid-March through May. Kentucky bluegrass and timothy spread their seed from May through July. Ragweed kicks up a fuss in mid-August and continues through September—although most parts of Maine have little if any at all.

Mid-Atlantic states. Oak, birch, hickory, and walnut trees blossom from March through May. Kentucky bluegrass, redtop, timothy, and salt grass release their pollen from May through July. Ragweed, goosefoot, pigweed, and plantain reign supreme during August and September.

South. Oak, sweetgum, pecan, box elder, ash, and cottonwood blossom from mid-January through May. Bermuda grass, Kentucky bluegrass, Johnsongrass, orchard grass, and wild rye shake their tassels from May through September. All are a problem in northern Florida all year round. Ragweed, marsh elder, pigweed, and goosefoot release their pollen during August and September, although ragweed has been known to start in June in Florida and not end until October or November in South Carolina, Tennessee, Louisiana, and northern Florida.

Moms Can Give Kids Allergies

Babies born to moms who smoke are four times as likely to develop an allergy within the first 18 months of life as babies born to moms who don't, report Swedish researchers.

The chemicals in tobacco smoke circulate between the mother and her unborn child and apparently trigger the baby's immune system before he or she is even born. Then when mom lights up after birth, she knocks out more of her baby's natural defenses and opens the child to an allergy.

Do You Have Allergy Symptoms?

Every part of the body can and will react to an allergen in its own way. Here are the symptoms that try men's—and women's—souls. (Because many of these symptoms may have other causes besides allergy, be sure to check with your doctor.)

▼ Runny nose

▼ Itchy eyes, lips, mouth, throat

▼ Swollen eyes, lips, mouth, throat

▼ Hives

▼ Nausea

▼ Vomiting

▼ Cramps

▼ Gas

▼ Diarrhea

▼ Migraines

▼ Stuffy ears

▼ Bed-wetting

▼ Constricted airway

▼ Dark circles under eyes

▼ Watering eyes

▼ Abdominal pain

▼ Abdominal bloating or swelling

▼ Rash

▼ Eczema

▼ Irritability

▼ Restlessness

▼ Hyperactivity

▼ Fatigue

▼ Depression

▼ Cough

▼ Recurrent croup

▼ Feeling of tightness in chest

▼ Ear infection

▼ Popping and clicking sounds in ears

▼ Anemia

▼ Arthritis

▼ Wrinkled, "old-looking" skin around eyes

▼ Blurred vision associated with eating certain foods or smelling certain odors

▼ Sinus headache

▼ Ringing or buzzing in the ears

▼ Difficulty swallowing

▼ Chronic sore throat

▼ Chronic dry feeling in mouth or throat

▼ Sudden change of voice

▼ Chemical taste in mouth

▼ Stiff neck

▼ Chest pain

▼ Irregular heartbeat

▼ Recurrent pneumonia

▼ Swelling in both breasts

▼ Aches and pains in muscles and joints

▼ Loss of sex drive

▼ Mouth ulcers

A Bath for Your Stuffy Nose

Israeli scientists asked 102 patients with the stuffy noses of allergic rhinitis to inhale humidified warm air for two 30-minute periods separated by a 90-minute break. They repeated the experiment a week later.

The result? Seventy percent of the patients said they were breathing easier after the first week. Ninety percent claimed their breathing was easier after the second.

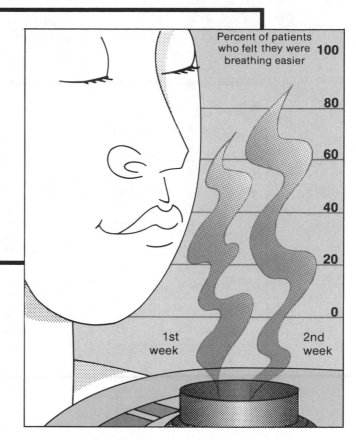

Collagen implants used in cosmetic surgery can occasionally trigger an allergic reaction. Fortunately for those getting the implants, the reactions seem to subside without treatment.

Never Underestimate the Power of Afternoon Tea

A group of scientists may have found an inexpensive way to rid your home of allergy-causing dust mites —those microscopic creatures who reside in couches and carpeting even after the gale force winds of a ferocious vacuuming.

The scientists sprayed a 3 percent solution of tannic acid—a common ingredient found in tea—over four dusty carpets and a couch to see how the solution would affect the carpets' resident population of mites.

The result? The solution killed almost every single mite in the carpets. And it decimated the ones hiding in a couch.

Allergies can be triggered by sunlight and extremes in temperature as well as by specific allergens.

Do Air Cleaners Help?

Yes. Tests involving cigarette smoke—which has particles even smaller than those of pollen or dust —reveal that a number of commercial air cleaners can effectively clear the air of airborne allergens.

In this table, machines that removed 95 percent of the smoke from a typical room in under 30 minutes were rated *excellent*.

Product	Air-Cleaning Mechanisms*	Smoke Removal Time (min.) 95% Removal	Rating
F56A 1003	AC, ESP	25.5	Excellent
Air Techniques Cleanaire 300	AC, HEPA	27.0	Excellent
Trion Console II	AC, ESP	27.5	Excellent
Associated Mills, Pollenex 1801	AC, NG	37.5	Very good
Oster 404-06	AC, ESP	42.5	Very good
Bionaire Corp. BT-1000	ELEC, NG	43.0	Very good
Trion Tabletop	AC, ESP	49.0	Good
General Time Ecologizer 99005	AC, HEPA	54.7	Good
Air Techniques Cleanaire 150	AC, HEPA	56.5	Good
Teledyne WaterPik AF3-W	AC, ESP	57.3	Good
Five Seasons Air Duster 585 A1	AC, ESP, NG	79.0	Fair
Lasko 9152	AC, NG	94.0	Fair
North American Phillips Cam 50	AC, ESP	110.0	Fair
General Time Ecologizer 98005	AC, HEPA	120+	Poor
Oster 402-06	AC, ESP	120+	Poor

*AC—Activated carbon filter
ELEC—3M Electret filter
ESP—Electrostatic precipitator
HEPA—High-efficiency particulate air filter
NG—Negative ion generator

Some people are allergic to sex. How do they know? In at least one case study, the tip-off was a fit of sneezing one minute after intercourse.

Asthma Deaths on the Upswing

The number of deaths due to asthma have more than doubled over the last two decades.

Part of the problem, experts say, is that asthmatics are delaying heavy-duty treatment in serious situations because they have so much faith in the everyday drugs—bronchodilators for the most part—prescribed to control their condition.

Some asthmatics also use everyday medication to compensate for exposure to known allergens rather than trying to avoid the allergen. Other factors that may have led to the increased number of deaths—particularly among the elderly—include irregular heartbeats as a side effect of some of the newer drugs such as theophylline.

At least a part of the increase in asthma deaths may also be due to a change in the reporting procedures of health statistics.

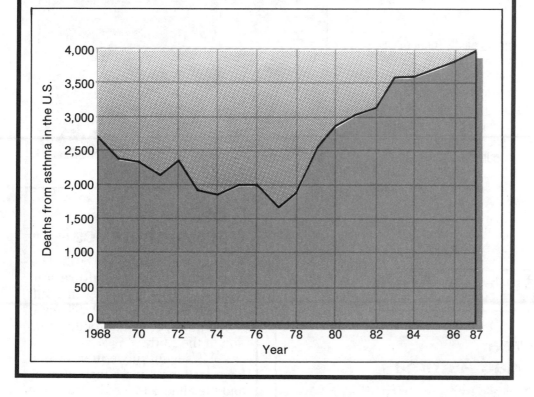

good allergic sneeze can throw water droplets 6 feet into the air at speeds of up to 100 miles per hour. Suppressing that sneeze can injure ribs, facial bones, cartilage, and ears.

What Triggers Asthma?

Sometimes it seems as though the answer could be almost anything. Here's a list of the most common asthma triggers:

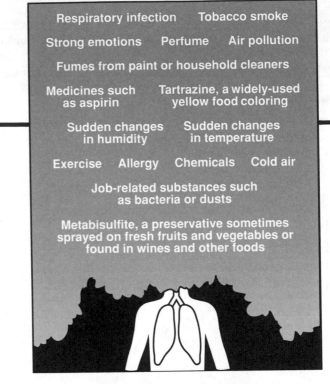

Respiratory infection   Tobacco smoke

Strong emotions   Perfume   Air pollution

Fumes from paint or household cleaners

Medicines such as aspirin   Tartrazine, a widely-used yellow food coloring

Sudden changes in humidity   Sudden changes in temperature

Exercise   Allergy   Chemicals   Cold air

Job-related substances such as bacteria or dusts

Metabisulfite, a preservative sometimes sprayed on fresh fruits and vegetables or found in wines and other foods

Asthma that is easily triggered by emotional stress can sometimes be prevented by hypnosis. Under hypnosis, the asthmatic learns to identify the people, places, or substances that may consciously or unconsciously provoke an attack, then develops post-hypnotic strategies to use when they are encountered.

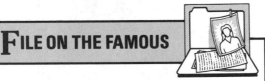

FILE ON THE FAMOUS

Superman Once Had Asthma

In his screen role as the man of steel, actor Christopher Reeve may be able to leap tall buildings in a single bound and fly faster than a speeding bullet. No one would guess that as a child, he had asthma.

Can Vitamin B$_6$ Help Asthmatics?

In a study conducted by the U.S. Department of Agriculture and Columbia University, seven adult asthmatics were given 100 milligrams of vitamin B$_6$ every day for the duration of the study.

All seven subsequently had fewer asthma attacks than normal, and the attacks that did occur were shorter and less severe. The bodies of some asthmatics may not be able to properly use B$_6$, concluded the researchers, thus creating an apparent deficiency.

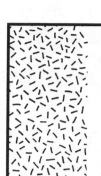

6

ANGINA

Angina. It's a pain, literally, right smack in the middle of the chest. It can press, choke, suffocate, or squeeze. It can radiate into the neck, jaw, teeth, shoulders, arms, or hands. It can affect one side or both sides of the body. It's more likely to occur in the morning than the afternoon, often during periods of exertion or emotional upset, or after eating, and it usually lasts for less than 10 minutes.

Angina is actually a symptom of myocardial ischemia, a condition in which the heart does not get enough blood. Ischemia is generally caused by the narrowing of blood vessels around the heart. The vessels become so clogged with cholesterol and other arterial debris that the flow of blood—with its precious oxygen cargo—is drastically reduced.

If you have ischemia, you may not notice the reduced blood flow when you're sitting, but when you make demands on your heart—running to catch a bus, arguing with a friend—the lack of blood may trigger angina.

But that's stable angina. Unstable angina is, as its name implies, not quite so predictable. It comes on more quickly and with less provocation, and is more difficult to relieve. And, left untreated, there's a good chance that it can escalate into a heart attack.

Fortunately, most angina can be treated with drugs that either increase the supply of oxygen to the heart muscle or reduce the heart's demand for oxygen. When that doesn't work, doctors may recommend bypass surgery: A blood vessel from the leg or chest is used to construct a detour around the clogged blood vessels in the heart. Or doctors may recommend balloon angioplasty, a kind of surgical plumbing procedure in which a thin plastic tube is threaded through an artery into the heart. Inside this first tube is a second tube with a balloon tip which is then inflated to stretch the artery walls and widen the passage. The result is often an improved flow of blood. And less angina.

Who Has Angina?

More than 7 million Americans, as this chart shows, develop ischemia that can lead to angina. The number jumps significantly after the age of 45.

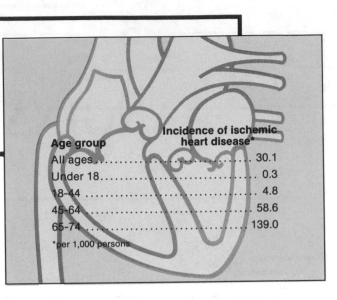

Age group	Incidence of ischemic heart disease*
All ages	30.1
Under 18	0.3
18-44	4.8
45-64	58.6
65-74	139.0

*per 1,000 persons

Only 25 percent of men and 12 percent of women with stable angina will have a heart attack within five years after the onset of ischemia.

When Angina Is Most Likely to Strike

Twenty-eight people with stable angina kept a diary of their mental states as a portable heart monitor recorded angina attacks for 48-hour periods. Taking into account the relative amounts of time spent per day in each type of activity, researchers concluded that ischemic episodes were most likely to prevail while the individuals were under mental stress.

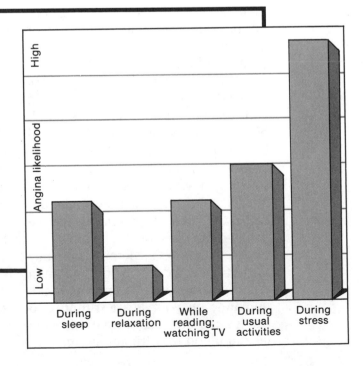

Where Do They Live?

Angina is a serious nationwide problem, but it's particularly prevalent among men in the South where, some scientists suspect, a high-fat diet of red-eye gravy and other regional specialties contributes to the build-up of cholesterol. The map shows the number of chronic angina conditions in each region.

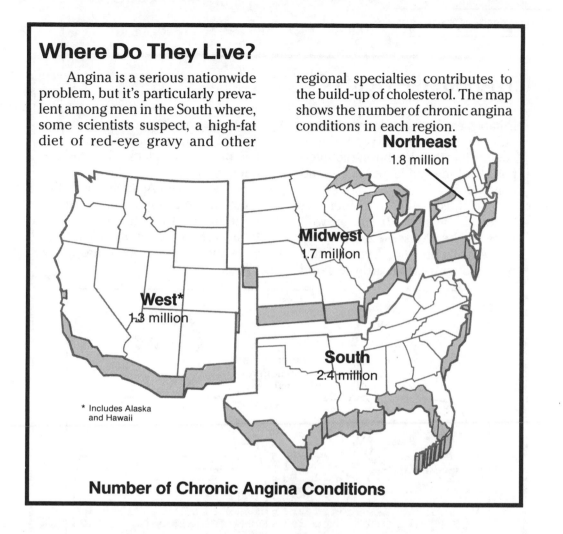

Northeast
1.8 million

Midwest
1.7 million

West*
1.3 million

South
2.4 million

* Includes Alaska and Hawaii

Number of Chronic Angina Conditions

I S THAT A FACT?

People with angina that's brought on by exertion shouldn't exercise.

No. Studies indicate that judiciously exercising right up until the onset of chest pain carries no risk, says Mayer M. Bassan, M.D., of the Jerusalem Heart Clinic. Studies have shown that exercising until the onset of pain, stopping until it subsides, then resuming the exercise actually improves exercise tolerance.

Cardiac arrest or heart attack are rarely the result of exercise, scientists report. In fact, cardiac rehabilitation programs that included exercise reduced the risk of death by 20 percent.

The Hostile Heart

Male heart patients who are irritable, easily angered, or argumentative are more likely to experience angina than their less hostile counterparts, a study conducted in Finland concluded.

Scientists asked 316 men between the ages of 40 and 59 with ischemic heart disease to complete a questionnaire that revealed how hostile they were toward the world around them. Then, based on their level of hostility, the men were divided into four groups and the number of angina attacks was subsequently tallied.

The results? As shown here, the most hostile group reported nearly three times as much chest pain as their least-hostile counterparts. They were also three times more likely to die.

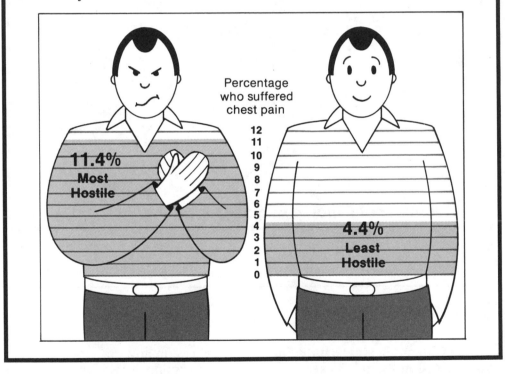

Men who are apparently healthy who choose diets relatively poor in linoleic acid—an essential fatty acid commonly found in safflower oil, sunflower oil, and corn oil—for a year or more may predispose themselves to the development of angina or a heart attack, report scientists at the University of Edinburgh.

Nifedipine, propranolol, and atenolol are all drugs given to control angina. In an eight-week study of 10 smokers with angina, British scientists found that cigarette smoking significantly interferes with the action and effectiveness of all three drugs.

Angina pain can frequently cause a decrease in saliva secretion. That's not a problem unless, of course, you try to dissolve a nitroglycerin tablet under your tongue to stop the pain. The solution? A squirt of salt water to moisten your mouth. Or ask your doctor to prescribe the new spray form of nitroglycerin.

When Nitroglycerin Fails—Try, Try Again

Sublingual (under-the-tongue) nitroglycerin tablets are frequently prescribed by doctors to halt an angina attack in its tracks.

Unfortunately, a British study revealed that 62 percent of people for whom the drug was prescribed didn't know what to do if they slipped a pill under their tongue and it didn't work.

What *should* you do? Take a second tablet 5 minutes after the first, doctors say. And if that doesn't do the job, try a third pill 5 minutes after the second.

But three pills is the maximum dose, doctors caution. If that doesn't work, call your doctor immediately.

The Best Nitro Delivery System

Nitrate drugs have been the mainstay of angina treatment for years. You can pop or squirt them under your tongue, smear them over your arm like paste, or simply apply an adhesive patch.

Which is the best? Many doctors feel it's the patch. In a study of 4,444 people with angina, doctors found that people with the patch had fewer angina attacks, fewer side effects, and less limitation of their activities.

The only drawback other than cost seems to be that the longer you wear the patches, the less effective they tend to be. Fortunately, that's easily overcome, doctors say, by removing them at night.

Can Aspirin Block a Heart Attack?

Doctors divided 479 people who had had an episode of unstable angina (the pre-heart-attack variety) within the preceding 24 hours into four groups. One group intravenously received a blood-thinning drug called heparin. A second group received aspirin plus heparin. A third group received just aspirin tablets. A fourth group received nontherapeutic (placebo) tablets.

As the chart indicates, the intravenous treatment—which can only be done in the hospital—of heparin or heparin plus aspirin was the best at preventing a subsequent heart attack.

But the strong showing of aspirin alone led the researchers to suggest that people who have unstable angina may be significantly helped by taking aspirin on a regular basis.

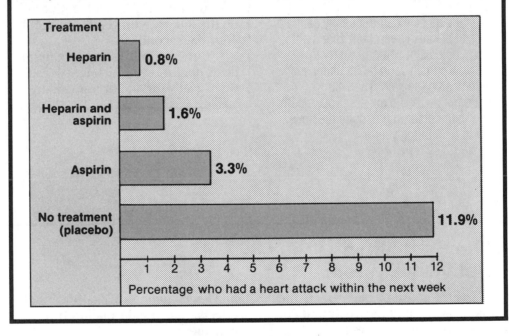

Treatment	
Heparin	0.8%
Heparin and aspirin	1.6%
Aspirin	3.3%
No treatment (placebo)	11.9%

Percentage who had a heart attack within the next week

Bypass surgery may be overused, concluded researchers at the Center for the Health Sciences, University of California at Los Angeles. In a study of 386 patients they conducted for the Rand Corporation, the researchers concluded that 14 percent of the bypasses were performed for "inappropriate" reasons, while another 30 percent were done for "equivocal reasons."

High-Tech Treatments Are on the Rise

The numbers of heart bypasses and balloon angioplasty procedures performed in the United States are dramatically increasing.

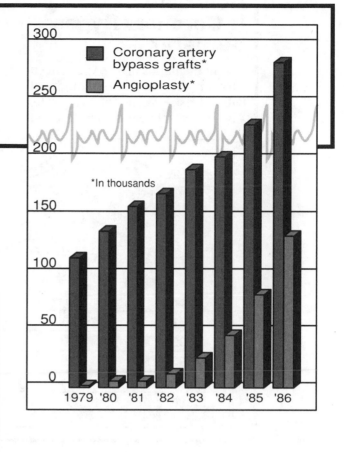

The Best Candidate for a Bypass

The angina patient who seems to be in the worst shape—or as doctors put it, the one at "increased risk"—has probably the best chance of benefiting. Such a patient would have:

▼ Angina that cannot be controlled by drugs

▼ Disease in all three major coronary blood vessels

▼ A blocked left main coronary artery

▼ A left lower heart chamber that isn't doing its job

A Harvard School of Public Health study reveals that 84 percent of patients who sought a second opinion after being scheduled for a heart bypass were told that they didn't need it.

Of those who subsequently cancelled their surgery and simply continued medical therapy, none died during the study's two-year follow-up.

How Safe Is Coronary Bypass Surgery?

In the hands of an experienced surgeon, the operation—though not without risk—can be relatively safe. And it can achieve complete relief of angina in 80 percent of patients and partial relief in another 10 percent.

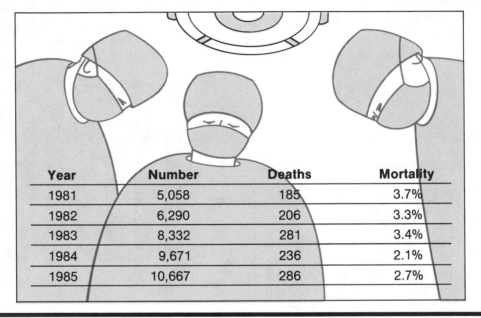

Year	Number	Deaths	Mortality
1981	5,058	185	3.7%
1982	6,290	206	3.3%
1983	8,332	281	3.4%
1984	9,671	236	2.1%
1985	10,667	286	2.7%

How Safe Is Balloon Surgery?

Data from the National Heart, Lung, and Blood Institute Registry involving 1,802 people who had angioplasty indicate the procedure's mortality rate is relatively low. But serious complications can occur during the course of the operation.

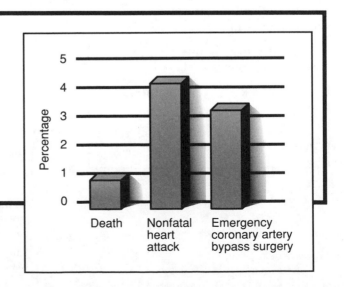

The Best Candidate for Balloon Surgery

According to the American College of Cardiology and the American Heart Association, balloon surgery is most likely to be successful if you:

▼ Are a man

▼ Are less than 65 years old

▼ Have normal function in the lower two chambers of your heart

▼ Have only one coronary blood vessel that's partially, not totally, blocked

▼ Have a procedure that only deals with a single area that is accessible to the surgeon

▼ Have a blood vessel that's flexible—not hardened, for example, by arteriosclerosis

Fish Oil Prevents Repeat Treatment

A group of doctors at the University of Texas Health Science Center at Dallas have discovered that fish oil can cut chances of needing a second artery-opening balloon procedure—a common occurrence—almost in half.

The doctors divided 82 men into two groups. One was treated with standard postballoon therapy and the other was treated with capsules of fish oil. Both groups started treatment a week before their surgery and continued it for six months afterward.

The results are shown below.

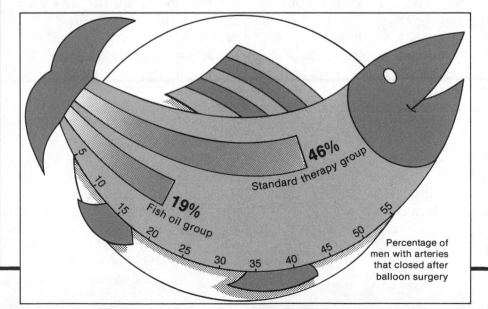

46% Standard therapy group

19% Fish oil group

Percentage of men with arteries that closed after balloon surgery

7

ARTHRITIS

Arthritis is generally a disease of aging: If you live long enough, you'll probably get some kind of arthritic pain or stiffness somewhere, like the 37 million Americans who have arthritis right now. If one kind doesn't get you, there are more than 100 others skulking about looking for joints, muscles, ligaments, or tendons to invade. The National Institute of Arthritis and Musculoskeletal and Skin Diseases estimates that serious arthritis hinders the daily lives of 4.4 million Americans, partially disabling 1.5 million, and completely disabling another 1.5 million. This disability robs the country of 70 million days of work each year.

Arthritis can be caused by injury to joints. It may also come along with an infection like Lyme disease. Or, as in the case of drug-induced lupus, it can be a by-product of medication. But most of the time, the cause is unknown. Why should joints wear out, as in osteoarthritis? Is there some kind of microbe that makes the immune system attack the very body it's supposed to defend, as in rheumatoid arthritis? Could arthritis be an allergic reaction to certain foods? Can you inherit a susceptibility to it? Is it a nervous system malfunction? Or is it perhaps not a single disease at all, but a group of symptoms, each with a different cause?

All of these theories, and more, backed by rigorously researched evidence, have been advanced in the search for a cause, and thus a cure, for arthritis. The search continues; there is no known cure. But treatment for all types of arthritis is constantly improving, and people with arthritis generally live much more comfortable lives than a generation ago.

The Major Types of Arthritis

Type	Incidence in United States	Symptoms	Prognosis
Osteoarthritis	15.8 million, mostly elderly. More common in women.	Pain, loss of mobility in one or more joints.	Progressive joint degeneration if untreated. May be halted by prescribed rest, exercise, and medication.
Rheumatoid arthritis	2.1 million. Often strikes between ages 20 and 45. Hits women three times as often as men.	Symmetric joint pain, inflammation, swelling, possible deformity, morning stiffness, fatigue, weight loss.	Chronic degenerative disease with periodic remissions. May be crippling if not treated promptly with comprehensive program of medication, rest, exercise, and other therapy.
Juvenile rheumatoid arthritis	250,000 children. May begin before age 7.	Knee or other joint pain and stiffness. Sometimes starts with high fever, rash, and no joint symptoms.	Can cause eye inflammation, growth abnormalities. Treatment generally prevents damage. Seventy percent outgrow the disease.
Ankylosing spondylosis	2.5 million. Seventy-five percent of victims are men. May strike in teens to 20s.	Gradual onset of pain and severe morning stiffness in spine; rest aggravates, exercise relieves.	Progressive loss of movement in back, legs, collarbone; abnormal curvature of spine; vertebrae may fuse. Generally controlled by medication, postural training, and exercise.
Gout	1.6 million, 80–90% men. Usually strikes after age 40; usually strikes women after menopause.	Sudden onset of extreme pain, swelling, and inflammation in a single joint, often the big toe; occasional fever, headache.	Can cause joint damage, destroy kidney cells. Controlled with medication and diet.
Scleroderma	300,000, mostly women in their 30s–50s.	Thickening and hardening of skin— especially over fingers, face, and arms—limits flexibility.	Attacks connective tissues, so can affect joints, blood vessels, internal organs. No specific medications, although aspirin, high blood pressure drugs, and antacids are helpful. Exercise to maintain flexibility.
Systemic lupus erythematosus	300,000. Women outnumber men 10 to 1; incidence higher in blacks. Begins anywhere from teens to 50s.	May start with fever, weakness, weight loss; rash on arms, neck, and face. Joint pain and symptoms of organ damage may follow.	Course of disease depends on amount of internal organ involvement. With medication, rest, exercise, and protection from sunlight, five-year survival now exceeds 90%.

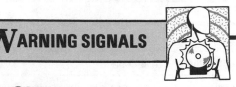

WARNING SIGNALS

Seven Signs of Arthritis

Arthritis has seven major warning signs.

▼ Swelling in one or more joints

▼ Early-morning stiffness

▼ Recurring pain or tenderness in any joint

▼ Inability to move a joint normally

▼ Obvious redness and warmth in a joint

▼ Unexplained weight loss, fever, or weakness combined with joint pain

▼ Symptoms like these lasting for more than two weeks

The Price We Pay for Arthritis

Arthritis has a cost that goes beyond pain and hits all of us in the pocketbook. Somebody must treat, care for, and insure the nurse whose arthritic hands can't hold a syringe, the pilot whose arthritic spine can't tolerate hours in the cockpit, the baseball player whose arthritic shoulder silences his bat. It all adds up, says the Arthritis Foundation, to billions of dollars annually, and it's getting costlier every year.

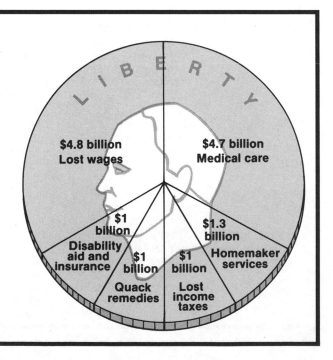

Where Osteoarthritis Strikes

Osteoarthritis most often hits the body's weight-bearing joints—hips, knees, feet, and spine (especially the neck and lower back)—and the hands. The joints at the base of the big toe and base of the thumb, and the finger joints closest to the tips, are especially vulnerable. Yet often osteoarthritis will attack only one or two joints, sparing others.

Bacterial food poisoning from poultry may cause arthritis in some people. Researchers think the bacteria's genes may even become incorporated into human cells, permanently altering the cell's DNA.

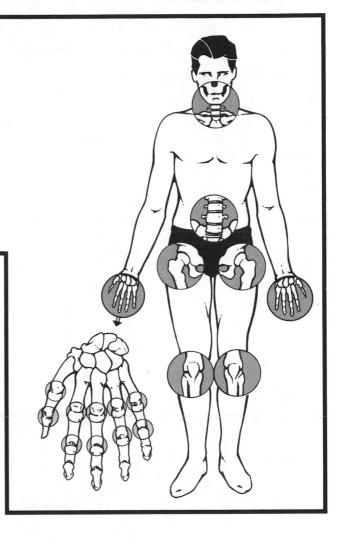

IS THAT A FACT?

People with arthritis can predict the weather by how their joints feel.

True. Several studies have confirmed that many people with arthritis feel more pain when humidity levels rise and barometric pressure drops—two hallmarks of approaching storms. Conversely, lower humidity and higher air pressure generally mean better weather, so a person with arthritis can often tell from lessening pain that the storm is passing. It's also been shown that arthritis pain drops as the temperature rises and increases as the mercury drops.

Where Rheumatoid Arthritis Strikes

In contrast to osteoarthritis, rheumatoid arthritis (RA) usually invades several joints at a time. And the attack is often symmetrical, involving the corresponding joints in each hand, foot, arm, or leg. Knees, hands, and feet are commonly the first sites to be affected. And unlike osteoarthritis, RA frequently strikes the elbows and wrists.

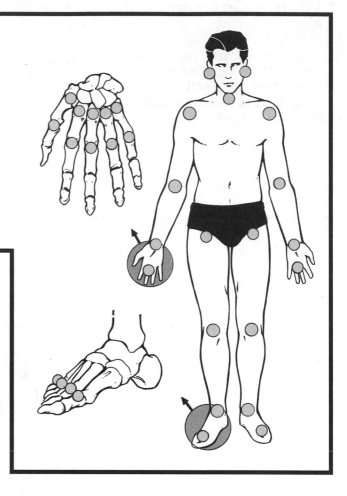

One of the best medications for rheumatoid arthritis and lupus originally was prescribed for malaria. It's a quinine-derived compound called hydroxychloroquine. More than 30 years ago it was found to bring about a remission in these severe forms of arthritis. Yet after all these years, doctors still don't know how it works.

IS THAT A FACT?

Rheumatoid arthritis is an infectious disease.

The answer isn't in, but some fascinating research indicates it may indeed be caused by some kind of infection. Rheumatologists have found evidence of RA in the skeletons of 6,500-year-old American Indi-ans excavated from the Tennessee River banks in northwestern Alabama. Yet they've been unable to find a trace of RA in Europe or Africa before the late 1600s. That leads researchers to think that some kind of microorganism or allergen native to the New World was carried to the Old World by traders or products.

The Arthritis Fact Sheet

Rank of opening medicine packages on a list of main problems of everyday life encountered by people 55 and older: 1.

Rank of fastening buttons, snaps, or zippers: 4.

Percentage of people with arthritis who say they see a physician regularly: 70.

Percentage who say they've seen a physician in the last six months: 45.

Percentage who have seen a doctor in the last six months whose quality of life worsened: 65.

Percentage who have *not* seen a doctor in the last six months whose quality of life improved: 71.

Percentage of arthritis sufferers who say, "Most arthritics feel sorry for themselves": 41.

Percentage who admit they sometimes feel sorry for themselves: 10.

Percentage of arthritis sufferers who waited less than a month to see a doctor after symptoms appeared: 30.

Percentage who waited more than a year: 33.

Between a white woman and a black woman, the odds that it is the black woman who has osteoarthritis of the knee: 2:1.

Between a 35-year-old woman and a 45-year-old woman, the odds that it is the 45-year-old who has osteoarthritis of the knee: 3:1.

Between a married man and an unmarried man, the odds that it's the bachelor who has osteoarthritis of the knee: almost 2:1.

Between a normal weight man and an obese man, the likelihood that it's the obese man who has osteoarthritis of the knee: 50 percent more likely.

Between a normal weight woman and a very obese woman, the likelihood that it's the very obese woman who has osteoarthritis of the knee: 75 percent more likely.

In the Framingham Osteoarthritis Study, percentage of nonsmokers with severe osteoarthritis: 19.7.

Percentage of light smokers: 13.5.

Percentage of heavy smokers: 11.8.

Number of hip joint replacements in 1987: 212,000.

Number of knee joint replacements in 1987: 210,000.

Amount spent by the National Institutes of Health on arthritis research, 1988: $119.7 million.

Amount spent by the federal government on interest on the national debt, fiscal 1987, *per day:* $534.2 million.

70

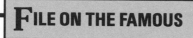

FILE ON THE FAMOUS

Living with the Pain

People whose careers have continued despite arthritis:

▼ Lynn Adams, 29, women's national racquetball champion; diagnosed with rheumatoid arthritis at age 16; still experiences flare-ups in her hands, feet, and knees; has never withdrawn from a tournament due to arthritis.

▼ Oscar Peterson, jazz pianist; diagnosed in 1979 with osteoarthritis in his hands, shoulders, and knees; uses exercise and medication; continues to record and play concerts.

Arthritis Remedies You Don't Need

A lot of people—sometimes even doctors—claim they have the cure for arthritis. That claim is your first hint you're being quacked at. Other giveaways: The "cure" is "secret" or "exclusive"; testimonials; hard-sell advertising; the treatment "cleanses" the body of "toxins"; no evidence is offered of reliable clinical testing. Here are a few remedies that have been promoted by these methods and found scientifically wanting.

▼ Sitting in a uranium mine for 2 hours a day

▼ Copper bracelets

▼ Seaweed bracelets

▼ WD-40 lubricant sprayed on joints

▼ Vibrating chairs and beds

▼ Elimination diets (except for gout)

▼ Bee, ant, or snake venom

▼ Injections of turtle blood

▼ Aloe vera

▼ Mussel extract

▼ Radioactive uranium mittens or bracelets

▼ DMSO (dimethyl sulfoxide)

▼ Counterirritants (menthol or camphor ointments)

▼ Self-administered hormones or steroids

▼ Covering your body with cow manure twice a day

▼ Standing naked in the full moon

IS THAT A FACT?

People with arthritis should avoid exercise because of pain and possible damage to joints.

No. The Arthritis Foundation says that people with arthritis need to exercise their joints daily. The benefits? Joint flexibility, muscle strength, overall stamina, a positive self-image, and a sense of accomplishment. Here are six tips to help you exercise safely and effectively.

1. Consult with your doctor to set up an exercise program.

2. Start at a comfortable level and gradually increase repetitions.

3. Be sure to get enough rest between exercise periods. Sleep and nap as much as you need.

4. Plan to exercise twice a day for the rest of your life.

5. Choose a time and place for your daily workout, and then stick to them.

6. Exercise when you have the least pain, stiffness, and fatigue.

When Drugs and Nutrients Don't Mix

Some vitamins and minerals interfere with arthritis drugs, although most often it's an arthritis drug that interferes with vitamins and minerals. Because of your medication, it may be necessary to take a supplement, or to stop taking one. Check with your doctor first.

Penicillamine. This drug may increase your need for vitamin B_6 and zinc.

Zinc. Supplements of this mineral can make drug-induced lupus worse.

Too much vitamin D. In patients with gout and rheumatoid arthritis, excess vitamin D can lead to deposits of calcium on already damaged joints.

Colchicine. This gout drug can inhibit your ability to absorb vitamin A and may adversely affect potassium levels.

Probenecid. Another gout drug, probenecid decreases the body's absorption of riboflavin (vitamin B_2) and may adversely affect potassium levels.

Cortisone drugs. These drugs, such as prednisone, interfere with your calcium balance and cause you to lose zinc. They may also adversely affect potassium levels.

Anti-inflammatory drugs. Combined with rheumatoid arthritis inflammation, these drugs may increase the need for vitamin C.

The Most Popular Pain Relief Remedies

When the Upjohn Company surveyed the lifestyles of 501 arthritis sufferers, 98 percent responded with information about the remedies they use. Medication to relieve pain and inflammation leads the way. But heat can also ease the morning stiffness arthritis brings and increase blood circulation to ailing joints. Exercise keeps joints mobile and also helps circulation. Resting a hurting joint is an easy, commonsense remedy. Cold water or ice packs reduce inflammation, while paraffin baths are a particularly good treatment for sore hands.

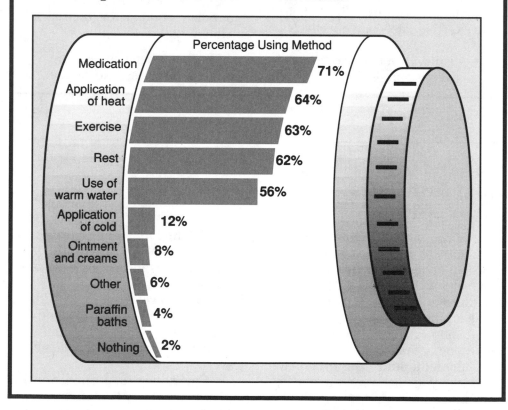

Percentage Using Method

Method	
Medication	71%
Application of heat	64%
Exercise	63%
Rest	62%
Use of warm water	56%
Application of cold	12%
Ointment and creams	8%
Other	6%
Paraffin baths	4%
Nothing	2%

Whipple's disease, a fat malabsorption disorder, often hides behind arthritis, a major symptom. One study found patients had arthritis for up to 26 years before doctors realized they actually had Whipple's disease and put them on antibiotics, saving their lives and often curing the disease.

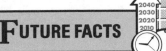

FUTURE FACTS

Brave New (Arthritic) World

These are some of the products you'll be seeing more and more of as America ages and a larger proportion of the population comes down with arthritis.

There will be fewer knobs on doors, cabinets, and sinks, and more **levers.** Instead of having to push windows open and pull them closed, you'll be able to use a **crank.** Back zippers will have **long-handled grips** for ease of closing. To wash dishes you'll have **lightweight, motorized scrubbers.**

Bathtubs will be constructed of a **soft material** that's safer and more comfortable and keeps water hotter longer. Bathtubs and showers will have **built-in seats.**

Public transportation will have **lower steps** and **lifting platforms. Slower-changing traffic lights** and **pedestrian islands** in the middle of wide streets will let you cross the street safely. More and more **microcars** will help you get around town and through the shopping malls.

On the medical front, more people with arthritis will be able to have joints, bones, ligaments, tendons, and even muscles replaced with **bionic parts.** Twenty or more years down the road, laboratory-created **mono-clonal antibodies** will target immune cells that have run amok, contributing to the inflammation of rheumatoid arthritis and lupus. Doctors will be able to switch on and off different parts of the immune system. They'll be able to **alter or block infective agents** that trigger some types of arthritis—much of this therapy will be based on research gained from studying Lyme disease. Advances in **genetic therapy** will enable doctors to identify people at high risk and treat them before arthritis gets a foothold. Arthritis treatments will be **less toxic.**

Cancer research has yielded new possibilities for arthritis treatment. Be ready for futuristic drugs like **spirogermanium** and **radiopharmaceuticals.** By 1992, humans may be test subjects for the anti-cancer drug spirogermanium, which stops inflammation by suppressing the immune system's attack on healthy cells. And radiopharmaceuticals like **dysprosium 165**—when attached to a special carrier—have already been shown to stop the overproduction of synovial tissue, reducing swelling. Researchers are now investigating the long-term effectiveness and safety of these drugs.

BACK PROBLEMS

Four out of five backs were made wrong. The 33 vertebrae, 23 disks, 31 pairs of nerves, and countless muscles and ligaments that are arranged into four gentle curves around the spinal cord just didn't come out the way they were intended.

Fortunately, these congenital oddities rarely cause problems. The primary causes of back problems are everyday muscle stresses and strains. They occur so frequently that—aside from the common cold—back pain is the most common affliction known to man. It strikes 80 percent of all adults, with nearly half of the adult population in pain at any given moment.

An estimated $5 billion is spent on diagnosis and treatment every year. One study found that 40 percent of Americans with back pain tried to get rid of it by visiting a doctor of medicine or doctor of osteopathy. Thirty percent visited a chiropractor. Those visiting doctors averaged 2.8 visits per year, while those visiting chiropractors averaged 8.2. Interestingly, no matter who you do—or do not—visit, 45 percent of all back pain disappears in one week, 80 percent disappears in four weeks, and 90 percent disappears in eight weeks.

Most back pain can be relieved by a combination of bed rest and anti-inflammatory medication followed by gentle exercise. But 300,000 people undergo surgery to relieve back pain every year. Doctors are beginning to suspect that much of it is unnecessary.

Where You Live Affects Your Back

Statistics suggest you have a much better chance of living without chronic back problems if you live in the northeastern United States. Your risk increases by almost 45 percent if you live in the West.

Here are the actual rates of chronic back problems per thousand people in the United States.

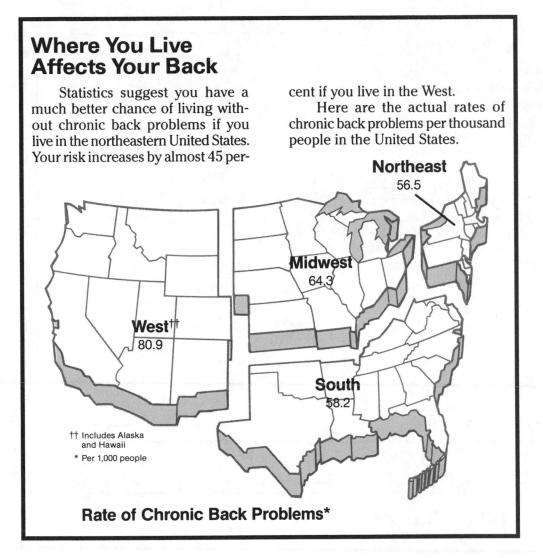

Northeast
56.5

Midwest
64.3

West††
80.9

South
58.2

†† Includes Alaska and Hawaii

* Per 1,000 people

Rate of Chronic Back Problems*

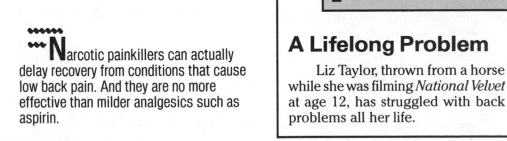

Narcotic painkillers can actually delay recovery from conditions that cause low back pain. And they are no more effective than milder analgesics such as aspirin.

File ON THE FAMOUS

A Lifelong Problem

Liz Taylor, thrown from a horse while she was filming *National Velvet* at age 12, has struggled with back problems all her life.

Where's the Pain?

The most common cause of acute back pain is an injury to the joint between the lumbar vertebrae and the sacrum in your lower back. The joint acts as a fulcrum and supports your weight when you lift or bend. If you twist your back while lifting—or perhaps heave something before your back muscles are braced —it's this joint and its overlying muscles that are likely to cry out in pain. It may take them a day or two to start screaming, but once stretched or strained you can be sure that they're going to let you know how they feel about this kind of abuse.

The most common cause of chronic low back pain, particularly in those over the age of 50, is degenerative disk disease. It's characterized by the narrowing of the space between the vertebrae, placing destructive stress on the spine.

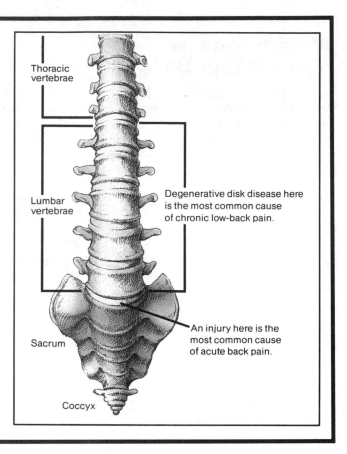

Thoracic vertebrae

Lumbar vertebrae

Degenerative disk disease here is the most common cause of chronic low-back pain.

Sacrum

An injury here is the most common cause of acute back pain.

Coccyx

When Surgery Makes Sense

Back surgery is reserved for those few people who:

▼ Have evidence of actual or impending nerve damage that does not respond to conservative medical treatment

▼ Have a numbness that progresses to a definite loss of feeling in the skin

▼ Have muscular weakness in the area affected by the damaged nerve

▼ Have loss of bowel or bladder function

Pain is *not,* doctors say, a reason to have surgery.

The Pressures of Everyday Life

Since most back pain is caused by stretched, strained, or torn back muscles, a Swedish doctor decided to investigate the amount of physical stress everyday activities such as laughing and lifting placed on the back.

Using a pressure gauge, he literally measured the amount of pressure (in pounds) on a woman's spine for each of 13 activities. Here's what he found.

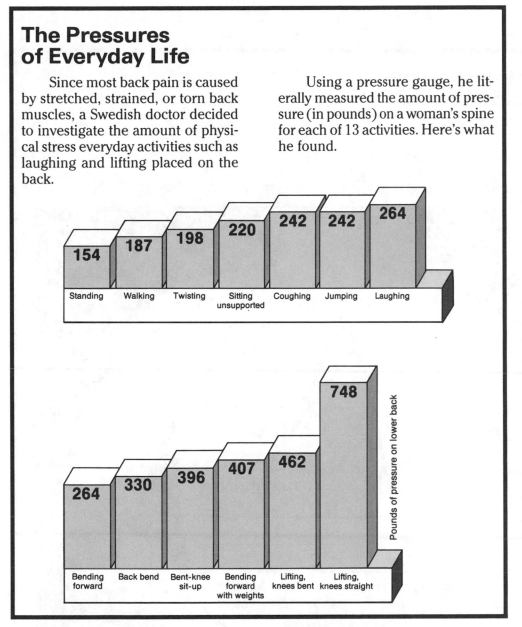

154	187	198	220	242	242	264
Standing	Walking	Twisting	Sitting unsupported	Coughing	Jumping	Laughing

Pounds of pressure on lower back

264	330	396	407	462	748
Bending forward	Back bend	Bent-knee sit-up	Bending forward with weights	Lifting, knees bent	Lifting, knees straight

Back pain is primarily a man's problem—partly because men are more likely to be involved in heavy-duty labor, and partly because they are more susceptible than women to infections, tumors, and diseases affecting the back.

Who Gets a Sprained Back?

Everyone. Between the ages of 17 and 45, though, it's mostly men. After the age of 65, it's mostly women. And everybody's highest risk occurs between the ages of 25 and 55.

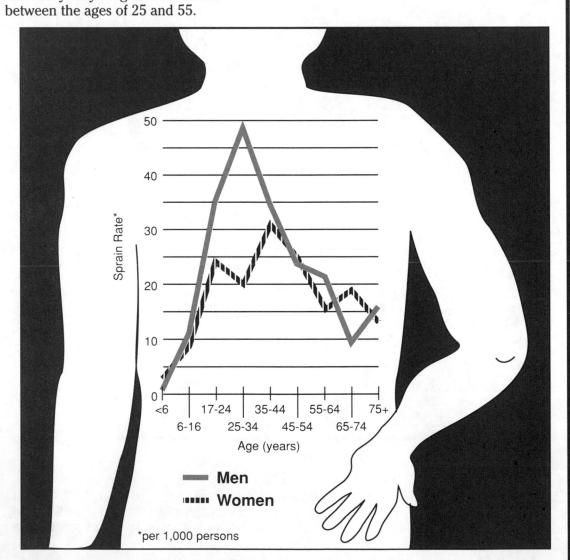

Sprain Rate*

Age (years)

━━━ **Men**
▪▪▪▪▪ **Women**

*per 1,000 persons

What Kinds of Doctors Treat a Bad Back?

Any doctor you visit will probably be willing to treat your back. But some can provide more specialized services than others. Here's a list of whom you're likely to see or be referred to:

▼ Family practitioner—specializes in general medicine

▼ Neurologist—specializes in treating the nervous system

▼ Neurosurgeon—specializes in using surgery to treat the nervous system

▼ Orthopedist (including orthopedic surgeon)—specializes in treating damaged muscles, bones, and joints

▼ Osteopathic physician—specializes in manipulating muscles and joints to treat problems

▼ Physiatrist—specializes in using physical therapy to treat problems

▼ Chiropractor—specializes in manipulation and adjustment of the spinal column

Getting Back to Work

A team of doctors, nurses, and physical therapists at the University of Texas Health Science Center (UTHSC) in Dallas were concerned because a significant number of workers who injure their backs never return to work.

So the UTHSC team compared two groups of back-injured people. One group received several weeks of intensive rehabilitation including exercises, personal counseling, and work simulation. A second group received regular medical care as needed, but did not participate in the intensive rehabilitation program.

Two years later the UTHSC team evaluated both groups. Their findings are summarized in the chart.

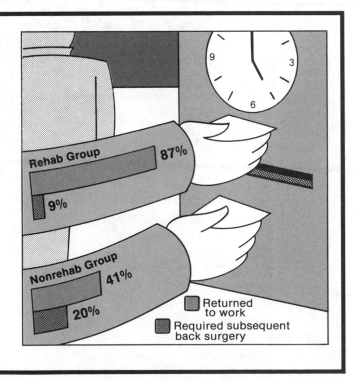

Rehab Group 87%
9%

Nonrehab Group 41%
20%

■ Returned to work
▨ Required subsequent back surgery

What You're Most Likely to Be Doing When You Sprain Your Back

Lifting. A survey of 903 workers by the U.S. Department of Labor revealed that 77 percent of back sprains were the result of lifting—generally while bending.

How can such injuries be avoided? Bend your knees and keep any object you're lifting close to your body, experts advise.

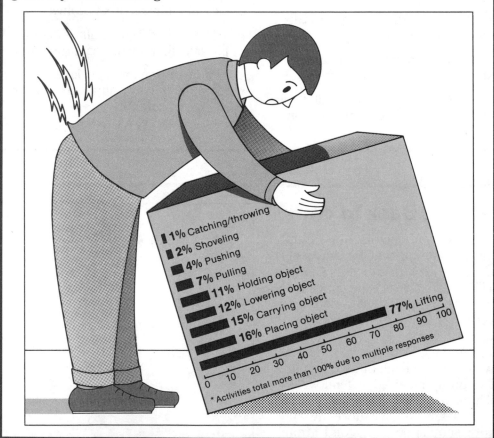

1% Catching/throwing
2% Shoveling
4% Pushing
7% Pulling
11% Holding object
12% Lowering object
15% Carrying object
16% Placing object
77% Lifting

0   10   20   30   40   50   60   70   80   90   100

* Activities total more than 100% due to multiple responses

Smokers are more likely to have unsatisfactory back surgery results than nonsmokers. The reason? Smoking robs the vertebrae of nutrients and lowers the available oxygen supply needed for proper fusion and healing.

Treatments for Back Problems

Most back problems seem to respond to a combination of bed rest and anti-inflammatory medications, followed by gentle movement. Here's a rundown of treatments your doctor is likely to recommend for specific problems.

Problem	Character of Pain	Possible Treatments
Arthritis	Ache	Exercise; nonsteroidal anti-inflammatory drugs (NSAIDs) such as ibuprofen; antirheumatic drugs; corticosteroids
Broken back	Sharp	Set broken bones; use cast or brace to immobilize spine; spinal fusion if fracture doesn't heal properly
Diskitis	Severe, sharp	Antibiotics; immobilization
Gout	Sharp (acute) or ache (chronic)	Colchicine; NSAIDs; corticosteroids; uricosurics; xanthine oxidase inhibitors
Herniated disk	Sharp with numbness	Rest; NSAIDs; steroid shots; no lifting over 50 lbs.; progress to exercises; surgery if pain continues
Herpes zoster (shingles)	Burning	Analgesics; corticosteriods
Infection	Sharp	Antibiotics; bed rest with plaster body cast or brace to rest spine; surgery to drain an abscess (rare)
Muscle strain	Sharp or ache	Controlled physical activity; NSAIDs
Osteoporosis	Acute (fracture) or dull (chronic)	Calcium; vitamin D; estrogens; calcitonin; fluoride
Osteomalacia	Diffuse ache	Vitamin D; calcium; phosphate
Scoliosis	None	No active treatment if mild; brace if moderate; spinal fusion if severe

A Caution about Rub-On Relief

Those warm-but-smelly topical painkillers—Ben-Gay, Icy Hot, Tiger Balm, and oil of wintergreen—stimulate the circulation of blood to an aching back and can bring relief.

But exercise some common sense in using them. Never use a heating pad after any of these rubs, and never cover the area afterward with anything other than normal clothing. Covering or heating could dangerously increase absorption of these painkillers and cause serious injury to the skin.

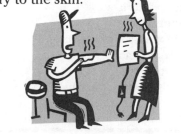

The Best and Worst for an Aching Back

A bad back can make you feel as though you'll never be comfortable again. You shift in your seat, lean forward, lean back, sit on one buttock, then the other, cross and uncross your legs. Nothing helps. It may be that your problem is being complicated—and exacerbated—by the way in which your back is supported. Here's a list of the best and the worst supports for a bad back.

Item	The Best	The Worst
Chair	Firm recliners with contoured support and an adjustable, lower-back cushion	Soft, cushy chairs that don't adjust
Car seat	Japanese and Swedish models—they usually support the curve of the spine	American models—they often lack contoured support
Bed	An adjustable waterbed that doesn't make too many waves	Any bed with a soft, saggy mattress

Back Pain Relief—Who's Got the Knack?

Who is most likely to provide relief from back pain? An orthopedist? A neurologist? How about a neurosurgeon?

The answer—at least in one survey of 492 back pain sufferers from 10 to 90 years old—is none of the above.

Practitioner	Moderate to Dramatic Long-Term Relief (%)	Temporary Relief Only (%)	No Relief (%)
Yoga instructors	96	4	0
Dance instructors	90	0	0
Physiatrists	86	0	7
Physical therapists	65	8	17
Acupuncturists	36	32	28
Chiropractors	28	28	33
Osteopathic physicians	28	15	46
Orthopedists	23	9	61
Neurosurgeons	26	8	51
Family practitioners and internists	20	14	54
Massage therapists	10	63	27
Neurologists	4	4	76

Fit Backs Don't Get Hurt

A study of 1,652 firefighters reveals that people who keep their backs in shape don't suffer from back problems like the rest of us.

Based on tests of muscular strength, flexibility, and cardiovascular endurance, the firefighters were divided into three groups: most fit, moderately fit, and least fit.

The results? Firefighters in the "most fit" group were least likely to injure their backs, while almost 80 percent of the firefighters in the "least fit" group actually did.

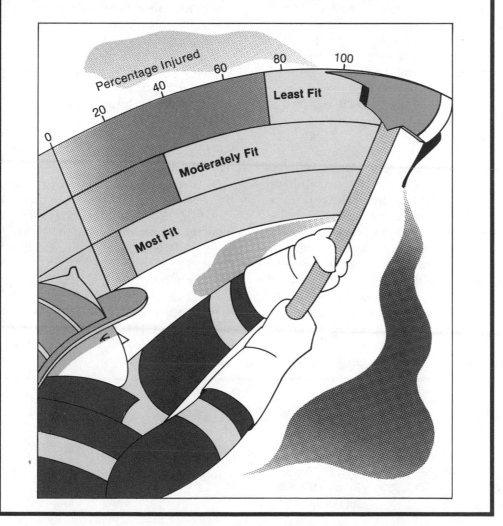

Percentage Injured
0 20 40 60 80 100

Least Fit

Moderately Fit

Most Fit

The Best Back Strengtheners

Ninety percent of back pain is due to weak, inflexible muscles. Here are seven back exercises that will build both strength and flexibility.

Pelvic tilt. Stand with your back and shoulders against a wall, your feet at shoulder width and your heels about 8 inches from the wall. Bend your knees slightly, then tighten your buttocks and pull in your stomach. Try to make the small of your back touch the wall. Hold for a count of six. Relax upward, then repeat. Once you've got the hang of it, do it without the wall. This simple stance instantly relieves lower back strain when lifting and standing.

Arm and leg raises. Lie face-down on a mat, with two pillows under your abdomen. Keep your arms at your sides. With your knee straight, lift one leg off the floor until it is even with the level of the pillows. Hold 6 seconds. Drop, and repeat with the other leg. Next, extend your left arm straight forward overhead. Simultaneously, lift your right leg, keeping your knee straight, until it is level with the pillows. Hold 6 seconds. Alternate arms and legs.

Curls. Lie on your back and bend both knees. Begin to exhale slowly while lifting first your head, then your shoulders, off the mat. With your arms outstretched, hold for 6 seconds.

Side-to-side sit-ups. Lie on your back with knees bent and feet on the floor. Touch your chin to your chest, stretch your arms forward, and slowly curl up, reaching toward the right (or left) knee. Hold for 6 seconds.

"Cat" pose. Get on your hands and knees, with lower back relaxed. Drop your head, pull in your stomach muscles, and make your back as rounded and high as possible. Hold 6 seconds.

Butt-tucks. Lie on your back, knees bent and feet flat. Push down and lift buttocks off the floor. Shoulders should remain on the mat. Hold 5 seconds, then slowly return to the floor.

Side-lying leg lifts. Lie on your right side, your bottom leg slightly bent, your top leg straight. Slowly lift your top leg up, keeping the kneecap facing forward and your body straight.

Just slipping on a pair of cushioned running shoes or sticking a spongy dime-store insert into regular shoes relieved chronic low back pain in 80 percent of one study's participants.

9

BODY CYCLES

iming is everything. Each of the more than 200 lashes on each of your eyes is shed every three to five months. The life span of a taste bud is ten days. About a quart of blood flows through your brain every minute. It takes 72 seconds for an ovary to push an egg cell into a fallopian tube, but an entire day for your brain to produce half a quart of cerebrospinal fluid.

Every part of your body is affected by a number of inner cycles, or circadian rhythms, each with its own particular ebb and flow. Some cycles control the way your body uses food. Others control the way you eat. Still others control your mood, fertility, sleep, even your ability to make love.

What normally keeps these cycles moving to a regular inner beat? The coordinator is believed to be a "master clock," which becomes activated in the seventh month of gestation. Most scientists believe it is located in a special part of the brain's hypothalamus and is "set" by your mother's master clock while you're still growing in the womb. Sunlight hitting the retina after you're born transmits signals directly to the hypothalamus, keeping your body in sync.

Time for Your Personal Best

Many of the body cycles that ebb and flow throughout the day affect your ability to do various kinds of jobs. Your ability to think reaches a peak around noon, for example, then bottoms out suddenly and rises again somewhere around 3:00 P.M. And it's not an occasional variation. It's a cycle you can count on day after day—a cycle you can use to reach your highest levels of emotional, intellectual, and physical performance.

Here's a round-the-clock overview of when several body cycles make your personal bests most likely to occur. Exact timing may vary from person to person.

Time	Activity
9 A.M.–Noon	You think best in the morning. Complex analyses and decisions are most likely to demonstrate peak mental performance right up until noon.
1 P.M.	Your alertness takes a sudden drop after noon. But a lunch that is high in protein, low in both fat and calories, and devoid of alcohol will help counter your body's natural after-lunch droop.
2 P.M.	Your physical flexibility peaks in the early afternoon—making this a good time for yoga, stretching exercise, or even a gymnastic workout.
3 P.M.	You learn best in the afternoon. That means you should study for tests, take tennis lessons, or hold instructional staff meetings between the hours of 3 P.M. and 5 P.M.
4 P.M.	You work with your hands best at midafternoon. Whether you're making a piece of

Time	Activity
	furniture, practicing a new sonata, or typing a letter to mom, you're more likely to do it best right about this time.
5 P.M.	Your senses are most acute in the late afternoon. This is the time to sniff your roses, stroke your cat, or listen to a Bach cantata. You'll experience them all much more intensely before the evening gets started.
6 P.M.–10 P.M.	Your body is ready for peak physical performance. You can catch any ball that comes your way because your reaction time and your coordination is highest right about now.
11 P.M.–4 A.M.	Your body's best time to sleep is when it's dark.
4 A.M.–6 A.M.	You're least alert either mentally or physically. This is an especially dangerous time to drive.
7 A.M.–8 A.M.	You make love best in the morning, when sex hormones are at their peak.

Most women will have over 400 menstrual cycles between menarche and menopause.

〜〜〜
Irregular periods are associated with a near-doubling of a woman's risk of heart attack.

What's Best for Shift Workers

A perfect shift rotation—perfect for you, not necessarily your employer—would rotate shifts clockwise (example: the 3:00 P.M.-to-11:00 P.M. shift would follow the 7:00 A.M.-to-3:00 P.M. shift) and require a minimum of 18 days between shift changes. This approach keeps sleep-wake cycle disruptions at a minimum.

IS THAT A FACT?

There's more violence on the streets and in mental institutions when the moon is full.

This one's light years away from the truth. A review of 37 studies that attempted to correlate the moon's phases with violent crime, suicide, crisis center hotline calls, psychiatric disorders, and mental hospital admissions found that there is absolutely no relation between moon and mind.

〜〜〜
Premenstrual Syndrome—PMS—is a cyclical disorder with a confusing array of symptoms. Everything from noise sensitivity to indecisiveness—as well as weight gain, bloating, and a stiff neck—has been labeled as an indication of the problem.

The Reproductive Cycle

Most girls enter puberty roughly around the age of 11 and are biologically mature and ready to produce babies four years later. Boys start puberty about six months after the girls, but finish the job a little more quickly: in 3½ years. Scientists don't know exactly what triggers puberty itself, but they do know that the timing is determined by genes.

After age 35, female sex hormones begin a very gradual decline until, somewhere in a woman's late forties, the decline accelerates and menopause begins. Menopause itself is a transitional period that can take 10 or 15 years to complete.

Men follow a similar pattern, so that by age 45 the amount of male sex hormones secreted by the testes is significantly reduced. By the time a man is 60 his hormone levels have sunk to where they were before puberty.

A Headache
for All Seasons

A number of scientific studies have demonstrated that seasonal variations can trigger headaches in large numbers of people.

A group of Italian researchers studied 495 people who suffered from a variety of headaches to see if they could figure out what kinds of headaches were most likely to be triggered in which seasons. They discovered that seasonal influences were more likely to trigger headaches in those who suffered from migraines—especially in the spring.

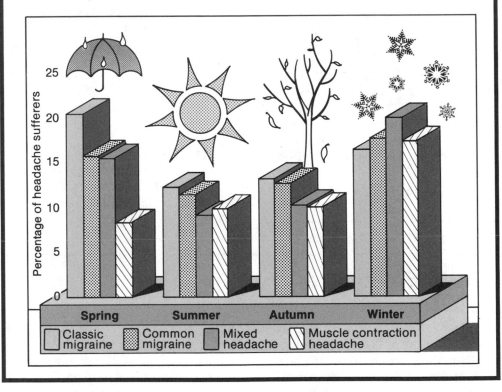

Stefania Follini, a young Italian interior decorator, spent 131 days alone in a New Mexico cave to see what effect light deprivation would have on her body cycles. The result? She lost 17 pounds, her menstruation ceased, and her sleep/wake cycles altered until she was staying awake 20 to 25 hours at a time.

When Should You Get a Tooth Filled?

In the afternoon. Because that's when your tooth's pain threshold—as determined by the time it takes to react to severe cold—is highest. It's also the time when the numbness caused by anesthesia lasts the longest.

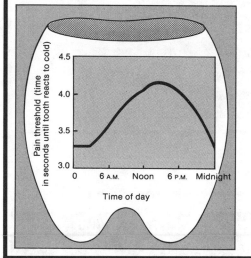

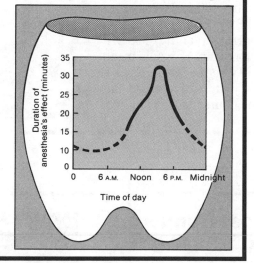

A Year in the Life of Vitamin D

Because vitamin D generation depends on sunlight striking the skin, the amount of this nutrient in your bloodstream rises and falls with the seasonal availability of sunshine.

Here's how the levels of vitamin D fluctuated between seasons in a British study of 912 elderly men and women.

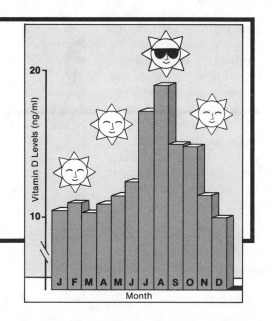

Do You Really Have a Fever?

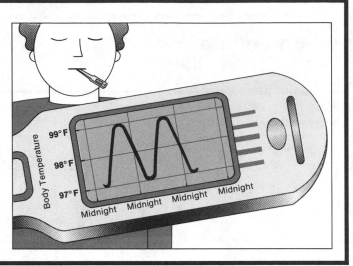

It depends on when you take your temperature. That's because normal body temperature rises and falls throughout the day, reaching a high of 99°F by 5:00 or 6:00 P.M. and a low of 97°F by 3:00 or 4:00 A.M.

So a "normal" reading of 98.6°F at 3:00 A.M., for example, would mean that, yes, you've got a fever. Here's a look at how your temperature can vary over the course of a day or two.

The Most Dangerous Drink of the Night

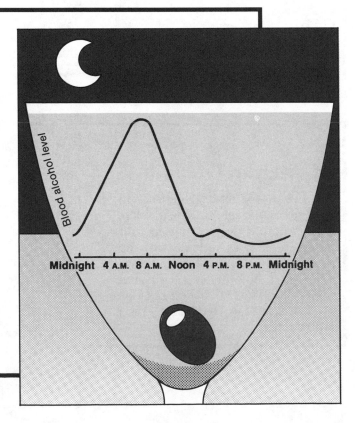

An enthusiastic group of volunteers has demonstrated that an early evening cocktail is far less likely to affect you than a wee-hours nightcap.

Why? Your body breaks down alcohol more slowly in the hours after midnight than it does earlier in the evening. So late-night alcohol stays in your blood longer and depresses your mental ability far more than at any other time. That's why "one for the road" after a late party can be the most dangerous drink all night.

The chart indicates how long alcohol stays in the blood after regular hourly intakes of equal amounts.

Where People Are SAD

Seasonal Affective Disorder (SAD) and its milder variant, the winter blues, are conditions that affect nearly one-quarter of the American population every winter. SAD is characterized by depression and a tendency to overeat and oversleep to the point that both work and relationships are impaired.

Some scientists feel that abnormally timed circadian rhythms—brought on by short winter days with their limited sunlight—may influence this condition. Fortunately, 60 to 80 percent of those who are treated by daily exposure to intense artificial light seem able to overcome the problem and return to a life of normal eating, sleeping, and feeling.

Here's a map of where people who suffer from SAD in the United States are most likely to live. As you can see, people who live in the sunnier areas of the country are least likely to have the condition.

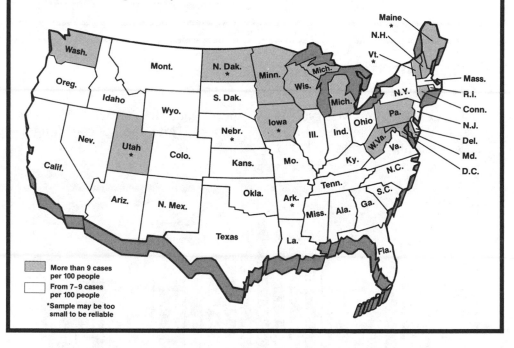

More than 9 cases per 100 people

From 7–9 cases per 100 people

*Sample may be too small to be reliable

The amniotic fluid that surrounds a baby in the womb is completely replaced every 3 hours. No wonder pregnant women are always running to the bathroom!

When Hearts Beat Fastest

Perhaps regulated by the rhythmic output of adrenaline and similar hormones from the adrenal gland, your heart has a regular daily rhythm that speeds up during the day and slows down at night.

The variation amounts to a difference of 20 to 30 beats per minute —not an insignificant amount when you consider that the average number of beats per minute is only around 85.

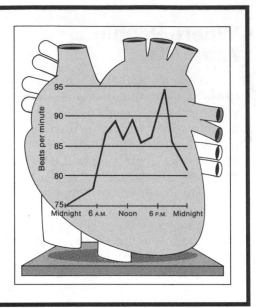

Some Mornings Can Kill You

Here are the times when you're most at risk for a sudden, fatal heart attack, according to a study of 2,203 people at the Harvard Medical School. Note the special danger period from 9:00 to 11:00 A.M.

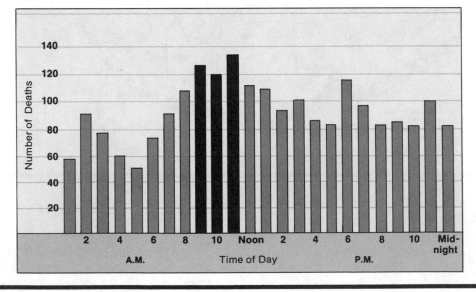

The Highs and Lows of Cholesterol

A study of 1,446 men with high cholesterol levels reveals that cholesterol levels are highest in the winter and lowest in the summer.

Following participants over a four-year period, the scientists found that cholesterol levels were 7.6 points higher in December and January of each year than in June and July. Heavy holiday eating might account for at least some of the variation, scientists suspect, as might an increase in enzyme activity triggered by long winter nights. At least one preliminary study indicates that seasonal cholesterol changes may be offset by a daily dose of vitamin C.

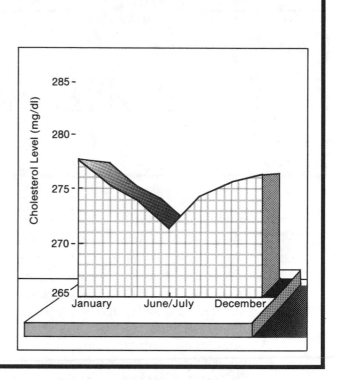

Even our craving for certain types of foods follows a seasonal cycle. A study conducted in a cafeteria at the National Institutes of Health revealed that people generally buy salads, cottage cheese, yogurt, and skim milk in the spring and summer, but switch to a heavy carbohydrate load of starchy foods and cooked vegetables during the fall. It may be this pattern, scientists say, that makes it easiest to lose weight in the spring—and hardest to lose weight in the fall.

FUTURE FACT

Time for Your Medicine

Instead of merely prescribing medication once, twice, or four times a day, doctors of the future will probably be able to tell patients the *exact* time to take their medicine. Synchronizing a particular drug with the body's absorption rhythms will allow doctors to reduce the unpleasant side effects of some medications and maximize the beneficial effects of others.

10

BONE HEALTH

Your skeleton is not just a bunch of bones; a stiff, unyielding, and unchanging scaffold to hang your organs, muscles, skin, and the latest fashions on. Well supplied with blood, your 206 bones are dynamic, living tissue, constantly being broken down and built up in a process known as remodeling. Cells called osteo*clasts* absorb bone; other cells, the osteo*blasts,* create bone by laying down a web of protein and filling in the spaces with calcium. By the time you've reached your first birthday, your entire skeleton has been remodeled. During each of your young-adult years, between 15 and 30 percent of your skeleton is remodeled again. By about the time you reach age 35, your skeleton has reached its peak mass, when your bones are most dense and strong, tough enough to bear a pressure of 24,000 pounds per square inch.

Then things start going downhill. After your mid-thirties, your bones start losing more substance than they create, and bone mass begins dropping. As women approach age 45 and men near 60, they begin absorbing less calcium from food. Aging also makes people less active, so they eat less, including less calcium. And after menopause, the loss of estrogen accelerates women's loss of bone.

No one knows for certain why all this happens. The bottom line, however, is certain: Bone mass drops about 0.5 percent a year. Bones become more porous and more fragile—a condition called osteopenia, which is reversible. At some still ill-defined point, however, fractures develop: Osteopenia has become osteoporosis, which with current standard treatment is harder to reverse. It afflicts 15 to 20 million Americans (one-third to one-half of them postmenopausal women), including close to 100 percent of all elderly Americans.

More fragile bones mean more broken bones. The figures are daunting: 1.3 million fractures a year, 247,000 hip fractures (fatal for one in six), and a cost ranging from $7 billion to $10 billion a year. Because of the nation's aging population, the annual number of hip fractures is projected to rise to more than 500,000 by 2030.

Risk Factors for Osteoporosis

When it comes to avoiding bone-weakening osteoporosis, doctors still don't have all the answers. Here risk factors have been ranked in groups according to scientific certainty. While some risks are unavoidable, you *can* control others, especially diet, exercise, and smoking.

Well-Established Evidence		Moderate Evidence		Inconclusive or Inadequate Evidence	
Risk Factors	Protective Factors	Risk Factors	Protective Factors	Risk Factors	Protective Factors
Elderly	Obesity	Heavy alcohol use	Heavy exercise	Diabetes	Progestin use
Postmenopausal	Black ethnicity	Cigarette smoking		Asian ethnicity	Drinking fluoridated water
Removal of ovaries	Estrogen use	Low dietary calcium		Thiazide diuretic use	Moderate physical activity
Corticosteroid use				Caffeine use	Motherhood
Extreme immobility (bedridden)				Drinking soda	

Who Gets Osteoporosis?

A majority of American women over the age of 55 do. This chart documents the evidence from a spinal x-ray study of 2,000 women. Men also get osteoporosis, but the main impact—broken bones—is less obvious because men have bigger, stronger bones to begin with.

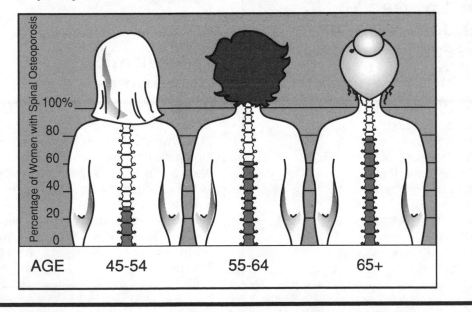

Percentage of Women with Spinal Osteoporosis

AGE 45-54 55-64 65+

Which Bones Break Most Often?

The spine, wrists, and hips are the bones people with osteoporosis most often break. Falls are the usual way osteoporotic wrists and hips break, while weakened spines can suffer so-called crush fractures when a person bends forward or lifts heavy objects.

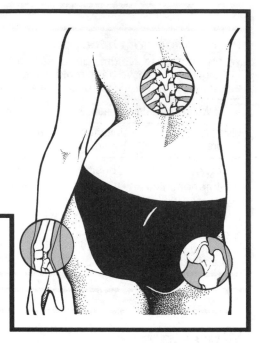

If you're a woman in your fifties with osteoporosis, research shows you're three times more likely to need dentures than a nonosteoporotic woman is.

Alcoholism is a leading cause of osteoporosis in men. In one study of 96 alcoholic men, researchers found 45 of them—two-thirds under the age of 50—had evidence of bone loss.

FILE ON THE FAMOUS

Toulouse-Lautrec Transcended Bone Disease

Henri-Marie-Raymond de Toulouse-Lautrec was born in 1864 to one of France's most aristocratic families. As an athletic adolescent, he broke each thigh bone on separate occasions. Because of a crippling bone disease, his legs never healed; his upper body grew to maturity while his legs remained boy-size.

Toulouse-Lautrec began painting during his convalescence, and by the time he was 30 he was recognized as a great artist.

The Shrinking Syndrome

One of the most common effects of osteoporosis is shrinking in height. This shrinkage happens when spinal crush fractures produce "dowager's hump." An Australian study found an elderly woman with osteoporosis may lose up to 16 percent of her height, meaning a woman who reached 5 feet, 5 inches at maturity could shrink 10 inches to 4 feet, 7 inches.

Screening for Osteoporosis

You don't need to include screening for osteoporosis as part of your regular health checkups unless you're at risk. With a few exceptions, younger women don't benefit from screening. Those exceptions include such factors as hormone disorders, premature menopause, anorexia, removal of the ovaries, and unexplained fracturing of bones.

Tests of bone density can be expensive, they may need to be repeated, and their reliability is not what some doctors would like to see. The tests are improving, however.

Test	Measures	Advantages	Disadvantages	Comments
Single Photon Absorptiometry (SPA)	Density of forearm or heel bones	Low-dose radiation, ⅙ of standard chest x-ray	Not a good predictor of bone loss at hip and spine	Most useful in people over 75, and to measure large changes in bone density due to medical treatments
Dual Photon Absorptiometry (DPA)	Density of hip, spine, forearm, heel, other sites	Low-dose radiation, ½ of chest x-ray; best for middle-aged women	Not a good predictor for those with calcium deposits or bone degeneration around the spine	Less useful for those over 75; new developments reduce time needed to several minutes and increase reliability to high levels
Quantitative Computed Tomography (QCT)	Cross-sectional images of vertebrae, other sites	Measure spongy bone in vertebrae's forward side	High-dose radiation, averages 3 times chest x-ray	Useful for any age; new developments reduce time needed and increase reliability to high levels
Bone biopsy	Spongy bone	No radiation exposure	Invasive	Best for those under 50 who have osteoporosis
Dual energy radiography	Density of hip, spine, forearm, heel, other sites	Better precision, lower radiation, lower cost	Unknown	Still being researched
Ultrasound	Speed that sound waves travel through bone	Faster (takes less than a minute), lower cost, no radiation exposure	Unknown	This new test may detect bone fragility unrelated to bone mass; sensitive to mild or early cases of osteoporosis

The Leading Osteoporosis Treatments

Medical treatments for osteoporosis vary according to the goals, which also vary according to the specific problem. The problem could be fractures, low bone mass, insufficient calcium, low estrogen levels. This table presents the leading medical treatments, plus the two main non-medical therapies.

Therapy	Advantages	Disadvantages	Comments
Sodium fluoride	Only current drug that can bring spinal bone mass up to normal and so reduce fractures; ideal for men, who can't be treated with estrogen	Small minority get digestive upsets, joint pain; may thin cortical bone if sufficient calcium isn't also given	Widely used, but not federally approved, for osteoporosis in the United States; enteric coating helps prevent digestive upsets; monofluorophosphate has fewer side effects than sodium fluoride
Estrogen replacement	Female sex hormone that slows down or halts bone loss; best available preventive if taken early enough, especially in women at high risk; can cut fractures by 50%; available as tablet, cream, patch, or implant	Quadruples risk (to 4 in 1,000) for uterine cancer; some increase in risk for blood-clot formation; abnormal bleeding in women who still have uterus; possible increase in risk for breast cancer	Widely used, approved therapy; best for women who lose bone quickly; acts directly on bone cells; may not work for women who begin taking it after age 70; often combined with progesterone for patients who still have uterus
Etidronate disodium	Slows bone loss; slightly increases bone density	None known	Major treatment for Paget's disease; promising for osteoporosis prevention
Calcitonin	Slows bone loss; slightly increases bone density; relieves pain; very safe	Mild facial flushing in almost all patients; rash; nausea and anorexia in 1 per 1,000 patients; requires injection daily; very expensive	Should be taken with at least 1,000 mg of calcium daily; acts directly on bone cells; may work for men, who can't be treated with estrogen
Calcitriol (active form of vitamin D)	Lowers fracture rate substantially; helps absorption of calcium	Can cause overdose of vitamin D, toxic elevation of blood calcium	Not officially available in the United States for osteoporosis
Thiazide	Reduces bone loss slightly; helps body conserve calcium by preventing its excretion	Diuretic used to control high blood pressure, can cause adverse reactions in people with normal pressure	Promising drug; increases estrogen effectiveness; useful mainly for those who excrete too much calcium
Calcium	Maintains bone health; helps prevent bone loss; cheap, readily available; reduces need for estrogen	Can cause constipation, digestive upset	Most effective as preventive when gotten in sufficient amounts before age 35; not a substitute for estrogen; in elderly, supplements are best way to ensure adequate intake; greatly increases effectiveness of estrogen
Exercise	Strengthens bones; increases bone mass and volume	Risk of injury; inhibited by fractures	Weight-bearing exercise formerly thought essential, but swimming also helps

"Where Were You When You Broke Your Hip?"

People break their hips in their own homes more often than in all other places combined. That's probably because elderly women are far more likely to have osteoporosis than men, and they're more likely to be at home.

While breastfeeding is best for babies, too long at the nipple may promote osteoporosis in mothers by robbing them of bone mass. Calcium supplements and exercise may counter the bone losses.

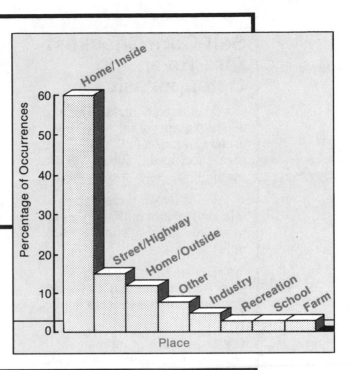

Ranking the Treatments

Ask a dozen doctors to rank the effectiveness of osteoporosis therapies, and you'll get a dozen different answers, says Robert Heaney, M.D., professor of medicine at Creighton University and a leading researcher in osteoporosis. Because their patients vary widely in age, background, other medical conditions, and severity of osteoporosis, doctors can't prescribe the same treatments for them all. Dr. Heaney, however, ventures the following ranking:

1. Sodium fluoride

2. Estrogen replacement

3. Etidronate disodium

4. Calcitonin

5. Calcitriol (active form of vitamin D)

6. Thiazide

Exercise and calcium supplements are prerequisites for any therapy, Dr. Heaney says, because porous bones must be rebuilt. If broken bones are also part of the problem, physical therapy and pain relief are also necessary therapeutic ingredients. And hip replacement surgery for osteoporosis is becoming common.

Self-Care Checklist for Preventing Osteoporosis

▼ Maintain an intake of at least 800 milligrams of calcium daily, preferably more. (1,000 milligrams premenopausal, 1,500 milligrams postmenopausal without estrogen.)

▼ Drink two or three glasses of milk daily (skim milk supplies the same amount of calcium as whole milk).

▼ Eat foods high in calcium (especially milk products, yogurt, sardines, collards, tuna, tofu, nuts, sunflower seeds).

▼ Use a calcium supplement if not securing an adequate amount of calcium daily.

▼ Take a calcium supplement with meals for optimum absorption.

▼ Eat calcium and fiber foods at separate times. (Fiber may decrease calcium absorption.)

▼ Maintain adequate vitamin D (400 international units daily) or secure at least 15 minutes of sunlight daily.

▼ Avoid high protein consumption. (High-protein diets remove calcium from body.)

▼ Use vinegar to marinate meats and prepare stock. (Vinegar helps to move calcium from bone to meat.)

▼ Use low-cholesterol cheese instead of butter. (Cheese is high in calcium.)

▼ Use hard water if possible. (Hard water contains more calcium than soft water.)

▼ Sleep 7 to 8 hours each night. (This is a recommended health-protective behavior.)

▼ Do abdominal and back exercises regularly.

▼ Participate in weight-bearing exercises such as walking the equivalent of 2 miles three to four times each week. This is a very important step.

Note: If you are at high risk at menopausal age, seek medical advice regarding estrogen replacement. Do not take calcium supplements when taking diuretics if you have a history of renal stones or have been diagnosed as hypertensive, unless you consult with a physician.

Soda pop may more than double your risk of breaking your bones. One study links the phosphorus in carbonated beverages with bone fractures in women after age 40.

How Exercise Can Mineralize Your Bones

Washington University medical researchers studied exercising and nonexercising women, ranging in age from 55 to 70, to learn how walking, jogging, and stair climbing affected the mineral content of their bones. In nine months nonexercisers lost about 1 percent of their bone mineral content. But after an average 17 months of workouts, the exercisers had increased their mineral content average by 6.2 percent, a significant gain.

Researchers measured the exercisers again 13 months after they stopped working out. Their average bone mineral content had *dropped* 4.8 percent, although it was still better than when they began the study.

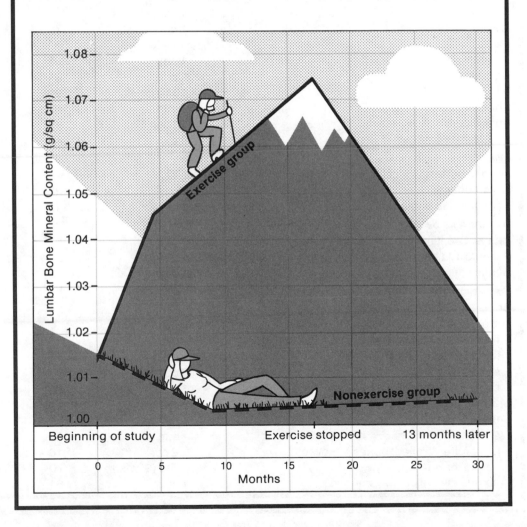

Where to Find Calcium

Although calcium is found in a vast number of foods, it is found in large amounts in only a few. Dairy products are the best source. The calcium in milk is easily absorbed by most people. Sardines and salmon are also good sources if you eat the bones. Green leafy vegetables contain considerable calcium, but their high fiber content may cut down on absorption. Meats are generally poor sources, while fruits are not rich sources but can be a tasty contribution to a varied diet.

Food	Portion	Calcium (mg)
Dairy Products		
Buttermilk	1 cup	285
Cheese		
Cheddar	1 oz.	204
cottage, small curd	1 cup	126
pasteurized process spread, American	1 oz.	159
Swiss	1 oz.	272
Ice cream, hardened	1 cup	176
Milk		
nonfat (skim)	1 cup	302
whole	1 cup	291
Milk shake, chocolate	10.6 oz.	396
Sherbet	1 cup	103
Sour cream	1 Tbsp.	14
Yogurt, fruit-flavored	8 oz.	343
Eggs		
Fried in butter	1	26
Hard-cooked	1	28
Scrambled in butter (milk added)	1	47
Legumes, Nuts, Seeds		
Beans, Great northern, cooked	1 cup	90
Peanuts, roasted in oil, salted	1 cup	125
Sunflower seeds	1 cup	168
Meat, Poultry, Fish		
Beef		
ground, broiled	3 oz.	10
liver	3 oz.	9
roast, relatively lean	3 oz.	11
steak, lean	3 oz.	9
stew, with vegetables	1 cup	29
Bluefish, baked with butter or margarine	3 oz.	25
Chicken		
à la king	1 cup	127
half broiler, broiled, bones removed	6.2 oz.	16
potpie, baked	⅓ pie (9″ dia.)	70
Crabmeat, white or king, canned	1 cup	61

Food	Portion	Calcium (mg)
Ham, light cure, lean	3 oz.	5
Lamb chop	3 oz.	16
Pork chop, lean	3 oz.	4
Salmon, pink, canned	3 oz.	181
Sardines, Atlantic, canned in oil	3 oz.	351
Shrimp, french fried, 10% fat	3 oz.	57
Vegetables		
Asparagus, canned, spears	4 spears	11
Beans, lima, thick-seeded	1 cup	32
Beans, green, frozen, cut	1 cup	61
Beets, canned, diced or sliced	1 cup	26
Broccoli, cooked	1 stalk	205
Cabbage, raw, coarsely shredded or sliced	1 cup	33
Carrots, raw,	1 (7½" × 1⅛")	19
Cauliflower, raw	1 cup	29
Celery, raw	1 stalk	14
Collards, cooked	1 cup	357
Lettuce, iceberg, chopped	1 cup	10
Onions, raw, chopped	1 cup	40
Peas, frozen, cooked	1 cup	38
Potatoes		
baked, peeled	1	8
mashed, with milk	1 cup	55
Potato salad	1 cup	48
Sauerkraut, canned	1 cup	71
Spinach, chopped, frozen	1 cup	277
Squash, summer, cooked	1 cup	49
Sweet potatoes, baked in skin, peeled	1	32
Tomatoes		
raw	1	9
juice	1 cup	22
Miscellaneous		
Soups		
cream of chicken, prepared with milk	1 cup	181
cream of mushroom, prepared with milk	1 cup	179
tomato, prepared with water	1 cup	12

Calcium Intake: The Ideal vs. the Reality

Your bones are about 25 percent calcium by weight. And that represents 99 percent of your calcium reserves. So if you don't get enough calcium in your diet, your body takes what it needs from your bones. Although osteoporosis is a complex disease, it can be induced in laboratory animals by feeding a calcium-deficient diet.

The amount of bone capital you build in your youth can determine how susceptible you are to osteoporosis in later life. And if you do get osteoporosis, calcium combined with medication and exercise may help control it. This chart shows how vast the gap is between what most American women are getting and what experts say they need.

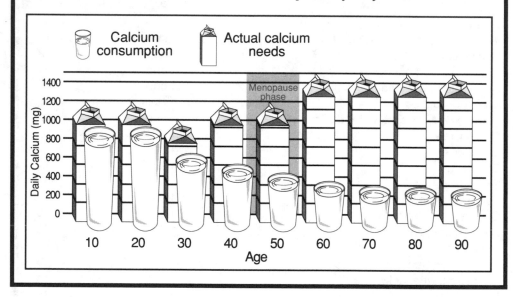

Boron Is Bone-Friendly

Boron is more than a handcleaner, laundry softener, and cargo of 20-mule teams. It seems to harden bones, says the U.S. Department of Agriculture's Agricultural Research Service. A small study of postmenopausal women on a very-low-boron diet found quick and dramatic changes when they were put on a 3-milligram-per-day supplement, the amount you would get in a wellbalanced diet. Within eight days, the women were losing 40 percent less calcium, one-third less magnesium, and slightly less phosphorus.

Calcium Supplements Compared

Though there are individual differences among calcium supplements, experts say the best one is the one you can take every day without problems. You can improve absorption if you break up your daily dose into smaller amounts and take them throughout the day, especially with meals. Calcium levels in the blood decline with inactivity, so it may make sense to take some calcium just before bed.

Supplement	Percentage of Calcium	Advantages	Disadvantages
Calcium carbonate	40	Cheap; high percentage of calcium; readily absorbed; main ingredient in Tums; available in wide range of dosages and forms	Insoluble in water, so not good for those with little or no stomach acid (take with meals); possible nausea, gas, constipation; high doses can cause stomach acid "rebound"
Calcium lactate	13	Nonconstipating; soluble in water; nonirritating	Low percentage of calcium means numerous tablets must be taken daily, leading to greater expense and inconvenience
Calcium gluconate	9	Nonconstipating; soluble in water; nonirritating	Low percentage of calcium means numerous tablets must be taken daily
Calcium citrate	18	More efficient absorption, especially in those with little or no stomach acid	Expensive
Dibasic and tribasic calcium phosphate	23–39	Little or no gas produced; found in calcium-fortified foods; provides phosphorus in good balance to calcium; some antacid activity	Insoluble in water, so not good for those with little or no stomach acid (take with meals)
Chelated calcium	Varies	Manufacturers claim it is better absorbed	Very expensive; no solid evidence of better absorption; solubility varies among brands, so those with little or no stomach acid must read labels to check claims of solubility; proportion of calcium varies among brands; no information on side effects

niffing your calcitonin may be better than getting shots of it. This osteoporosis-fighting hormone has unpleasant side effects when injected. A prescription-only calcitonin nasal spray has been found to be superior.

Where We Get Our Calcium

This pie chart tells you what you probably suspected all along: Dairy products are by far America's favorite choice of calcium-rich food.

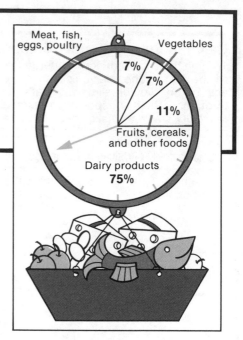

Meat, fish, eggs, poultry

Vegetables

7%

7%

11%

Fruits, cereals, and other foods

Dairy products
75%

You exercise and eat fiber to keep yourself healthy. But if you also have exercise-induced menstrual irregularity, too much fiber may lead to bone loss. Excess fiber has been linked to greater fecal excretion of estrogen and calcium.

FUTURE FACT

2040
2030
2020
2010

Boning Up on the Future

Someday—seven to ten years from now—you may be taking OIF and TGF to stimulate your osteoporotic bones into new growth. OIF is Osteoinductive Factor, a protein discovered by scientists at Collagen Corporation in Palo Alto, California. TGF is Transforming Growth Factor, a natural growth hormone. When it's given with TGF, OIF sets off a chain reaction: Connective tissue cells produce a webbing of cartilage (collagen protein), which is subsequently transformed into bone.

This new bone is as strong as the person's own natural bone, says physiologist and pharmacologist Bruce Pharriss, Ph.D., senior vice president of Collagen. OIF can also stop the natural tearing-down phase of bone remodeling, Dr. Pharriss says.

OIF can't be taken orally because it's a protein that would be broken down by digestion. It could be administered in a skin patch, as an injection, or as a nasal spray. And it could be made into a putty and surgically applied right on a broken bone to speed healing and strengthen the mend.

Other researchers believe that someday osteoporotic bones may be treated with biostimulation, also known as pulsed electromagnetic fields (PEMFs). A wire coil encased in a plastic disk could send weak electromagnetic "messages" through the skin to bone cells, telling them to start making more bone. Biostimulation is generally recognized as safe, though its effectiveness for osteoporosis is unproven.

11

CAFFEINE AND COFFEE

Meeting a friend for a hot cup of coffee has been one of life's pleasures since the year A.D. 1,000. So whether it's called *gahwah, kahveh, cafe, kaffee,* or *coffee,* a cup now and then is a cultural rite that none of us is likely to give up. And we really shouldn't have to.

Caffeine is the naturally occurring ingredient that gives coffee its punch. It's most often used as a stimulant to keep late-night drivers and last-minute students on the alert. It hits your brain about 30 minutes after the first sip and stays on the job for the next 2 to 8 hours.

Caffeine stimulates the nervous system by blocking adenosine, a naturally occurring brain chemical that slows you down. Too much caffeine, however, can *over*stimulate the system and result in a bad case of the jitters, a feeling of irritability, increased urination, or even a faster heartbeat.

But how much is too much? The answer varies. It's not unusual for heavy coffee drinkers to build up a tolerance to caffeine and its effects, while a 12-ounce mug of freshly brewed coffee might make someone who never drinks the stuff bounce off the walls. For most people, however, moderation is the key.

Do coffee and caffeine cause any more serious problems than "coffee nerves"? Probably not. Scientists have been sniffing suspiciously around the edges of this issue for more than a decade without managing to prove much in the way of negative effects. Yes, coffee can boost your blood pressure a couple of points, and it may knock your cholesterol level up one or two notches. But no, it doesn't cause breast cancer, birth defects, or fibrocystic breast disease.

How Much Coffee Do You Drink?

Probably less than you did a few years ago. America has cut its per capita coffee consumption in half over the past couple of decades.

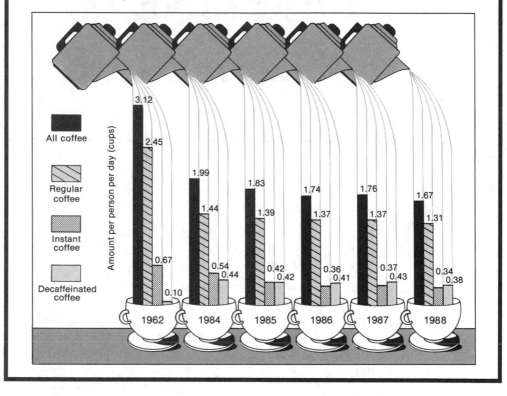

The Stimulating Effects of Caffeine

Caffeine hits your brain within a half hour after you drink a cup of coffee. It blocks the path of adenosine, a naturally occurring brain chemical that slows you down both mentally and physically. The result is that you think quicker, react faster, work more accurately, and stay on top of things longer.

How long does this effect last? Individuals vary. But generally, an effective dose of coffee remains in the body for 2 to 8 hours. Now you know why that after-dinner cup of coffee can keep you awake until 3:00 A.M.!

Young People Have Kicked the Habit

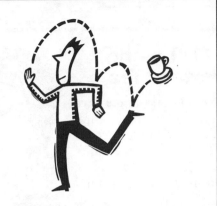

A major reason that coffee consumption is declining in the United States is that fewer young people are developing the habit. In 1962, 81 percent of those in their twenties drank coffee. By 1988 that figure had plummeted to 31.9 percent.

Age	Percentage of Coffee Drinkers						Percentage of Change
	1962	1984	1985	1986	1987	1988	1962–1988
10–19	25.1	8.9	7.1	4.6	5.3	4.7	−20.4
20–29	81.0	41.4	40.5	38.4	33.1	31.9	−49.1
30–59	90.8	73.4	70.6	67.1	67.2	63.5	−27.3
60+	88.4	84.4	78.7	77.8	77.8	76.9	−11.5

Caffeine ingested 30 minutes before a meal causes men to eat almost 25 percent less food, say Canadian researchers. The same effect, unfortunately, does not hold true for women.

Who Drinks the Most Coffee?

We're the champs. The United States imports about a third of the world's coffee. West Germany, France, Japan, Italy, the Netherlands, Spain, the United Kingdom, Sweden, and the USSR are runners-up that trail far behind. Here's a list showing the world's top ten importers of coffee.

Country	Share of World Coffee Imports
United States	30.0%
West Germany	13.6%
France	9.1%
Japan	8.4%
Italy	7.2%
Netherlands	4.2%
United Kingdom	3.8%
Spain	3.8%
Sweden	2.8%
USSR	2.8%

England Is Losing Her Thirst for Tea

Even the English no longer have time for afternoon tea, a cultural ritual introduced by Anna, seventh Duchess of Bedford, in the nineteenth century and adopted as a mark of civilization by countries around the world.

Of course, that doesn't mean that they've stopped sipping from teacups altogether. According to market reports, tea drinking has dropped from about 2,000 cups a year per person (5½ cups a day) to about 1,200 (3½ cups a day). That's still ten times the per capita tea consumption in the United States.

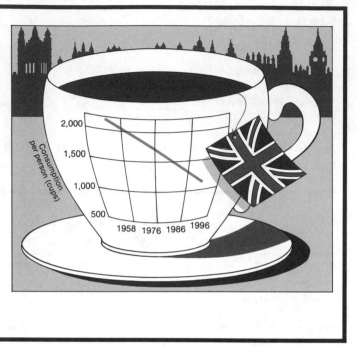

How Much Caffeine Is Okay?

More than 300 milligrams of caffeine a day can overstimulate your central nervous system, experts say, causing an increased heart rate, insomnia, nervousness, headache, irritability, diarrhea, and frequent urination. But limiting your intake to three 6-ounce cups of regular coffee, six cups of tea, or six cans of soda should give you a buzz without the ill effects.

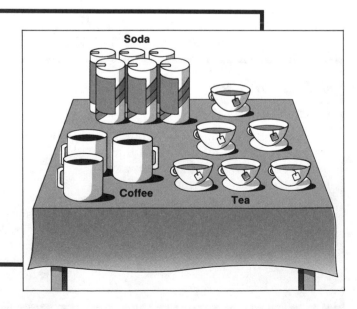

How They Get the Caffeine Out

There are two methods generally used to decaffeinate coffee. In the first, coffee beans are placed in a rotating drum and softened by steam for 30 minutes. Then they're rinsed in a chemical solvent such as methylene chloride for about 10 hours. When the chemical has absorbed the caffeine, both caffeine and chemical are drained away, and the beans are steamed for another 8 to 12 hours so any remaining solvent evaporates. A minute amount of the chemical—approximately 0.1 parts per million—remains in the beans.

The second method used to decaffeinate coffee is frequently referred to as the "water process." Green coffee beans are soaked in hot water until the caffeine dissolves out of the beans and into the water. The water and caffeine are drained away, treated with a chemical such as methylene chloride to absorb the caffeine, then heated until the chemical and the caffeine evaporate. The remaining water is returned to the beans, which—coffee experts claim—regain most of their flavor.

How Much Kick to the Cup?

It depends largely on how you make it. Dripped coffee, for example, has almost twice the caffeine of some instants, as this table shows.

Coffee	How It's Made	Caffeine (mg) in a 6-oz. Cup
Chock Full O'Nuts	Drip	105
Shop Rite	Drip	101
Savarin	Drip	98
Nescafe Brava	Instant	66
Folgers	Instant	64
Stop & Shop	Instant	63
Shop Rite	Instant	63
Melitta, extra fine	Drip	61
Food Club	Instant	61
Maxwell House	Instant	23

Coffee may boost your ability to perform complex mental tasks more easily—provided you have a specific type of personality. Extroverted, impulsive people are aided by a morning shot of caffeine, say researchers. Thoughtful introverts are hindered by it.

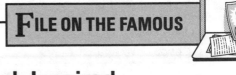

FILE ON THE FAMOUS

Bach Inspired by Coffee

Johann Sebastian Bach, known more for his counterpoint than his coffee, apparently loved coffee so much that he combined it with comedy and counterpoint in a one-act operetta called—are you ready for this?—the *Coffee Cantata*.

Where's the Caffeine?

Up to 90% of the caffeine in our lives comes from coffee. But many sodas, teas, chocolate-based products, and drugs also contain a significant amount of the stimulant.

Sodas	Caffeine (mg) in a 12-oz. Can
Jolt	67.2
Mountain Dew	56.6
Dr. Pepper	50.6
Diet Coke	46.0
TAB	44.6
Pepsi Light	36.9
Pepsi-Cola	36.2
Diet Pepsi	36.0
RC Cola	35.0
Coca-Cola Classic	33.6
Coca-Cola	33.0
Diet Rite Cola	0
Diet Sprite	0

Chocolate-Based Products	Caffeine (mg)
Milk chocolate, 1 oz.	15
Dark semisweet chocolate, 1 oz.	13
Baker's German sweet chocolate, 1 oz.	8
Chocolate milk, 8 oz.	8
Chocolate-flavored syrup, 1 oz.	5
Cocoa beverage, 5 oz.	4

Teas	Caffeine (mg) in a 6-oz. Cup
Salada	49
Bigelow English Teatime	47

Teas	Caffeine (mg) in a 6-oz. Cup
Lipton	46
Boston's Darjeeling Blend	38
Tetley	38
Salada, "naturally caffeine reduced"	22
Tetley, decaffeinated	6
Lipton, decaffeinated	5
Celestial Seasonings	0

Drugs	Purpose	Caffeine (mg) per Tablet or Capsule
Vivarin	Alertness	200
Dexatrim	Weight control	200
Nō Dōz	Alertness	100
Aqua-Ban	Diuretic	100
Cafergot	Headaches	100
Excedrin	Pain relief	65
Norgesic Forte	Muscle relaxant	60
Fiorinal	Headaches	40
Anacin, Maximum Strength	Pain relief	35
Vanquish	Pain relief	33
Darvon	Pain relief	32
Dristan	Decongestant	16

Cost of a cup of coffee at New York City's Waldorf Astoria hotel in 1897: $0.25. Cost in 1989: $1.65.

A Protective Role against Asthma

Regular coffee consumption may actually help prevent the onset of asthma. During an Italian National Health Survey of 72,284 people, for example, a group of doctors in Milan found that those folks who drank three cups of regular coffee per day were about 28 percent less likely to have asthma than nondrinkers. Two-a-day drinkers were 23 percent less likely to be asthmatic. Even those who drank only one cup a day reduced their risk of wheezing by 5 percent.

How does coffee prevent asthma? Caffeine, which is chemically related to a potent asthma drug called theophylline, is known to relax the bronchial tubes in the lungs. That may, scientists suspect, prevent the life-threatening airway constriction that occurs in asthmatics.

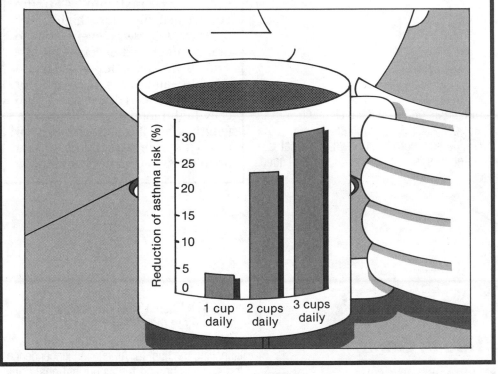

In Turkey, coffee is so important that bridegrooms were at one time required to promise during the marriage ceremony that they would keep their brides supplied with the brew. The price of failure? Running out of coffee was considered "grounds" for divorce.

Does Caffeine Affect Fertility?

Yes. In a study of 104 women at the National Institute of Environmental Health Sciences, women who drank more than a cup of brewed coffee each day were half as likely to get pregnant as women who drank less.

The first coffee break on the moon took place on July 20, 1969, at 7:27 P.M. (CDT), when an astronaut from the Eagle spacecraft sat down to a meal that included bacon squares, sugar cookie cubes, and good old-fashioned java.

IS THAT A FACT?

The caffeine in a cup of coffee will raise your blood pressure.

Yes. But that doesn't mean it causes high blood pressure. Here's what we mean: A study of 5,147 Australians between the ages of 20 and 70 reveals that people with normal blood pressure consumed just as much caffeine over the course of a day as people with high blood pressure. Translation? Caffeine doesn't actually cause high blood pressure. Otherwise everyone who drank caffeinated beverages in the study would have developed it.

But—and this is a big "but" for people with heart disease or chronically high blood pressure—the caffeine in a cup of coffee *will* raise your blood pressure two to four points for up to three hours after you drink it.

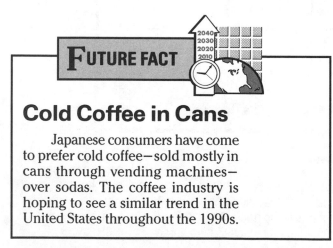

FUTURE FACT

Cold Coffee in Cans

Japanese consumers have come to prefer cold coffee—sold mostly in cans through vending machines—over sodas. The coffee industry is hoping to see a similar trend in the United States throughout the 1990s.

The Boston Tea Party was significant for more than the dumping of 343 chests of tea into Boston Harbor and launching the fight for American independence. It also launched coffee as our national drink. After Sam Adams led his raiding party to the docks, it became downright unpatriotic to drink tea. It's no coincidence that the fundamentals of our republic were formulated in early colonial coffeehouses rather than tearooms.

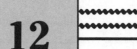

12

CANCER

Today 5 million Americans have cancer. Approximately 500,000 people will die of the disease in the next year—9,600 people this week, 1,370 by the end of today, 57 in the next hour, one in the next 63 seconds. All told, about 76 million Americans who are alive today will eventually encounter cancer. Experts say that three out of every four families will be affected by one form of the disease or another. It's the price we pay for living in a society that smokes, drinks, lies out in the sun, eats a lot of fatty foods, and works with hazardous substances that are incompatible with human life.

And the price is going up. The annual number of cancer deaths among men has increased by 16 percent over the past 30 years, an increase that is almost totally due to the epidemic proportions of lung cancer. Eighty-five percent of all those lung cancer cases are directly attributable to cigarettes.

Women are in better shape. Largely due to a drop in uterine, stomach, and bladder cancer, deaths due to cancer among women have actually dropped by 5 percent over that same 30-year span. This may change in the near future, however, since the number of women dying from lung cancer —75 percent of which is directly attributable to cigarettes—has accelerated by more than 300 percent.

Is cancer survivable? In many cases, yes. The American Cancer Society estimates that 49 percent of those with cancer are still alive five years after the disease is diagnosed. Fortunately, the odds for *preventing* the disease are even better. It's estimated that 66 percent of all cancers could be prevented by avoiding cigarette smoke and making the simple dietary changes summarized in this chapter.

115

What Causes Cancer?

The sad truth is that to a large extent, cancer is a self-inflicted disease. Tobacco use and bad diet account for almost two-thirds of all cases, while where we work, where we live, who we sleep with, and whether or not we drink alcohol and fry in the sun pretty much account for the rest. Here's a complete breakdown.

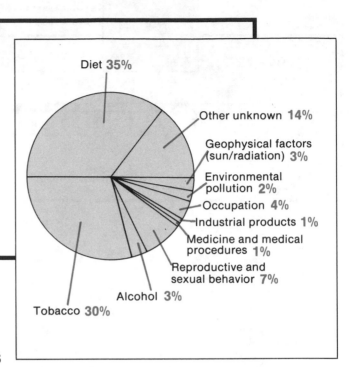

Diet 35%
Other unknown 14%
Geophysical factors (sun/radiation) 3%
Environmental pollution 2%
Occupation 4%
Industrial products 1%
Medicine and medical procedures 1%
Reproductive and sexual behavior 7%
Alcohol 3%
Tobacco 30%

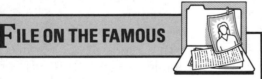

In a study of 3,271 women, cervigrams (photographs of the cervix) detected five times as many potentially cancerous conditions as Pap smears did.

Spreading the Word

Former First Lady Betty Ford, who developed breast cancer in 1973, launched a spirited one-woman public education campaign against breast cancer after her own cancer was removed. Her efforts were so effective that they caused an upsurge in breast cancer detection and reporting that skewed the statistics of cancer scientists for several years.

Walk away from cancer. A study of 613 adults indicates a significant reduction in colon cancer for those who keep physically active. The reason? Researchers speculate that body movement stimulates bowel movement. And that decreases the time that carcinogens have to make trouble in your intestines.

It Matters Where You Live

You are most likely to die of cancer if you live in the District of Columbia, followed by Delaware, Maryland, New Jersey, Ohio, Rhode Island, Michigan, Alaska, Pennsylvania, and Massachusetts.

You are least likely to die of cancer if you live in Utah, followed by Wyoming, Colorado, Texas, Idaho, New Mexico, North Dakota, Kansas, Nebraska, and South Dakota.

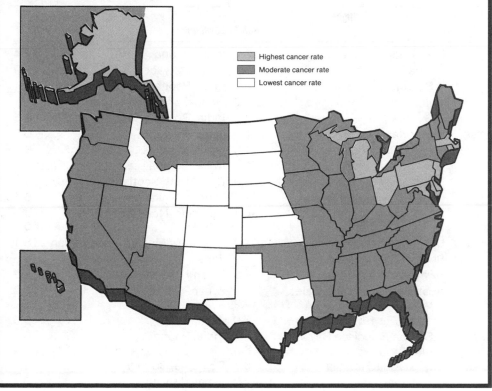

- Highest cancer rate
- Moderate cancer rate
- Lowest cancer rate

Age spots—those patches of darkened skin that form in response to years of sun exposure—are the source of 60 percent of all squamous cell carcinomas. Fortunately, the spots may fade and disappear if shielded from the sun before they turn cancerous.

Worldwide Cancer Rates—The Best and the Worst

Japanese men living in Nagasaki have the highest incidence of stomach cancer in the world, while non-Jewish women living in Israel have the lowest. Black men living in New Orleans have the highest incidence of lung cancer, while Spanish women living in Navarra have the lowest. Hawaiian women living on the island of Hawaii have the highest rate of breast cancer, while Japanese women living in the countryside around Osaka have the lowest.

Why is one particular kind of cancer concentrated in one region but not another? The answer is a complex mix of diet, environment, lifestyle, and genetics that scientists are only beginning to sort out. This table highlights the highest and lowest incidence of selected cancers from around the globe.

Cancer	Men			
	Highest		Lowest	
	Location	Rate*	Location	Rate*
Bladder	Switzerland, Geneva	30.2	India, Poona	2.4
Brain	Australia, South	8.2	Japan, Miyagi	0.9
Colon	U.S., Connecticut	32.3	India, Poona	3.1
Esophagus	Shanghai	24.7	Hungary, Szabolcs, rural	1.1
Gallbladder	U.S., New Mexico, Amerindian	7.7	India, Bombay	0.5
Hodgkin's disease	Switzerland, Vaud, urban	4.9	Japan, Miyagi	0.5
Hypopharynx	France, Bas Rhin, rural	11.0	Israel, all Jews	0.2
Kidney, etc.	U.S., Hawaii, white	11.2	India, Bombay	1.3
Larynx	Italy, Varese	16.0	U.K., North Scotland	1.8
Lip	Canada, Newfoundland	22.8	Japan, Osaka	0.1
Liver	Hong Kong	34.4	Australia, New South Wales, rural	0.6
Lung and bronchus	U.S., New Orleans, black	107.2	U.S., New Mexico, Amerindian	8.1
Lymphatic leukemia	Switzerland, Neuchâtel	7.9	Japan, Fukuoka, urban	0.5
Lymphosarcoma	Switzerland, Geneva	8.5	Poland, Warsaw, rural	1.2
Melanoma	Australia, New South Wales, urban	17.2	Japan, Osaka	0.2
Mouth	France, Bas Rhin, urban	13.0	Japan, Miyagi	0.5
Multiple myeloma	U.S., San Francisco Bay area, black	8.4	India, Poona	0.6
Myeloid leukemia	U.S., Hawaii, Hawaiian	8.7	Romania, County Cluj	0.7
Nasopharynx	Hong Kong	32.9	Japan, Miyagi	0.3
Oropharynx	France, Bas Rhin, urban	13.4	Norway	0.3
Pancreas	U.S., San Francisco Bay area, black	18.3	India, Bombay	2.0
Penis	Jamaica, Kingston	5.7	U.S., Los Angeles, white	0.2
Prostate	U.S., Alameda, black	100.2	Shanghai	0.8
Rectum	Canada, Northwest Territory and Yukon	22.6	Israel, non-Jews	3.1
Stomach	Japan, Nagasaki	100.2	U.S., Atlanta, white	5.7
Testis	Switzerland, Vaud, rural	10.5	Cuba	0.3
Thyroid gland	U.S., Hawaii, Chinese	7.8	India, Poona	0.4
Tongue	India, Bombay	10.2	Romania, County Cluj	0.5

Cancer	Women			
	Highest		**Lowest**	
	Location	*Rate**	*Location*	*Rate**
Bladder	U.S., New Orleans, white	6.5	Hungary, Szabolcs, rural	0.5
Brain	Poland, Warsaw City; U.S., Hawaii	6.6	Japan, Miyagi, rural	0.6
Breast	U.S., Hawaii, Hawaiian	87.5	Japan, Osaka, rural	8.9
Cervix	Colombia, Cali	52.9	Israel, non-Jews	2.1
Colon	U.S., San Francisco Bay area, Japanese	27.4	India, Poona	2.8
Esophagus	India, Bombay	10.7	U.S., Utah	0.4
Gallbladder	U.S., New Mexico, Amerindian	22.2	India, Bombay	0.7
Hodgkin's disease	Switzerland, Vaud, rural	4.3	Japan, Osaka	0.3
Hypopharynx	India, Bombay	2.2	Canada, British Columbia	0.1
Kidney, etc.	Canada, Northwest Territory and Yukon	15.3	India, Poona	0.6
Larynx	India, Bombay	2.6	Norway	0.2
Lip	Romania, County Cluj	2.3	U.K., Birmingham	0.1
Liver	Shanghai	9.1	Norway, rural	0.4
Lung and bronchus	New Zealand, Maori	48.8	Spain, Navarra	2.6
Lymphatic leukemia	U.S., New Mexico	3.3	Japan, Fukuoka	0.4
Lymphosarcoma	U.S., Hawaii, Hawaiian	6.3	Poland, Katowice	0.5
Melanoma	Australia, New South Wales, rural	19.1	Japan, Osaka	0.2
Mouth	India, Bombay	5.8	Yugoslavia, Slovenia	0.2
Multiple myeloma	U.S., Hawaii, Hawaiian	5.9	Poland, Katowice	0.4
Myeloid leukemia	New Zealand, Maori	5.4	Hungary, Szabolcs	0.8
Nasopharynx	Hong Kong	14.4	U.K., Trent	0.1
Oropharynx	U.S., Hawaii, white	2.7	Japan, Osaka	0.1
Ovary	Israel, Jews born in Europe and America	17.2	Japan, Osaka, rural	2.1
Pancreas	U.S., New Mexico, Amerindian	10.4	India, Bombay	0.9
Rectum	Switzerland, Neuchâtel	13.4	Israel, non-Jews	1.5
Stomach	Japan, Nagasaki	51.0	Israel, non-Jews	2.4
Thyroid gland	U.S., Hawaii, Hawaiian	17.6	Poland, Warsaw, rural	0.7
Tongue	India, Bombay	4.1	Czechoslovakia, W. Slovakia	0.2
Uterus	U.S., Alameda, white	38.5	Japan, Fukuoka, rural	1.0

*per 100,000 persons

Who's at Risk?

Here's a rundown of risk factors for the 11 most frequently occurring cancers in the United States.

This . . .	Can put you at risk for this . . .	This . . .	Can put you at risk for this . . .
Smoking	Lung cancer Oral cancer Bladder cancer Pancreatic cancer	First child after age 30	Breast cancer
Smokeless tobacco	Oral cancer	Early age at first intercourse	Cervical cancer
Exposure to workplace chemicals such as asbestos, rubber, tar, or pitch	Bladder cancer Skin cancer Lung cancer Leukemia	Multiple sex partners	Cervical cancer
Personal or family history of cancer	Colon and rectal cancer	Failure to ovulate	Endometrial cancer
Inflammatory bowel disease	Colon and rectal cancer	Prolonged estrogen therapy	Endometrial cancer
High-fat or low-fiber diet	Colon and rectal cancer Breast cancer Pancreatic cancer Prostate cancer	Obesity	Endometrial cancer Breast cancer
Over age 30	Pancreatic cancer	Alcohol	Oral cancer
Over age 50	Breast cancer Ovarian cancer Prostate cancer	Black skin	Prostate cancer
		White skin	Skin cancer
		Sun exposure	Skin cancer
Never had children	Breast cancer Endometrial cancer Ovarian cancer	Hereditary abnormalities such as Down's syndrome	Leukemia

꩜**B**reast cancer is almost six times more likely to recur if a woman is under severe stress. "Severe stress" is defined as a threatening life event with long-term consequences—divorce, death of a loved one, or other breakdown of family relationships.

꩜**T**hree years after the nuclear disaster at Chernobyl, cancer rates of residents reportedly doubled.

Smoker's Roulette

The average cigarette smoker is 10 to 15 times more likely to develop lung cancer than his non-smoking counterpart. And his risk increases as the number of cigarettes per day increases. A man who smokes two or more packs per day, for example, is 20 to 25 times more likely to develop lung cancer than a nonsmoker.

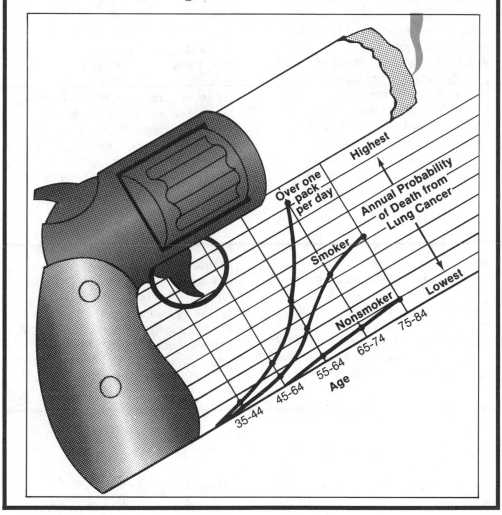

Quitters are winners. Those who have smoked for less than 20 years can cut their risk of lung cancer in half within a decade after they stop smoking.

Food and Cancer: The Facts

Scientists estimate that 35 percent of all cancer is caused by what we do or do not eat. Here are the facts about diet and cancer.

Overall Cancer Protection

▼ The less beta-carotene or vitamin A in your diet, the higher your risk of just about any cancer. Several studies indicate that diets high in beta-carotene or vitamin A may lower the risk of larynx, esophagus, and lung cancer. Other studies suggest a protective effect in the stomach, colon, and cervix. And animal studies indicate that vitamin A inhibits precancerous changes—and in some cases, cancer itself—in the prostate, bladder, and breast.

▼ Fruits and nuts—particularly strawberries, grapes, and Brazil nuts—contain ellagic acid, a compound that seems to block the effects of several of the carcinogens found in cigarette smoke and bacon. The fruits and nuts must be eaten just before or during carcinogen exposure to be effective.

▼ Fish oil may block the formation of cancer-causing agents from dietary fats.

▼ A study of more than 21,000 men linked a high blood level of vitamin E to a reduced overall risk of cancer.

▼ A study by the National Cancer Institute of 622 women revealed that those who ate more than 17 servings a week of whole-grain breads and cereals reduced their risk of cancer.

▼ Frying and broiling are the two cooking methods that encourage foods to produce the most cancer-causing chemicals. Stewing, boiling, pressure cooking, and microwaving produce less toxic fare.

Breast Cancer

▼ Italian scientists report that a diet rich in animal protein and fat—cheeseburgers, french fries, and ice cream, for example—increases a woman's risk of breast cancer threefold. Reducing animal proteins to less than 6 percent of calories while lowering total fat consumption to less than 30 percent eliminates the increased risk.

▼ Fish may also protect women from breast cancer. A comparison of breast cancer and diet in 32 countries indicates that countries with the highest consumption of fish as a percentage of total diet have the lowest incidence of breast cancer. Countries with the lowest consumption of fish have the highest incidence of breast cancer.

▼ Most studies of selenium have linked higher dietary levels of the mineral with a lower risk of breast and colon cancer.

Stomach Cancer

▼ A study of 3,000 Japanese indicates that daily consumption of fresh fruit and green tea may prevent the development of stomach cancer.

▼ A Chinese study of 1,695 people reveals that the more garlic and onions people eat, the less likely they are to develop stomach cancer.

Colorectal Cancer

▼ A survey of 106,203 men and women found that people who consume three or more alcoholic beverages a day have a significantly higher risk of developing rectal cancer than those who abstain.

▼ A high-fat, low-fiber diet doubles your risk of colon cancer.

▼ Studies suggest a link between higher calcium intake and lower rates of intestinal cancer. In one study, men who ate more foods containing calcium and vitamin D (vitamin D helps the body absorb calcium) had about one-third the risk of those who didn't.

▼ Vitamins C and E reduced the recurrence of colorectal polyps in a study of people who had had benign polyps removed. Colon cancer usually develops from polyps which go undetected.

▼ Cruciferous vegetables—broccoli, brussels sprouts, and cabbage, for example—may reduce the risk of cancer throughout the gastrointestinal tract.

Mouth and Throat Cancers

▼ A study of 629 men, 207 of whom had esophageal cancer, determined that men who smoke and drink are more likely to develop throat cancer than men who don't. The study also found that the risk of cancer was increased even further among men who consumed the lowest amounts of vitamins A and C as well as the least amount of fiber in the study.

▼ A study of South American tea drinkers reveals that very hot beverages can injure the throat and lead to esophageal cancer.

Lung Cancer

▼ Folate and vitamin B_{12} appear to reduce lung cell abnormalities that lead to cancer in men who smoke.

▼ The risk of lung cancer is three times higher among people who turn up their noses at carrots than among those who eat at least one serving a week.

▼ A study of 1,500 Chinese men and women indicates that people who inhale oil vapors while frying food are more likely to get lung cancer than those who don't.

Cervical Cancer

▼ Folate appears to stabilize or improve precancerous cervical abnormalities.

Pancreatic Cancer

▼ Regular consumption of Cajun-style pork and rice may increase your chance of developing pancreatic cancer. The problem may be caused either by the carcinogenic potential of capsaicin—the active ingredient in hot peppers—or the tendency of Cajun cooks to mix their rice with flour, oil, butter, and pork fat. Fortunately, consumption of fruits or other sources of vitamin C seems to exert a protective effect.

What the Experts Recommend

The major scientific institutions involved in cancer research in the United States have reached a consensus about how to reduce the risk of cancer through diet. Here's a summary of their recommendations.

Factor	National Academy of Sciences	Agency National Cancer Institute	American Cancer Society
Total fat (% of calories)	Reduce to 30%	Reduce to 30% or below	Reduce to 30%
Fiber (vegetables, fruit, whole grains)	Eat daily	Increase to several servings per day	Eat more
Vitamin A/Beta-carotene foods	Eat frequently	Eat daily	Eat daily
Vitamin C foods	Eat frequently	Eat daily	Eat daily
Cruciferous vegetables	Eat frequently	Eat several servings per week	Include in diet
Charred or smoked foods	Minimize	Choose less often	Moderation in smoked foods only
Alcohol	Moderation	Moderation	Moderation
Nitrites (cured/preserved foods)	Minimize	—	Moderation
Obesity	—	—	Avoid

Whole-Grain Protection from Prostate Cancer?

Two California researchers have discovered that nonsoluble fiber—the kind found in whole wheat cereals and breads, for example—binds with more than half of the male hormone circulating throughout a man's body.

This reduction in circulating testosterone, they suspect, reduces a man's chances of prostate cancer —perhaps by as much as two-thirds.

Animal studies suggest that the daughters of moms who eat a high-fat diet during pregnancy are more than twice as likely to develop reproductive system or pituitary tumors as daughters of mothers on a low-fat diet.

More than 70 percent of breast cancers are discovered by the woman herself, not a doctor.

50 Cancer-Fighting Foods

What foods protect against cancer? Here's a list of foods that are either extremely high in at least one factor believed to prevent cancer, a good source of several anti-cancer nutrients, or—since high-fat diets are known to cause cancer—a low-fat substitute for a common high-fat food.

Food	Protective Factor	Cooking Tips
Apricots	Vitamin A, fiber	Rehydrate dried fruit with a small amount of warm orange or apple juice, add a little grated orange rind for extra flavor, then grind into a spread. Use on toast or muffins instead of butter.
Bran cereal	Vitamin A, fiber	Use instead of low-fiber breakfast cereals, crush and sprinkle on casseroles, or coat chicken for baking.
Brazil nuts	Vitamin E, selenium, fiber	Crush and sprinkle on casseroles, muffins, vegetables.
Broccoli	Vitamin A, vitamin C, fiber	Skip the butter sauce. Use corn sauce. Use corn oil, lemon juice, and tarragon or thyme to taste.
Brown rice	Fiber, selenium	Combine with carrots, red peppers, and raisins for a super salad. Top with canola oil and raspberry vinegar. Chill.
Brussels sprouts	Vitamin C, fiber	Steam, then marinate for 30 minutes with cherry tomatoes and mushrooms in 1 tsp. low-sodium soy sauce, 1 tsp. vegetable oil, 2 Tbsp. lemon juice, 1 Tbsp. chopped parsley. Skewer vegetables and broil 5 minutes.
Butternut squash	Vitamin A, vitamin C, fiber	Puree cooked squash and toss with pineapple chunks instead of butter.
Cabbage	Vitamin C, vitamin E, fiber	For a crisp and sweet winter salad toss shredded cabbage with raisins and apples. Top with an herb vinaigrette or a dressing made of whipped nonfat yogurt, celery seed, and honey.
Cantaloupe	Vitamin A, vitamin C, fiber	To make a low-fat but creamy cooler, blend cantaloupe chunks with orange juice, nonfat yogurt, and crushed ice. Serve immediately.
Carrots	Vitamin A, fiber	To give pureed carrots a buttery consistency without fat, steam carrot chunks with pear chunks, then puree together.
Cauliflower	Vitamin C, fiber	Skip the cheese sauce. Steam and serve with light tomato sauce seasoned with oregano and basil.
Chard	Vitamin A, vitamin C, fiber	Boost the protective value of clear broth vegetable soups by adding chopped chard during cooking.

(continued)

50 Cancer-Fighting Foods—*Continued*

Food	Protective Factor	Cooking Tips
Chicken breast	Selenium	For a luscious and low-fat entrée, brush skinless, boneless breasts with an apple-cider/honey mixture and bake or broil. Baste frequently with the mixture during cooking.
Collard greens	Vitamin A, vitamin C, vitamin E, calcium, fiber	Use in stir-fries. Or puree steamed collards with low-fat cottage cheese and use to stuff onions. Bake at 350°F for 30–40 minutes.
Corn oil and canola (rapeseed) oil	Vitamin E	These mostly polyunsaturated and monounsaturated oils are rich sources of vitamin E. But since they are also fats, use them to replace (not in addition to) butter, lard, or other saturated fat in your diet.
Evaporated skim milk	Vitamin A, calcium, low fat	A boon to fat slashers. Use in place of cream in coffee, or whip and use immediately to top desserts. Flavor with a little maple syrup, if you like.
Figs (dried)	Fiber, calcium	To spice up brown rice, add ¼ cup chopped dried figs to 1 cup uncooked brown rice along with curry powder to taste. Cook the rice as usual.
Grapefruit	Vitamin C, fiber	Make a great seafood salad of canned salmon, grapefruit sections, and sliced cucumber. Drizzle with a dressing made of honey and citrus juices.
Great northern beans	Fiber, calcium	Use beans to replace some of the meat in meat loaf. You'll boost the fiber and cut the fat. Use about 1 cup of chopped, cooked beans per pound of meat in your recipe.
Kale	Vitamin A, vitamin C, vitamin E, fiber, calcium	For a delicious and moist fish dish, wrap fillets in steamed kale leaves and bake, basting frequently with chicken broth, until done.
Kidney beans	Fiber	For a tasty low-fat dip, blend 1 cup cooked kidney beans with chopped garlic, parsley, and scallions and add chili powder to taste. Thin to desired consistency with tomato juice or water.
Kiwis	Vitamin C, fiber	While kiwis are usually used as a garnish, you can get more of the goodness of kiwis by simply cutting them in half and eating with a spoon.
Mangoes	Vitamin A, vitamin C, vitamin E, fiber	Use chunks of mango in your favorite chutney recipe, then serve the chutney with meat, replacing fatty sauces and gravies.
Oatmeal	Fiber, selenium	Instead of butter, use figs, apricots, prunes, and sunflower seeds to dress up your oatmeal and make it extra-protective.

Food	Protective Factor	Cooking Tips
Oranges	Vitamin C, fiber	Combine chopped orange sections with a little honey and a little orange juice. Top fish fillets with mixture and bake. They'll be moist and flavorful without butter.
Papaya	Vitamin A, vitamin C, fiber	Puree ripe papaya into a sauce for poached chicken. Thin with a bit of water or fruit juice if necessary. Or combine pureed papaya with some nonfat yogurt and make frozen pops.
Peas (edible-podded)	Vitamin C, fiber	Stuff with herbed, nonfat yogurt cheese (see listing for nonfat yogurt cheese).
Popcorn	Fiber	Make in an air popper and season with your favorite herbs and spices instead of butter. Try adding chili powder for a savory snack, or honey, minced dried fruit, and minced nuts for a sweet one.
Potatoes	Vitamin C, fiber	Mix nonfat yogurt or low-fat cottage cheese with dill, chives, and pepper (or other herbs) and use instead of sour cream to top baked potatoes.
Prunes	Vitamin A, fiber	Make a nutrient- and fiber-packed compote: Mix prunes, raisins, apricots, grapefruit sections, and dried figs in a baking dish. Pour on enough orange juice to moisten and bake until warmed through, about 30 minutes.
Pumpkin	Vitamin A, fiber	Update your pumpkin pudding recipe for better health: Replace the whole milk with skim, and each egg with 2 egg whites. Add 2 or 3 Tbsp. of dry milk powder to boost the calcium content.
Raisins	Fiber	Sprinkle on salads to give a sweet fiber lift.
Salmon (canned)	Selenium, calcium, fish oil	Prepare a simple bisque by pureeing 1 can of salmon with 1 minced onion, 1½–2 cups of stock, a dash of lemon juice, and ½ cup of skim milk. Heat slowly until just simmering.
Sardines (canned)	Vitamin C, calcium, fish oil	Look for sardines packed in mustard or tomato sauce instead of oil. Try a nutrient-dense sandwich of sardines in mustard sauce with spinach on crusty whole wheat bread.
Skim milk	Vitamin A, low fat, calcium	Simply substitute for whole milk and you reduce fat from over 48% of calories to less than 3%.
Spinach	Vitamin A, vitamin E, fiber	Dress up a spinach salad with sliced strawberries and a vinaigrette of lemon juice, tarragon vinegar, honey, grated lemon rind, and a small amount of oil.
Strawberries	Vitamin C, fiber	Add pureed strawberries to applesauce for extra zip, as well as vitamin C and fiber.

(continued)

50 Cancer-Fighting Foods—*Continued*

Food	Protective Factor	Cooking Tips
Sunflower seeds	Vitamin E, selenium, fiber	Toss seeds in low-sodium soy sauce then toast at low heat in the oven or in a nonstick pan. Add to salads or yogurt.
Sweet peppers	Vitamin A, vitamin C, fiber	Roast some red peppers and cut them into strips. Toss with balsamic vinegar and a splash of olive oil for a tasty condiment.
Sweet potatoes	Vitamin A, vitamin C, fiber	Steam chunks of sweet potatoes with chopped dried apricots. Transfer to a baking dish, glaze with apricot nectar and bake for about 20 minutes.
Swordfish	Selenium, fish oil	Add chunks of swordfish to stir-fries in place of beef. Broccoli and red peppers go well with it.
Tofu	Calcium, fiber	Marinate in a small amount of low-sodium soy sauce mixed with oil. Stir-fry with vegetables.
Tuna (canned)	Selenium, fish oil	Prepare a low-fat version of tuna salad by combining a can of drained water-packed tuna with 1 Tbsp. red wine vinegar and chopped onions to taste.
Turnips, rutabagas	Vitamin C, fiber	Mash with orange juice concentrate and a dash of cinnamon, instead of butter.
Wheat germ	Vitamin E, fiber	Dip fillets of white fish in egg white, then dredge in a mixture of toasted wheat germ, cornmeal, and spices before baking. They will stay moist.
Whole wheat bread	Selenium, fiber	To make a simple bread-pudding dessert, combine 4 cups bread cubes, 2 egg whites, 1½ cups skim milk, and a dash of cinnamon and nutmeg in a baking dish. Bake for 45 minutes at 350°F.
Nonfat yogurt	Low fat, calcium	Use as a substitute for sour cream in sauces. To keep it from curdling when heated, add 1 Tbsp. cornstarch per cup.
Nonfat yogurt cheese	Low fat, calcium	A great substitute for cream cheese in cheese dips and spreads. The easiest way to make it: Use a coffee filter in a strainer positioned over a bowl. Pour nonfat yogurt into the filter and let drain (refrigerated) overnight. By morning the filter will contain yogurt cheese.

People living in communities with chlorinated water have almost twice the incidence of fatal bladder cancer as those residing in communities where water is disinfected by other methods.

Cancer Treatment Options

What kind of cancer treatment is most effective? It depends on the cancer. The table lists eight common cancers, their conventional treatments, and some of the experimental treatments that look promising.

Type of Cancer	Conventional Treatment	Experimental Treatment*	Type of Cancer	Conventional Treatment	Experimental Treatment*
Lung			**Prostate**	In early stages, surgery or radiation. In later stages, surgery and/or hormonal therapy to block activity of male hormones that stimulate cancer's growth.	New drugs and synthetic hormones to block the activity of male hormones. Radioactive pellets implanted in prostate. Chemotherapy using experimental drugs.
Small cell	Chemotherapy	Drugs or antibodies to suppress tumor growth. Chemotherapy plus radiation followed by surgery.			
Other	Surgery and radiation.	Chemotherapy			
Colorectal			**Uterus**		
Rectum	Surgery, sometimes followed by radiation.	Chemotherapy. Biological therapy using interferon, interleukin-2, and/or monoclonal antibodies.	Cervix	In early stages, surgery. In later stages, radiation.	Chemotherapy using experimental drugs. Radiation.
			Endometrium	In early stages, hysterectomy. In later stages, hysterectomy, radiation, and sometimes hormonal therapy.	Chemotherapy and hormonal therapy using experimental drugs.
Colon	Surgery	Chemotherapy. Biological therapy using interferon, interleukin-2, and/or monoclonal antibodies.	**Bladder**	In early stages, surgery or radiation. In later stages, chemotherapy and/or radiation.	High-dose chemotherapy before surgery. Standard-dose chemotherapy injected directly into the bladder.
Breast	In early stages, surgery sometimes with radiation. In later stages, surgery with radiation plus chemotherapy or hormonal therapy.	Chemotherapy or hormonal therapy used at early stages. High-dose chemotherapy.	**Melanoma (skin)**	Surgery	Surgery plus interferon, interleukin-2, and/or monoclonal antibodies to stimulate immune response.
Non-Hodgkins lymphoma	Chemotherapy	Chemotherapy and local radiation. Total body irradiation. High-dose chemotherapy.			

*Treatments listed are given both individually and in various combinations, and usually after conventional therapy.

Advanced Treatments Not Fully Utilized

A 1988 report from the General Accounting Office (GAO) revealed that large numbers of cancer patients who could benefit from state-of-the-art treatments—particularly radiation and chemotherapy as a surgical follow-up—were not getting them.

Here's a sample of the GAO's findings.

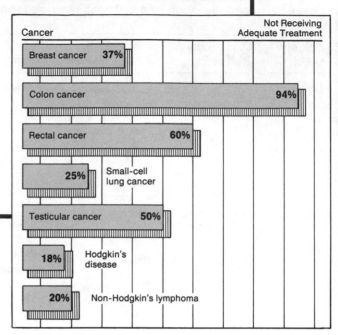

Cancer	Not Receiving Adequate Treatment
Breast cancer	37%
Colon cancer	94%
Rectal cancer	60%
Small-cell lung cancer	25%
Testicular cancer	50%
Hodgkin's disease	18%
Non-Hodgkin's lymphoma	20%

Y**our** significant other may be killing you. The Canadian government attributes 50 to 60 percent of all lung cancer deaths among nonsmokers to spousal smoking.

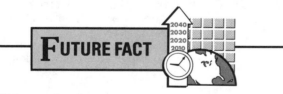

FUTURE FACT

Circulatory Submarines

A microscopic submarine, programmed by scientists and fueled by glucose, could someday patrol your bloodstream looking for cancer. If it finds any, the submarine may very well torpedo the tumor, then escort its remnants to the kidney for burial at sea.

Follow-Up Therapies Increase Survival

In a worldwide study, the likelihood of women over age 50 with breast cancer surviving more than five years after surgery increased 20 percent if they took an anti-estrogen drug called tamoxifen. Women under 50 increased their survival odds by 26 percent when surgery was followed by chemotherapy utilizing several different drugs. But 37 percent of all women who have breast cancer do not receive postsurgical treatment such as chemotherapy.

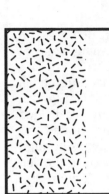

13

CHOLESTEROL

Every day millions of Americans inadvertently deposit harmful cholesterol along the arteries that distribute food and oxygen throughout their bodies, increasing the risk that they will eventually die of heart disease. When added to the 2,000 milligrams of cholesterol produced daily by the liver, the 450 milligrams of dietary cholesterol that the average adult puts in his mouth each day contributes to the gradual process of atherosclerosis that can literally seal arteries shut.

Just eating an extra 200 milligrams of cholesterol per 1,000 calories a day will take 3.4 years off the life of a middle-aged American man, scientists report. That much cholesterol is easy to find in a couple of eggs, a pile of bacon, or maybe a large piece of quiche.

On the plus side, researchers estimate that cutting much of the saturated fat and cholesterol out of our diets and lowering the cholesterol roaming our arteries to less than 200 milligrams per deciliter of blood would add another five years to the life span of the average middle-aged American man.

Defining the Problem

Cholesterol is a soft, waxy, fatlike alcohol that is used throughout the body to manufacture hormones, bile, and vitamin D. In excessive amounts, it also causes atherosclerosis, the artery-clogging disease that lays the foundation for a heart attack.

Blood cholesterol is cholesterol that is being transported through your blood. It's manufactured in the liver and absorbed through the intestine from the food you eat.

Dietary cholesterol is cholesterol that—after roaming the bloodstreams of other animals—becomes a key component of their tissues or by-products. It enters our bodies when we eat meat, eggs, milk, cheese, and other animal foods. There is no cholesterol in plants.

Fat is a nutrient that gives you energy and helps your body absorb vitamins. There are two types: saturated and unsaturated.

Saturated fat raises blood cholesterol levels even more than dietary cholesterol does. It's found in meat, poultry, and dairy products. It's also found in tropical oils such as coconut and palm. It's usually solid at refrigerator temperature.

Unsaturated fat is better. It's a type of fat that usually stays liquid at refrigerator temperature. It's divided into two types: *poly*unsaturated and *mono*unsaturated. Polyunsaturated fat is found in safflower, sunflower, corn, and soybean oils. Monounsaturated fat is found in olive and canola (rapeseed) oils. When substituted for saturated fat, both polyunsaturated and monounsaturated fats are known to reduce blood cholesterol levels.

Lipoproteins are protein-coated packages that transport cholesterol through the blood.

High-density lipoproteins (HDLs) carry cholesterol out of body tissues to the liver for excretion from the body. The more HDLs you have, the lower your risk of heart disease.

Low-density lipoproteins (LDLs) deposit cholesterol in artery walls. The more LDLs you have, the higher your risk.

How High Is Too High?

The National Cholesterol Education Program's Expert Panel has set these three classification categories based on risk for developing coronary heart disease.

More than half of all Americans have cholesterol levels that are too high—which means that their total cholesterol levels are over 200 mg/dl.

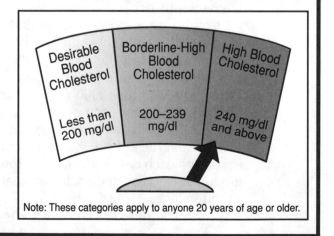

Desirable Blood Cholesterol — Less than 200 mg/dl

Borderline-High Blood Cholesterol — 200–239 mg/dl

High Blood Cholesterol — 240 mg/dl and above

Note: These categories apply to anyone 20 years of age or older.

Global Highs and Lows

Scientists first began to realize cholesterol's importance when they discovered that its levels vary widely from country to country, paralleling each nation's rate of heart disease. In a country where heart disease rates are sky-high, for example, so are cholesterol levels.

Here's a sampling of cholesterol levels from around the globe.

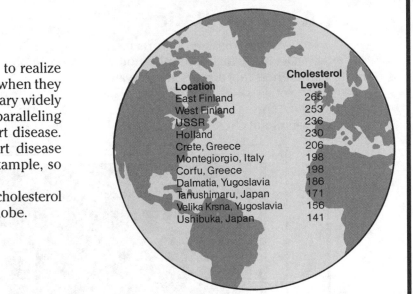

Location	Cholesterol Level
East Finland	265
West Finland	253
USSR	236
Holland	230
Crete, Greece	206
Montegiorgio, Italy	198
Corfu, Greece	198
Dalmatia, Yugoslavia	186
Tanushimaru, Japan	171
Velika Krsna, Yugoslavia	156
Ushibuka, Japan	141

Women "Win" in the End

Men in their late twenties through their early forties tend to have higher levels of cholesterol than women the same age. That changes around age 45, however, when women's cholesterol levels start to surge ahead.

The chart illustrates the relative positions of men's and women's cholesterol levels over an average life span.

Olive oil sales increased 28.8 percent in the United States from October 1988 to October 1989, according to Arbitron/SAMI, a New York–based market research concern.

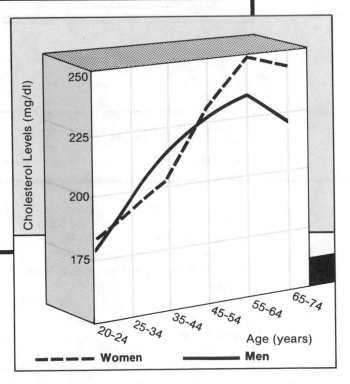

Cholesterol Levels (mg/dl)

250 — 225 — 200 — 175

Age (years): 20-24, 25-34, 35-44, 45-54, 55-64, 65-74

- - - - - Women ——— Men

A Healthy Ratio

Many cholesterol reports mention a ratio, which is simply another numerical tool doctors use to evaluate your risk of heart disease. The ratio expresses the relationship between total cholesterol and HDL. If your total cholesterol is 200, for example, and your HDL is 50, your ratio is $200 \div 50 = 4$.

The optimal ratio is 3.5 or lower. Anything higher and you're at increased risk for heart disease.

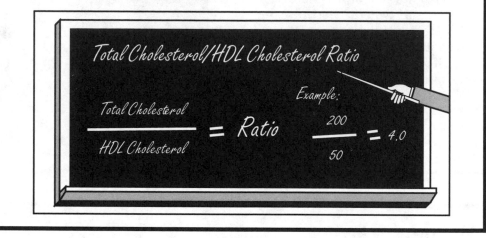

$$\frac{Total\ Cholesterol}{HDL\ Cholesterol} = Ratio \qquad \frac{200}{50} = 4.0$$

Total Cholesterol/HDL Cholesterol Ratio

Example:

LDL and HDL: What's a Good Number?

If your total cholesterol is above 200 mg/dl, your doctor may send a sample of your blood to the lab for a lipoprotein analysis. The lab will measure the amounts of low-density lipoproteins (LDLs) and high-density lipoproteins (HDLs) in each deciliter of your blood, and report the total for each.

When you read the report, keep in mind that an LDL reading under 130 is good. Over 130 and you'll be told to watch your diet. Over 160 and you may also be a candidate for a cholesterol-lowering drug.

Doctors don't worry about having too many HDLs. Just the opposite: Any HDL level under 35 mg/dl is considered too *low*.

When to Check Your Cholesterol

The National Cholesterol Education Program's Expert Panel recommends that all adults over 20 years of age should have their blood cholesterol measured at least once every five years.

Any test that shows a cholesterol level over 200 mg/dl should be repeated to verify the results. If cholesterol levels are between 200 and 239 mg/dl and you have coronary heart disease or two other risk factors for heart disease—being a man and smoking are two risk factors, for example—you should also have a lipoprotein analysis. The analysis will measure the amount of HDL and LDL in your blood—thus giving your doctor some idea as to what's going on inside your arteries and what your chances are of a heart attack. If you have a cholesterol level of 240 mg/dl or more, you should have the lipoprotein analysis done whether or not you have any other risk factors.

The American Academy of Pediatrics recommends that cholesterol levels be measured in children over two years of age who come from families with a history of high cholesterol or early heart attack.

Among those with high cholesterol levels, the risk of a heart attack can be reduced 2 percent for every 1 percent reduction in blood cholesterol.

High Cholesterol Kills

A study of 356,000 men in 18 cities across the United States reveals that the higher your cholesterol, the higher your risk of death due to coronary heart disease. Scientists calculate that 46 percent of the deaths in this study could be attributed to cholesterol levels of 180 mg/dl or above.

Serum Cholesterol (mg/dl)	Coronary Heart Disease Mortality	
	Deaths	Rate*
167 or less	95	3.16
168–181	101	3.32
182–192	139	4.15
193–202	149	4.21
203–212	203	5.43
213–220	192	5.81
221–231	261	6.94
232–244	272	7.35
245–263	352	9.10
264 or more	494	13.05

*per 1,000 persons

Are You at Risk?

Your risk of heart disease is directly related to your cholesterol level—particularly the "bad guy" LDLs. The higher your levels, the higher your risk.

Find your age, sex, and cholesterol levels in this table, then check out whether or not you're likely to be headed for trouble.

Age	Total Cholesterol (mg/dl)		LDL Cholesterol (mg/dl)	
	Moderate Risk	High Risk	Moderate Risk	High Risk
Men				
0–14	173	190	106	120
15–19	165	183	109	123
20–29	194	216	128	148
30–39	218	244	149	171
40–49	231	254	160	180
50+	230	258	166	188
Women				
0–14	174	170	113	126
15–19	173	195	115	135
20–29	184	208	127	148
30–39	202	220	143	163
40–49	223	246	155	177
50+	252	281	170	195

The Framingham Study: How HDL Protects

An ongoing study of residents between the ages of 49 and 82 in Framingham, Massachusetts, reveals that men and women with high levels of HDL have half the risk of developing coronary heart disease (CHD) of those with low levels of HDL.

That finding holds true even among study participants with total blood cholesterol levels under 200 mg/dl. At these ages, low blood cholesterol does not really protect against CHD unless HDL levels are over 40 mg/dl. Below 40 mg/dl, the incidence of heart disease soars.

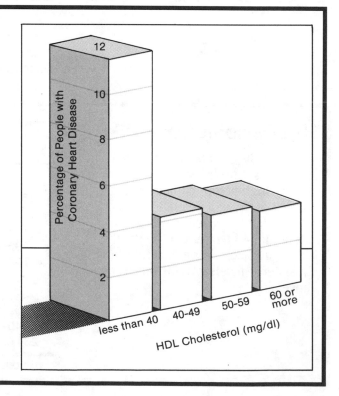

Can Heart Disease Be Stopped?

Yes. The Leiden Intervention Trial, a Dutch study of 35 men and 4 women who had at least one coronary artery that had been narrowed more than 50 percent by heart disease, clearly demonstrated that for some people a low-cholesterol diet can stop heart disease in its tracks.

For two years the Leiden participants ate a vegetarian diet that contained less than 100 milligrams of cholesterol a day. They also ate twice as much polyunsaturated as saturated fat. At the end of the study, a check of coronary arteries revealed that there was no progression of arterial disease in 46 percent of the study participants.

The major difference between those whose disease progressed and those whose disease did not was found in their total cholesterol and HDL levels. Those whose disease did not get worse had lower cholesterol/HDL total ratios than those in whom the disease progressed. Average HDL for those who showed no advance in arterial disease was 43 mg/dl. Average HDL for the others was 35 mg/dl. The chart shows the equally dramatic difference in total cholesterol levels between the two groups.

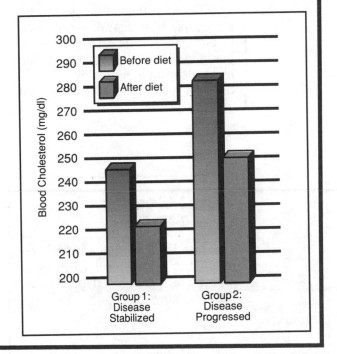

An Australian meat cutter has developed a mechanical process that not only lops visible fat off the edges of meat but also separates it out of the meat fibers themselves. The process, according to its inventor, can reduce fat levels in any meat by up to 96 percent, cholesterol by 30 percent, and calories by 50 percent.

A 1 mg/dl increase in HDL lowers the rate of death from heart disease by 3.7 percent in men and 4.7 percent in women.

Can Heart Disease Be Reversed?

On occasion. In a landmark study, researchers from the University of Southern California School of Medicine tested and monitored 162 men with heart disease who had previously had a bypass.

The investigators first took arterial x-rays of the men's diseased blood vessels to gauge the extent of damage. Then they gave half the men a low-fat diet plus two cholesterol-lowering drugs; the other half got just the low-fat diet. After two years, the researchers again took x-rays and compared them with the earlier ones.

The result? In 16 percent of the diet-plus-drugs group, the amount of heart disease was visibly less. In 2.4 percent of the diet-without-drugs group, the amount of heart disease was also visibly less. Clearly, in some cases heart disease can be reversed.

What Causes Low HDL?

The level of HDLs, which remove the cholesterol from your blood, can be reduced by the following factors.

▼ Cigarette smoking

▼ Obesity

▼ Lack of exercise

▼ Steroid drugs

▼ Beta-adrenergic blocking agents (frequently found in heart medication)

▼ High triglyceride levels

▼ A genetic predisposition to low HDLs

Studies indicate that men who smoke 20 or more cigarettes a day have HDL levels that are 11 percent lower than those of men who don't smoke. Smoking lowers women's HDL levels by 14 percent.

Weight loss can result in a sizable increase in "good" HDL cholesterol. A study at the Stanford University School of Medicine showed that a group of men who lost about 5 pounds of body fat over the course of a year, either by diet or exercise, had significant increases in HDL and a significant improvement in the ratio of total cholesterol to HDL. The authors conclude that more attention should be paid to weight loss and increased exercise as ways to reduce risk of coronary heart disease.

Which Diet Lowers Cholesterol the Most?

An Oxford, England, study of 3,277 men and women reveals that a vegan diet—one in which absolutely no food of animal origin is eaten—will lower both total cholesterol and LDLs far more than other diets which include eggs, dairy products, fish, or meat.

Cholesterol levels of vegans in the study were 24 percent lower than those of traditional meat eaters, 17 percent lower than those of people who included fish but no meat in their diet, and 14 percent lower than those of people on a vegetarian diet that included egg and dairy products.

Eating a lifelong vegan diet, researchers concluded, could lower the incidence of heart disease by 57 percent.

Diet	Total Cholesterol (mg/dl)
Vegan	166
Vegetarian	189
Fish eater	194
Meat eater	205

How Much Saturated Fat Is Too Much?

Many cholesterol-lowering diets advise you to eat only a certain percentage of calories as saturated fat. But what does "get no more than 10 or 7 percent of calories from saturated fat"—which is what the National Cholesterol Education Program's Step-One and Step-Two Diets suggest—actually mean?

The table shows you exactly how many grams of saturated fat you can have, depending on the number of calories you consume and the percentage of calories from saturated fat your physician decided is appropriate for you.

Caloric Need	10% of Calories as Saturated Fat	7% of Calories as Saturated Fat
1,000 calories	11 grams	8 grams
1,500 calories	17 grams	12 grams
2,000 calories	22 grams	16 grams
2,500 calories	28 grams	19 grams
3,000 calories	33 grams	23 grams
4,000 calories	44 grams	31 grams

How Much Saturated Fat and Cholesterol Are You Eating?

The following table will help you compare the amount of saturated fat and cholesterol in various foods. Remember, depending on the number of calories needed, most people on a cholesterol control program need to limit saturated fat to between 11 and 28 grams and dietary cholesterol to less than 300 milligrams per day.

Food	Saturated Fat (g)	Cholesterol (mg)
Dairy and Egg Products		
Cheese (1 oz., unless otherwise noted)		
American process cheese, pasteurized	5.6	27
American process cheese food, pasteurized	4.4	18
Blue	5.3	21
Brick	5.3	27
Brie	4.9	28
Camembert	4.3	20
Cheddar	6.0	30
Colby	5.7	27
Cottage cheese, creamed, 4 oz.	3.2	17
Cottage cheese, low-fat, 1% fat, 4 oz.	0.7	5
Cream cheese	6.2	31
Edam	5.0	25
Feta	4.2	25
Gouda	5.0	32
Gruyere	5.4	31
Monterey Jack	5.5	25
Mozzarella	3.7	22
Mozzarella, part skim	2.9	16
Muenster	5.4	27
Parmesan	5.4	22
Provolone	4.8	20
Ricotta, part skim, 4 oz.	5.6	25
Ricotta, whole milk, 4 oz.	9.4	58
Romano	4.9	29
Roquefort	5.5	26
Swiss	5.0	26
Eggs		
White	0	0
Whole	1.7	274
Yolk	1.7	274

Food	Saturated Fat (g)	Cholesterol (mg)
Ice cream and ice milk (1 cup)		
Ice cream, vanilla, hard	8.9	59
Ice cream, vanilla, rich, 16% fat	14.7	88
Ice milk, vanilla, hard	3.5	18
Ice milk, vanilla, soft serve	2.9	13
Milk (8 oz.)		
Buttermilk	1.3	9
Skim	0.3	4
Low-fat, 1% fat	1.6	10
Low-fat, 2% fat	2.9	18
Whole, 3.3% fat	5.1	33
Sour cream, 1 oz.	3.7	12
Yogurt (4 oz.)		
Plain	2.4	14
Plain, low-fat	0.1	2
Gravies (½ cup)		
Au jus, canned	0.1	1
Beef, canned	1.4	4
Chicken, canned	1.7	3
Meats and Seafood (3½ oz., unless otherwise noted)		
Beef		
Bologna, cured, 3–4 slices	12.1	58
Bottom round, lean only, braised	3.4	96
Brisket, whole, lean only, braised	4.6	93
Chuck, arm pot roast, lean and fat, braised	10.7	99
Chuck, arm pot roast, lean only, braised	3.8	101
Chuck, blade roast, lean only, braised	6.2	106
Corned beef, cured, brisket, cooked	6.3	98

Food	Saturated Fat (g)	Cholesterol (mg)	Food	Saturated Fat (g)	Cholesterol (mg)
Flank, lean and fat, choice, braised	6.6	72	Loin, fresh, sirloin, lean and fat, roasted	7.4	91
Flank, lean only, choice braised	5.9	71	Loin, fresh, sirloin, lean only, roasted	4.5	90
Frankfurter, cured, about 2	12.0	61	Sausage, cured, smoked link, grilled	11.3	68
Ground beef, lean, broiled medium	7.2	87	Sausage, Italian, fresh, cooked	9.0	78
Kidneys, simmered	1.1	387	Sausage, liver, cured, liverwurst	10.6	158
Liver, braised	1.9	389	Shoulder, cured, arm picnic, lean and fat, roasted	7.7	58
Round, full cut, lean and fat, choice, braised	7.3	84	Shoulder, cured, arm picnic, lean only, roasted	2.4	48
Salami, cured, cooked, smoked, 3–4 slices	9.0	65	Tenderloin, fresh, lean only, roasted	1.7	93
Sausage, cured, cooked, smoked, about 2	11.4	67	**Poultry**		
Short ribs, lean only, choice, braised	7.7	93	Chicken, broiler or fryer, dark meat without skin, roasted	2.7	93
T-bone steak, lean and fat, choice, broiled	10.2	84	Chicken, broiler or fryer, dark meat with skin, roasted	4.4	91
T-bone steak, lean only, choice, broiled	4.2	80	Chicken, broiler or fryer, light meat with skin, roasted	3.0	85
Tenderloin, lean only, broiled	3.6	84	Chicken, broiler or fryer, light meat without skin, roasted	1.3	85
Top round, lean only, broiled	2.2	84	Chicken, roaster, light meat without skin, roasted	1.1	75
Lamb			Chicken, roaster, dark meat without skin, roasted	2.4	75
Arm chop, lean only, braised	6.0	122	Chicken, stewing, light meat without skin, stewed	2.0	70
Leg, lean only, roasted	3.0	89			
Loin chop, lean only, broiled	4.1	94			
Pork					
Bratwurst, fresh, cooked	9.3	60			
Ham, fresh, shank half, lean only, roasted	3.6	92			
Ham, rump half, lean only, roasted	3.7	96			
Ham steak, cured, boneless, extra lean, unheated	1.4	45			

(continued)

How Much Saturated Fat and Cholesterol Are You Eating?—*Continued*

Food	Saturated Fat (g)	Cholesterol (mg)
Poultry—continued		
Chicken, stewing, dark meat without skin, stewed	4.1	95
Chicken frankfurter, about 2	5.5	101
Duck, domesticated, flesh only, roasted	4.2	89
Goose, domesticated, flesh only, roasted	4.6	96
Turkey, fryer-roaster, dark meat without skin, roasted	1.4	112
Turkey, fryer-roaster, dark meat with skin, roasted	2.1	117
Turkey, fryer-roaster, light meat without skin, roasted	0.4	86
Turkey, fryer-roaster, light meat with skin, roasted	1.3	95
Turkey bologna, about 3½ slices	5.1	99
Turkey frankfurter, about 2	5.9	107
Crustaceans		
Crab, blue, steamed	0.2	100
Lobster, northern	0.1	72
Shrimp, mixed species, steamed	0.3	195
Finfish		
Cod, Atlantic, baked	0.2	55
Grouper, mixed species, baked	0.3	47
Haddock, baked	0.2	74
Halibut, Atlantic and Pacific, baked	0.4	41
Herring, Atlantic, baked	2.6	77
Mackerel, Atlantic, baked	4.2	75
Perch, mixed species, baked	0.2	42
Pollock, walleye, baked	0.2	96

Food	Saturated Fat (g)	Cholesterol (mg)
Pompano, Florida, baked	4.5	64
Rockfish, Pacific, baked	0.5	44
Salmon, sockeye, baked	1.9	87
Sea bass, mixed species, baked	0.7	53
Snapper, mixed species, baked	0.4	47
Swordfish, baked	1.4	50
Trout, rainbow, baked	0.8	73
Tuna, bluefin, baked	1.6	49
Whiting, mixed species, baked	0.3	84
Mollusks		
Clam, mixed species, steamed	0.2	67
Mussel, blue, steamed	0.9	56
Oyster, eastern, steamed	1.3	109
Salad Dressings (1 Tbsp.)		
Blue cheese	1.5	—
French, low-calorie	0.1	1
French, regular	1.5	—
Imitation mayonnaise	0.5	4
Italian, low-calorie	0.2	1
Italian, regular	1.0	—
Mayonnaise	1.6	8
Russian, low-calorie	0.1	1
Russian, regular	1.1	—
Thousand Island, low-calorie	0.2	2
Thousand Island, regular	0.9	—
Sauces (½ cup)		
Barbecue	0.3	0
Bearnaise	20.9	99
Cheese	4.7	26
Hollandaise	20.9	94
Sour cream	8.5	45
Sweet and sour	trace	0
White	3.2	17

Which Fat Should You Reach for First?

The one with the monounsaturates. Studies indicate that "monos" —most readily available as olive oil— lower total cholesterol and LDLs while leaving the "good" HDLs intact. Experts are no longer quite as enthusiastic about polyunsaturates as a cholesterol-lowering agent because, although they can lower total cholesterol, they lower the protective HDLs as well.

Some experts suggest that for heart health, you should substitute— not add, but substitute—two or three tablespoons of olive oil a day for other fats in your diet. The fats you should substitute it for are the ones with the most saturated fat. The chart shows you, fat-by-fat, how to tell the good from the bad.

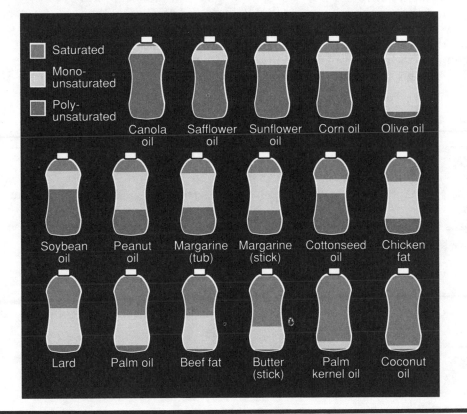

- Saturated
- Mono-unsaturated
- Poly-unsaturated

Canola oil · Safflower oil · Sunflower oil · Corn oil · Olive oil

Soybean oil · Peanut oil · Margarine (tub) · Margarine (stick) · Cottonseed oil · Chicken fat

Lard · Palm oil · Beef fat · Butter (stick) · Palm kernel oil · Coconut oil

In one study, a drop of 20 mg/dl in blood cholesterol was associated with a 16 percent drop in deaths due to heart disease.

Take a "CSI" Tally

CSI stands for Cholesterol-Saturated Fat Index, a formula that correctly weighs the effects of both a food's cholesterol and its saturated fat on blood cholesterol. Scientists have known for some time that both food constituents have a cholesterol-raising effect, but not until the CSI formula (developed by Sonja L. Connor, a registered dietitian, and William E. Connor, M.D., of Oregon Health Sciences University) was there a way of computing the combined effects of these two villains. The formula works as follows: A food's saturated-fat content, measured in grams, is multiplied by 1.01, while its cholesterol content, measured in milligrams, is multiplied by 0.05. The two products are then added to yield the food's CSI rating. The accompanying table lists CSI ratings for some selected foods.

The higher a food's CSI rating, the greater its tendency to raise levels of cholesterol in the blood—and hence your risk of heart disease. For optimum cholesterol-lowering results, your goal should be to eat foods totaling a CSI of no more than about 28 a day if you're a moderately active woman, and no more than about 36 a day if you're a moderately active man.

Food	Portion	CSI
Appetizers		
Liver pâté	2 Tbsp.	7
Soup, minestrone	1 cup	7
Sour-cream dip	¼ cup	8
Swedish meatballs	3	12
Baked goods		
Carrot cake	1 slice	14
Cheesecake	1 slice	22
Danish pastry	1	8
Doughnut, plain	1	4
Oatmeal cookies	3 (3")	4
Beans (cooked, no fat added)		
Lentils, split peas	½ cup	trace
Navy, pinto, kidney, black	½ cup	trace
Tofu (bean curd)	½ cup	<1
Beverages		
Coffee, black	1 cup	0
Coffee with ½ ounce half-and-half	1 cup	1
Fruit juice	1 cup	0

Food	Portion	CSI
Breads and tortillas		
Crescent roll	1	3
Corn tortilla, baked	1	trace
Taco, fried	1	1
White, whole wheat, raisin, rye, or pumpernickel bread	1 slice	trace
Breakfast dishes		
Omelet, plain	2 eggs	27
Omelet, with cheese	2 eggs	34
Omelet, made with egg whites only	½ cup	0
Pancakes, regular	3 (4")	8
Pancakes, made with oil, skim milk, no egg yolks	3 (4")	1
Cereals and grains		
Bran flakes	1 cup	trace
Granola, commercial, with soy oil	1 cup	3
Granola, commercial, with coconut oil	1 cup	17

Food	Portion	CSI	Food	Portion	CSI
Oatmeal, cooked	1 cup	trace	White fish (red snapper, sole, cod, and others)	3 oz.	3
Rice, white or brown	1 cup	trace			
Cheeses			**Frozen desserts**		
Cheddar, Monterey Jack, Colby, Havarti, Longhorn	1 oz.	8	Frozen yogurt, low-fat	1 cup	3
			Ice cream, 10% fat	1 cup	15
Cottage cheese, 1% fat	½ cup	<1	Ice cream, 12% fat	1 cup	19
Cream cheese, regular	1 oz.	8	Sherbet	1 cup	3
Cream cheese, reduced-fat	1 oz.	5	**Fruits and vegetables**		
Ricotta, part-skim	2 Tbsp.	2	Apple, pear, peach	1 med.	trace
Swiss	1 oz.	6	Carrots, celery, green beans, tomatoes, broccoli, cauliflower, raw	1 cup	trace
Dairy products					
Half-and-half	1 Tbsp.	1.5	Melon, berries	1 cup	trace
Nondairy creamer, powdered	1 Tbsp.	2	Peas, corn, potatoes, winter squash	½ cup	trace
Nondairy creamer, liquid	1 Tbsp.	<1			
Milk, whole	1 cup	7	**Meat (cooked, boneless)**		
Milk, 1% fat	1 cup	2	Beef, corned beef, pastrami	3 oz.	15
Milk, skim or powdered nonfat	1 cup	1	Flank	3 oz.	5
Sour cream, 20% fat	½ cup	18	Ground beef, 20% fat	3 oz.	11
Sour cream, light, 10% fat	½ cup	10	Ground beef, 10% fat	3 oz.	7
Yogurt, plain	1 cup	7	Lamb chop, shoulder	3 oz.	17
Yogurt, low-fat, plain	1 cup	3	Liver	3 oz.	22
Fats and spreads			Pork, tenderloin	3 oz.	5
Butter	1 tsp.	3	Pork sausage	4 links	12
Corn oil	½ cup	14	Spareribs	3 oz.	13
Coconut oil	½ cup	95	Sirloin tip	3 oz.	9
Margarine, stick	1 tsp.	<1	Tenderloin, porterhouse	3 oz.	15
Mayonnaise	1 Tbsp.	2.1	**Poultry (cooked and boneless)**		
Mayonnaise, light	1 Tbsp.	0.8	Chicken, Cornish game hen, or turkey, white meat, with skin	3 oz.	6
Olive oil	½ cup	15			
Palm oil	½ cup	54			
Rapeseed oil	½ cup	9	Chicken, Cornish game hen, or turkey, white meat, without skin	3 oz.	4
Safflower oil	½ cup	10			
Shortening, soft	½ cup	26			
Fish and shellfish (cooked)			**Salads**		
Clams, steamers	25 med.	3	Green salad, with 2 Tbsp. French dressing	1 cup	3
Lobster	1½ tails	7	Green salad, with 2 Tbsp. Italian dressing	1 cup	1
Salmon, canned	½ cup	3			
Sea scallops	8	2	Potato salad, German-style	1 cup	2
Shrimp	⅔ cup	9	Potato salad, with mayonnaise	1 cup	10
Tuna, canned, water-packed	½ cup	2			

Psyllium Sinks Cholesterol

Psyllium hydrophilic mucilloid — better known as the active ingredient in Metamucil—can dramatically reduce cholesterol. In a study of 26 men on typical high-fat American diets, one teaspoon of psyllium three times a day for eight weeks lowered their total cholesterol by 14.8 percent and their LDLs by 20.2 percent.

But what would happen, scientists wondered, if psyllium was given to people who were already on a cholesterol-lowering diet? Would the psyllium lower their cholesterol even more?

The answer is yes. Researchers at the University of Minnesota divided a group of 75 men and women who were on a low-fat, low-cholesterol diet. All continued on the diet, but half received a teaspoon of psyllium a day.

The result? Eight weeks later, total cholesterol levels of the psyllium group had dropped 4.8 percent *more* than the diet group, while their LDLs had plummeted 8.2 percent further.

Dinners with a Difference

The typical American diet that contributes to heart disease gets about 40 percent of its calories from fat. The kind of diet that reverses heart disease gets only about 18 percent of its calories from fat. Here's a sample dinner menu from each.

41% Calories from Fat	18% Calories from Fat
1 cup onion soup	1 serving pasta with red clam sauce (low-sodium tomato products used)
3½ oz. tenderloin steak, broiled	
1 baked potato	1½ cups tossed salad: romaine lettuce, grated carrot, sliced cucumber, red cabbage
1 Tbsp. sour cream	
½ cup green beans amandine seasoned with butter and salt	
	2 Tbsp. grated Parmesan cheese
lettuce wedge, ⅛ head	
1 Tbsp. Russian dressing	1 Tbsp. low-cal Italian dressing
1 cup coffee	1 slice whole wheat bread
1 Tbsp. half-and-half	1 tsp. soft tub margarine
1 piece pound cake	1 cup coffee
	1 Tbsp. skim milk
	1 strawberry fruit and juice bar
Total Calories: 876	Total Calories: 849
Cholesterol: 181 mg	Cholesterol: 45 mg

How Long Does It Take to Lower Cholesterol?

In most cases, both total cholesterol and LDL levels begin to drop soon after diet modifications are made. But maximum reductions are not achieved until several months later.

The Quaker Oat Company reported a 600 percent increase in sales of oat bran over the course of a single year.

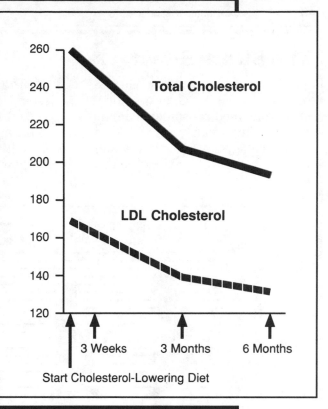

Total Cholesterol

LDL Cholesterol

3 Weeks   3 Months   6 Months

Start Cholesterol-Lowering Diet

Drugs That Drop Cholesterol

Some people inherit a tendency to develop high cholesterol—and sometimes diets don't lower it enough. They may be "hyperresponders," which means that their livers produce excess cholesterol.

In these cases, drug therapy and close medical supervision must be combined with a low-fat diet to get cholesterol out of the danger zone. Here's a breakdown of the drugs a doctor is most likely to recommend. Most work by reducing LDL.

Drug	Side Effects	Percentage of LDL Reduction
Cholestyramine	Constipation, abdominal pain, raises triglycerides	27
Colestipol HCl	Constipation, abdominal pain, raises triglycerides	27
Clofibrate	Gallstones	Not available
Gemfibrozil	Abdominal pain, nausea, diarrhea, myalgias	11
Lovastatin	GI upset, cataracts, myositis	31
Niacin	Flushing, itching, headache, ulcers	31
Probucol	Loose stools, decreases HDLs	12

The Stress Effect

Researchers at a Norwegian hospital measured the cholesterol levels of nine medical students on the day of an important exam and again on an average day two months later to see whether or not stress had an effect.

The result? The students' cholesterol levels were an average of 20 percent higher on exam day than on the average day. Here's a profile of each student's cholesterol level and how it changed under stress.

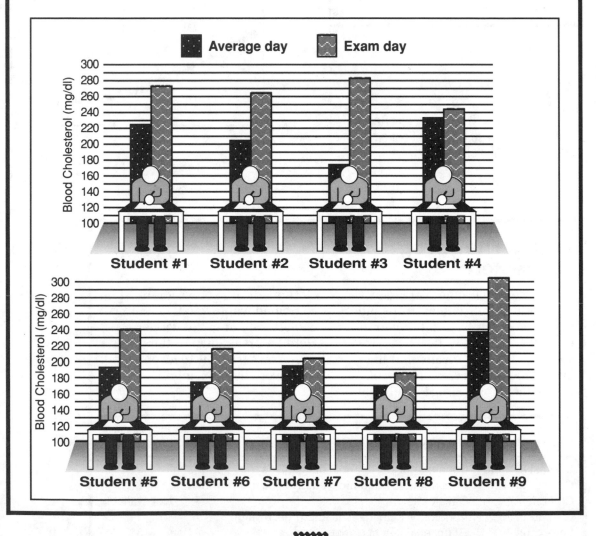

Laboratory studies using hampsters indicate that rice bran may be as effective as oat bran in lowering cholesterol levels.

Divers Have Their Ups and Downs

Several years ago a group of U.S. Navy psychologists in San Diego wanted to see if the rigorous training for an underwater demolition team had any effect on cholesterol levels of a random sample of the team's members.

The psychologists measured each man's cholesterol at regular intervals and discovered that levels peaked during particularly unpleasant activities that were loaded with anxiety. The two situations which seemed to stimulate the highest cholesterol increase were the men's introduction to scuba gear and underwater demolition team weapons, and their first drop from a helicopter into the waters below.

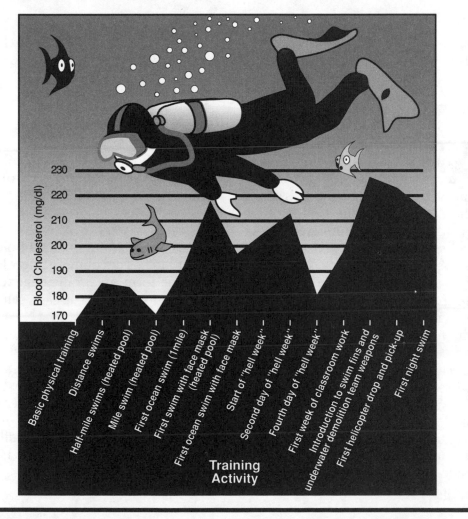

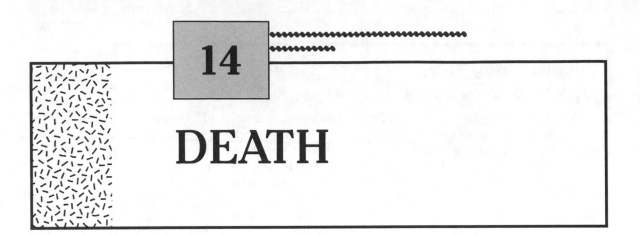

14

DEATH

Mortality statistics—the detailed scorecard of when and how we die—can tell us a lot about a society's health. The death rate in the United States, for instance, has plummeted 36 percent since 1950. Life expectancy has jumped seven years for women and five years for men, while the average life span now extends into the seventies and eighties. An American woman who turned 65 in 1983, for example, can expect to live until she's at least 83. Her male counterpart can expect to live until he's 79.

Why are we living longer? The answer is a tribute to the doctors and scientists who have battled the ancient plagues and other diseases that once made life into even the fourth or fifth decade a doubtful quest. Communicable childhood diseases and tuberculosis have been conquered. Viruses have been vanquished. Bacteria have been eradicated.

But as infectious diseases have receded as causes of death, an older population has encountered new killers in the form of chronic degenerative ailments like heart disease, cancer, and diabetes.

Fortunately, as scientists have determined what puts us at risk for these remaining modern-day diseases, we have made healthful lifestyle choices—decreasing smoking, increasing exercise, and modifying diet—until even deaths from such major killers such as heart disease and stroke have been cut in half.

The Ten Leading Causes of Death

Most Americans are likely to die from one of these ten conditions.

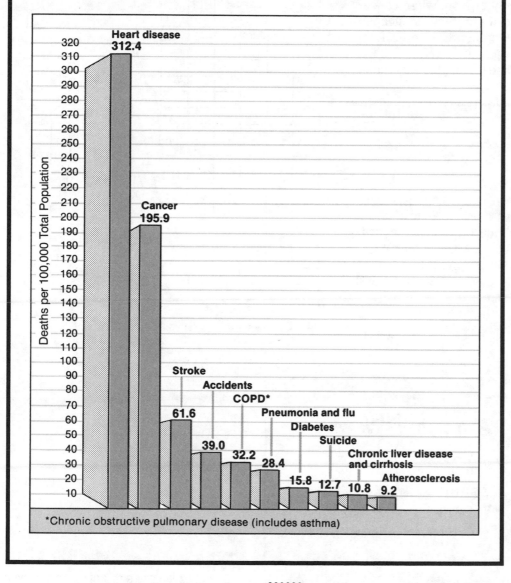

Deaths per 100,000 Total Population

- **Heart disease** 312.4
- **Cancer** 195.9
- **Stroke** 61.6
- **Accidents** 39.0
- **COPD*** 32.2
- **Pneumonia and flu** 28.4
- **Diabetes** 15.8
- **Suicide** 12.7
- **Chronic liver disease and cirrhosis** 10.8
- **Atherosclerosis** 9.2

*Chronic obstructive pulmonary disease (includes asthma)

A male smoker between the ages of 30 and 40 who smokes more than 40 cigarettes a day can expect to lose eight years of his life.

When Four Killers Reach Their Peak

Accidents are the leading cause of death until age 40, when cancer and heart disease begin to steepen their closely matched ascent. Heart disease surges ahead after age 60, peaking in the 80s at about the same time as stroke.

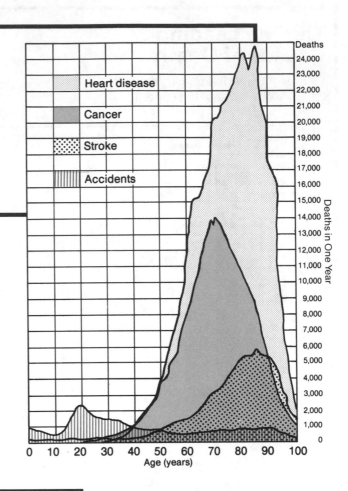

The number of childhood deaths due to injury decreased from 1980 to 1985 in every category except two: homicides and suicides. The increase in homicides was negligible, but the increase in suicides among children 10 to 14 was up a startling *112 percent.*

The New American War

54,246 Americans died in the Korean War.

58,012 Americans died in Vietnam.

116,708 Americans died in World War I.

407,316 Americans died in World War II.

978,542 Americans died from cardiovascular disease in 1986.

An ex-smoker's risk of death declines as the number of smoke-free years increases. It takes 15 years of not smoking for an ex-smoker's risk of death to equal that of someone who has never smoked.

The Decline of Heart Disease

Heart disease may be the leading killer in the United States, but the number of deaths due to this condition has been cut almost in half during the past two decades.

The reason? Decreased smoking, increased exercise, modified eating habits, more coronary care units, treatment advances, and better control of artery-damaging problems such as high blood pressure.

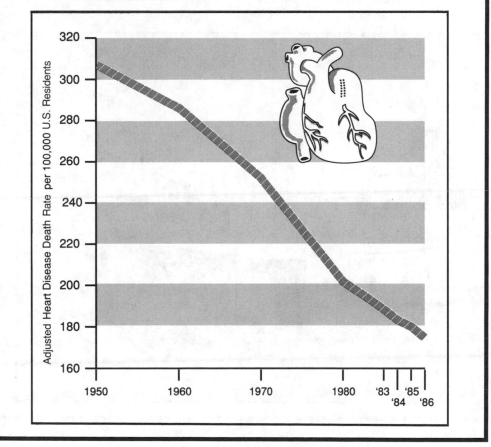

Nine out of ten premature deaths are linked to one of six behaviors: smoking cigarettes, overeating, misusing alcohol, failing to control high blood pressure, not exercising, or not wearing seat belts.

Where and When Lightning Kills

The map indicates the states in which the most lightning deaths have occurred over a 28-year-period, and the chart indicates the most dangerous months.

Most people who were killed by lightning were standing either in open fields (791 killed in the United States between 1959 and 1987), under trees (482 killed), on or near water (366), near tractors or other heavy equipment (172), on golf courses (111), or at telephones (31).

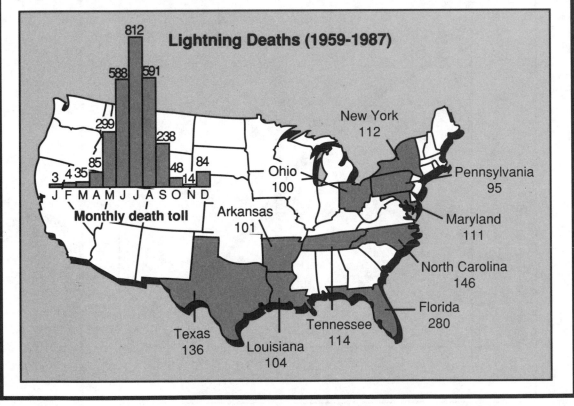

Lightning Deaths (1959-1987)

Monthly death toll:
J 3, F 4, M 35, A 85, M 299, J 588, J 812, A 591, S 238, O 48, N 14, D 84

New York 112
Pennsylvania 95
Maryland 111
North Carolina 146
Florida 280
Tennessee 114
Louisiana 104
Texas 136
Arkansas 101
Ohio 100

The major cause of death due to injury in children under the age of one is murder. It frequently occurs as the concluding act to a short life of physical and mental abuse.

What Are Your Odds of Being Murdered?

Of the 20,000 Americans who are murdered in an average year, 15 percent are killed by a family member, and another 40 percent are slain by people whom they knew at least casually. Alcohol is frequently involved, and arguments are the precipitating cause of about 40 percent of all such deaths.

Here are the odds of murder in your future, broken down by race and sex.

If You Are a:	Your Odds Are:
Black man	1 in 21
Black woman	1 in 104
White man	1 in 131
White woman	1 in 369

The Geography of Homicide

A study at the Johns Hopkins School of Hygiene and Public Health reveals that people in the South and West are more likely to be killed by a gun than those living in the North or East. The greater prevalence of firearms in the South is believed to be at least part of the reason.

A Deadly Society

In 1985, handguns killed:

▼ 5 people in Australia

▼ 5 people in Canada

▼ 8 people in Great Britain

▼ 18 people in Israel

▼ 31 people in Switzerland

▼ 46 people in Japan

▼ 8,092 people in the United States

The Ten Safest Cities

Of all the big cities in America, the ten with the fewest homicides in 1988 were:

▼ Pittsburgh

▼ Omaha

▼ Honolulu

▼ Tucson

▼ El Paso

▼ Tulsa

▼ San Jose

▼ Charlotte

▼ Austin

▼ Portland (Ore.)

The Ten Deadliest Cities

Of all the big cities in America, the ten with the greatest number of homicides in 1988 were:

- ▼ New York
- ▼ Los Angeles
- ▼ Chicago
- ▼ Detroit
- ▼ Houston
- ▼ Philadelphia
- ▼ Washington, D.C.
- ▼ Dallas
- ▼ Baltimore
- ▼ New Orleans

Is That A Fact?

Hair and nails keep right on growing after death.

Twelve to 18 hours after death the body begins to dry out. That causes the tips of the fingers and the skin of the face to shrink—thus creating the illusion that nails and hair have grown.

Every year, 2,000 Americans enter persistent vegetative (comatose) states.

What Are Your Chances of Dying This Year?

This table summarizes the statistical likelihood of a person's dying in the coming year, depending on age, sex, and race. Example: The chances are 1 in 172 that a 55-year-old white female will die this year.

Your Age	White Man	White Woman	Black Man	Black Woman
25	1 in 561	1 in 1,754	1 in 311	1 in 943
35	1 in 552	1 in 1,136	1 in 200	1 in 483
45	1 in 242	1 in 438	1 in 101	1 in 209
55	1 in 89	1 in 172	1 in 48	1 in 91
65	1 in 37	1 in 73	1 in 25	1 in 46
75	1 in 16	1 in 30	1 in 15	1 in 24

Where People Live the Longest

Barring catastrophic accident or illness, life in the United States usually extends into the seventh decade. On average, people in Hawaii live the longest, while those in Washington, D.C., have the shortest life expectancy. Check the listing to see how your state compares.

State	Life Expectancy	State	Life Expectancy
1. Hawaii	77.02	25. Wyoming	73.85
2. Minnesota	76.15	26. Indiana	73.84
3. Iowa	75.81	26. Missouri	73.84
4. Utah	75.76	27. Arkansas	73.72
5. N. Dakota	75.71	28. New York	73.70
6. Nebraska	75.49	29. Michigan	73.67
7. Wisconsin	75.35	29. Oklahoma	73.67
8. Kansas	75.31	30. Texas	73.64
9. Colorado	75.30	31. Pennsylvania	73.50
10. Idaho	75.19	32. Ohio	73.49
11. Washington	75.13	33. Virginia	73.43
12. Connecticut	75.12	34. Illinois	73.37
13. Massachusetts	75.01	35. Maryland	73.32
14. Oregon	74.99	36. Tennessee	73.30
15. New Hampshire	74.98	37. Delaware	73.21
16. S. Dakota	74.97	38. Kentucky	73.06
17. Vermont	74.79	39. N. Carolina	72.96
18. Rhode Island	74.76	40. W. Virginia	72.84
19. Maine	74.59	41. Nevada	72.64
20. California	74.57	42. Alabama	72.53
21. Arizona	74.30	43. Alaska	72.24
22. New Mexico	74.01	44. Georgia	72.22
23. Florida	74.00	45. Mississippi	71.98
23. New Jersey	74.00	46. S. Carolina	71.85
24. Montana	73.93	47. Louisiana	71.74
U.S. Average	**73.88**	48. Washington, D.C.	69.20

More than 7,000 people have filed "living wills" that order medical personnel not to prolong their lives by artifical means.

How Many of Your Classmates Are Left?

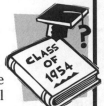

Ever wonder how many of those born in the same year as you are still alive? This list will tell you.

Your Age Now	Percentage of Men Surviving	Percentage of Women Surviving
1	98.8	90.0
20	97.7	98.4
30	95.9	97.8
40	93.8	96.8
50	89.9	94.9
60	80.9	89.4
70	62.8	77.7
80	34.7	55.5

Six Ways You Can Live after Death

▼ Bequeath your eyes to an eye bank.

▼ Bequeath your ear bones to a temporal bone bank.

▼ Bequeath your kidneys to a kidney bank.

▼ Bequeath your pituitary glands to the National Pituitary Agency.

▼ Bequeath skin to a local hospital or burn center.

▼ Bequeath your entire body to a medical school.

Where People Die

A National Institute on Aging study of 3,995 death certificates indicates that most people over 65 die in a hospital—although a substantial number die at home. Fifty-three percent of those studied died in their sleep.

Studies indicate that just 27 percent of all Americans have wills. But 70 percent of all adult Americans own life insurance policies.

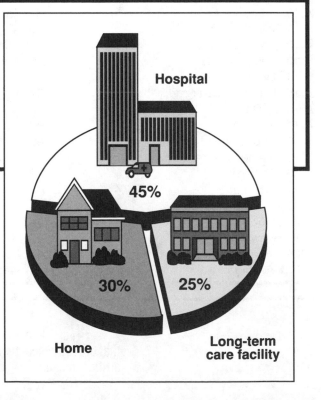

Hospital 45%

Home 30%

Long-term care facility 25%

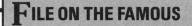

FILE ON THE FAMOUS

They Did So Much in So Little Time

Not everybody gets their fair four score years and ten. Some are cut down in their most productive years. What would have happened, for example, if the following people —politicians, musicians, artists, and adventurers who frequently shook the world—had managed to live out their lives? What would our world be like?

Famous Person	Age at Death	Famous Person	Age at Death
Attila the Hun	47	Stephen Foster	37
John F. Kennedy	46	Vincent van Gogh	37
Rasputin	45	Henri Toulouse-Lautrec	36
Billie Holliday	43	Wolfgang Amadeus Mozart	35
Franz Kafka	41	"Jeb" Stuart	31
John Lennon	40	Nat Turner	31
Martin Luther King, Jr.	39	Emily Brontë	29
Cleopatra	39	James Dean	24
Charlotte Brontë	38	Pocahontas	22
Amelia Earhart	38	Joan of Arc	19
Medgar Evers	38		

Do You Have the Right to Die?

Most people now do. In the wake of a 1976 New Jersey Supreme Court decision that allowed a ventilator to be removed from a comatose patient, 40 states plus the District of Columbia (as of February 1990) have passed laws that give patients the right to die naturally and without respirators, ventilators, tubes, paddles, syringes, and electrodes.

At the same time public support for the individual's right to die has swept the country. Public opinion polls report that 85 percent of the American public believe that life should not be prolonged by mechanical means. Seventy-eight percent of all physicians favor withdrawing life support systems from hopelessly ill or irreversibly comatose patients if they or their families request it.

15

DENTAL PROBLEMS

Among Americans, cavities are second only to colds as the most common disorder. Ironically, this wasn't true long ago—when dentists didn't even exist. In a study of several hundred skulls taken from Indian burial grounds in south Florida, tooth decay was found to be nearly nonexistent.

But by the 1940s, when the remaining Indians in Florida were more closely following the diet of modern civilization—eating a lot of sugar, for example—40 out of every 100 teeth examined were found to have been attacked by tooth decay.

Today the average American adult has 23 decayed or filled tooth surfaces. And since about 95 percent of all cavities have been filled, it's clear that Americans are visiting their dentists. In 1986, for example, Americans made more than 466 million dental visits.

Meanwhile, a national survey has found that since 1960, toothlessness among adults aged 55 to 64 has declined 60 percent. Unfortunately, 42 percent of Americans 65 and older already have lost all their teeth.

Periodontal (gum) disease is the primary cause of tooth loss in adults 35 and older. More than half of all people 18 and older are in the early stages of some type of periodontal disease.

Of course, people can do a lot to prevent tooth and gum problems by brushing and flossing regularly. And dental technology is constantly improving. Diagnostic methods are more advanced, as are treatment methods, which now include the use of lasers.

Dental Emergencies: What to Do

You probably know you should go to your dentist when you have a toothache or lose a filling, but what about if you lose or chip a tooth? Well, you still need to see a dentist, but you also need to take some immediate action. Check the chart.

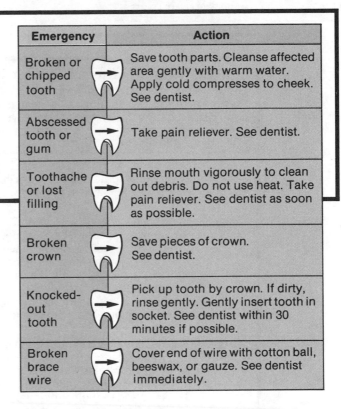

Emergency		Action
Broken or chipped tooth		Save tooth parts. Cleanse affected area gently with warm water. Apply cold compresses to cheek. See dentist.
Abscessed tooth or gum		Take pain reliever. See dentist.
Toothache or lost filling		Rinse mouth vigorously to clean out debris. Do not use heat. Take pain reliever. See dentist as soon as possible.
Broken crown		Save pieces of crown. See dentist.
Knocked-out tooth		Pick up tooth by crown. If dirty, rinse gently. Gently insert tooth in socket. See dentist within 30 minutes if possible.
Broken brace wire		Cover end of wire with cotton ball, beeswax, or gauze. See dentist immediately.

Dental patients who played electronic Ping-Pong or viewed comedy film clips while having their teeth filled experienced less stress than did patients who only listened to an audio tape of comedy skits, according to a study.

Cavities Are Commonplace

The National Institute of Dental Research's nationwide survey proved this—at least in grown-ups. Working adults and retirees both had a high number of decayed or filled crown surfaces (the part of the tooth above the gum line). Both groups had over 90 percent of those cavities filled. Meanwhile, the older group had three times as many root caries (cavities affecting the part of the tooth below the gum line, which becomes vulnerable as gums recede). These cavities were less likely to be filled.

	Employed			Seniors		
	Male	Female	Both	Male	Female	Both
Average number of decayed or filled crown surfaces	23	24	23	19	21	20
Cavities filled (%)	93	96	94	88	95	92
Average number of decayed or filled root surfaces	0.93	0.55	0.76	4.09	2.71	3.17
Cavities filled (%)	40	61	47	44	62	54

Dental Fillings—What's Right for You?

Getting a filling is not like competing in the Olympics—gold is not always better than silver. And silver, though better than bronze, may not always be better than composite resin. You need to consider several factors when choosing a filling.

Type	Advantages	Disadvantages
Gold	Expands and contracts more like natural tooth enamel. Less likely to crack. May last a lifetime.	Cost—four times more expensive than silver fillings. Conducts heat and cold, aggravating sensitive teeth.
Silver	Actually a mix of silver, mercury, copper, and tin. The most popular choice, silver fillings have been proven safe and effective over time. Many studies have found the mercury levels in these fillings pose no threat to patients or dentists. The most economical choice.	Not a long life span; may need to be replaced as often as every five years. And like gold fillings, they conduct heat and cold.
Composite resins	Can match your natural teeth in color. Composite resins adhere to a tooth's surface, thus requiring less drilling than metal fillings and reducing the chance of breakage later on. Better adhesion makes resins a good choice for filling shallow surface cavities. Do not conduct heat and cold.	Cost more than silver fillings and last about as long.

In 1978, nationwide dental school enrollment was 6,300. By 1988 it had dropped to 4,200. It is projected to go as low as 3,200 in the mid 1990s.

Worrying about Wisdom Teeth

Wisdom teeth, or third molars, are the last teeth to emerge, usually appearing in the late teens or early twenties. The question, of course, is whether or not wisdom teeth that fail to emerge should be pulled right away or left alone until they cause problems. Some dentists feel these impacted teeth should be pulled as soon as possible because they can damage other teeth, become infected or decayed, and create problems later for denture wearers. Ultimately, the dentist has to decide what's best on a case-by-case basis.

Children Are Getting Fewer Cavities

The incidence of cavities in U.S. children continues to decline. Half of all children aged 5 to 17 are completely free of cavities in their permanent teeth.

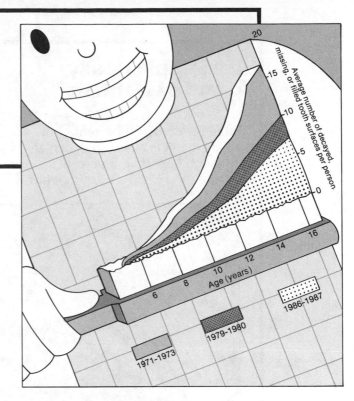

In a study of more than 800 adults who brushed twice daily with either a sodium-fluoride toothpaste or an identical toothpaste without fluoride, the fluoride group had 41 percent fewer crown-surface cavities and 67 percent fewer root-surface cavities than the nonfluoride group.

Blame It on Plaque

Cavities, gum disease, that foul taste in your mouth—plaque contributes to all of these.

But what, exactly, is plaque? It's the name given to the bacteria that colonize your mouth. At first, the buildup is invisible. But when these colonies of bacteria multiply (which is what happens when you don't clean your teeth regularly and effectively), you can eventually see a white, sticky film on your teeth.

When plaque hardens, forming a barnaclelike substance, it's called tartar. That's the stuff the dentist scrapes from your teeth periodically.

By the way, all plaque isn't the same. Bacteria in plaque above the gum line require oxygen to survive. And they need a steady diet of sugar and other carbohydrates. Unfortun-ately, that's just what the typical American diet delivers. The sucrose helps form a sticky substance that helps plaque adhere to the tooth surface, where it acidifies into tooth enamel and causes cavities.

Below the gum line, the bacteria do not need oxygen. The plaque here feeds on the proteins from gum tissue. Scientists are researching which of the microorganisms below the gums actually cause gum disease.

The best tactic against plaque is prevention. It's impossible to eliminate all plaque, but you can prevent it from growing out of control. Dentists advise brushing at least twice a day, flossing to remove food and plaque from between teeth, and having dental checkups about every six months.

Are People Really Afraid of Dentists?

According to a 1986 survey of Seattle residents, 50 percent of the public are not at all afraid of dental treatment. Less than 5 percent say they are "terrified." Of those who reported some level of fear, more than 65 percent of them said they began fearing dental treatment when they were children.

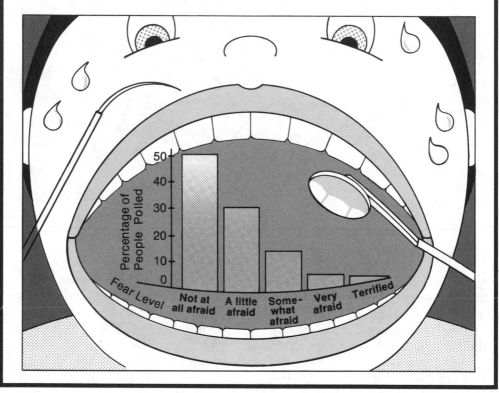

What's a Root Canal?

Root canal treatment is the only way to save a tooth when the pulp, which contains the blood supply and nerves, is damaged or diseased. This can be caused by an infection, abscess, or even a sharp blow.

After administering anesthetic, the dentist makes an opening and removes the pulp from the pulp chamber and root. The root canal is then cleaned and possibly medicated. When all evidence of infection is gone, the space is filled with a rubberlike material. The tooth usually needs a crown as well.

How Long Since Your Last Dental Visit?

The majority of people in the United States go to a dentist at least once a year, a major study suggests. But whites are more likely to have visited a dentist in the last year (60.8 percent) than are blacks (42.2 percent). By region, southwesterners were least likely to have visited a dentist within the last year (41.5 percent). About 1 percent of people say they have never been to a dentist.

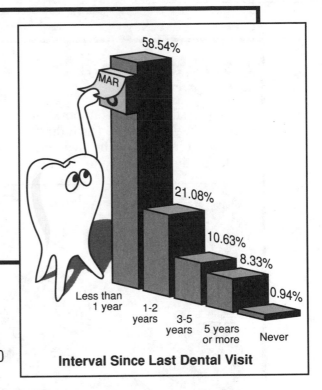

Interval Since Last Dental Visit

The United States has about 127,000 dentists. Rwanda has 1.

The Right Way to Brush and Floss

This technique is recommended for most effective brushing: With the bristle tips of your toothbrush set at a 45-degree angle to the plane of your teeth, gently scrub horizontally along the gum line using very small (¼-inch) strokes. Let the bristle tips do the work. Do the inner and outer surfaces of both your upper and lower teeth.

Also, don't forget to brush the chewing surfaces of your molars and premolars. Move slowly over these surfaces, taking time to clean each tooth separately.

Finally, brush the inside surfaces of the front teeth. Position the brush almost vertically and scrub with an up-and-down motion.

When flossing, you can use either waxed or unwaxed dental floss. The important thing is to floss every day to remove food particles and plaque you can't reach with a tooth-brush. Take about 18 inches of dental floss and wind most of it around the middle fingers of each hand, with about one inch of floss between your fingers. Draw the floss between the teeth and then, with a gentle sawing action, rub the sides of each tooth. Use a clean section of floss for each tooth.

How Many Teeth Are Left?

If you still have all your permanent teeth, you have 32 (including four wisdom teeth). The average working adult in the United States has only about 24 teeth in his or her mouth. People 65 and older, on average, have just 14.

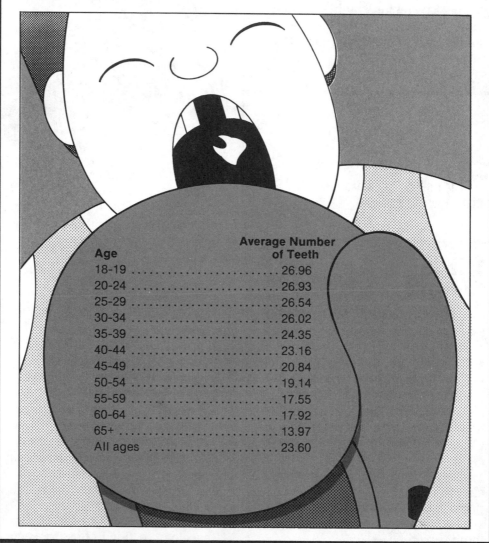

Age	Average Number of Teeth
18-19	26.96
20-24	26.93
25-29	26.54
30-34	26.02
35-39	24.35
40-44	23.16
45-49	20.84
50-54	19.14
55-59	17.55
60-64	17.92
65+	13.97
All ages	23.60

When Teeth Meet the Acid Test

Tooth enamel is tough, but overconsumption of foods with very low pH numbers (high acidity) may eventually cause it to wear away. Foods on the lower half of this list are most likely to contribute to dental erosion.

pH	
14	**Most alkaline**
7	**"Neutral"—pure water can range from 7–8.5**
6.8	Peas
6.6	Milk
4.6	Bananas
3.3	Apple Juice
3.1	Vinegar
2.9	Grapefruit juice, lime juice
2.7	Orange juice, lemonade, grapefruits
2.5	Cola drinks
2.4	Pure lemon juice
2.1	Lemons
0	**Most acid**

In a survey, 88 percent of Americans said they believe avoiding between-meal sweets is an important part of taking good care of their teeth.

IS THAT A FACT?

Braces aren't just for kids.

That's true. In 1986, 27 percent of the 1.3 million Americans receiving orthodontic treatment were over 18 years of age. Adults seek orthodontic help for a variety of reasons. Most just want to correct what should have been corrected long ago—crooked or crowded teeth that can lead to increased tooth decay and gum disease.

FILE ON THE FAMOUS

A Shipshape Smile on the Good Ship Lollipop

Question: When is a six-year-old girl—and movie star—no longer cute? Answer: When her mouth looks like she's just gone a couple of rounds with Joe Lewis. Of course, Shirley Temple was just doing what other six-year-old girls were doing—losing her baby teeth naturally.

To repair her smile, Hollywood dentist Charles Pincus was called upon. He fitted Temple with false teeth and facings to temporarily fill in the gaps in her smile. Dr. Pincus can probably be considered one of the pioneers of cosmetic dentistry.

16

DIABETES

Your body is a smoothly operating food processor, changing sugars, starches, and other components of the diet you eat into energy. Unless you're one of the 11 million Americans with diabetes.

Scientists don't know what causes diabetes, but they do know that when people have it, the body either doesn't make enough insulin, or it can't correctly use the insulin it does make. Insulin, a hormone produced by the pancreas, is needed to help move glucose, or blood sugar, into the cells where it can be changed into energy. Otherwise glucose levels in the blood build up, and sugar spills over into the urine.

Diabetes is a major killer. In 1989, an estimated 150,000 Americans died from diabetes and its complications.

The repercussions from the disease are enormous. Diabetes often leads to heart disease, stroke, gangrene, and kidney disease. The risk of heart disease is two to four times greater for people with diabetes; the risk of stroke is two to six times higher. Diabetes is also the number one cause of adult blindness in the United States. Each year, there are more than 5,000 new cases of blindness resulting from diabetes.

By age 65, a person's odds of developing diabetes are almost one in ten. But perhaps most disturbing is the fact that of the more than 11 million people with diabetes, 5 million have not yet been diagnosed—many may not even suspect that they have diabetes.

The Two Major Forms of Diabetes

There are two major types of the disease. Type I is insulin-dependent diabetes, sometimes called juvenile diabetes. It occurs most often in children and young adults.

Type II is non-insulin-dependent diabetes, sometimes called maturity-onset diabetes. About 90 percent of all people with diabetes have this form of the disease. It usually occurs in adults over 40 who are overweight.

Here are a few more facts about both types.

Insulin-dependent. This type tends to appear suddenly and progress quickly. Because the pancreas makes little or no insulin in this case, the insulin-dependent person must take daily injections of insulin—and follow a healthy diet—to stay alive. Before the isolation of pure insulin in 1921, people usually only lived a few years after diagnosis.

Non-insulin-dependent. Onset is usually gradual. It occurs when the body does not use insulin correctly. Often this form of diabetes can be controlled through diet and exercise. A few people also need either oral insulin or insulin injections to stabilize their blood-sugar levels. Doctors believe many people could avoid this form of diabetes by maintaining a normal body weight and staying physically active.

When researchers at the University of Minnesota School of Public Health traced the health histories of nearly 26,000 Seventh-Day Adventists, they found the death rate from diabetes was less than half that of other white Americans. Interestingly, the Adventists follow a low-meat or vegetarian diet.

Variations on a Theme

In addition to the two main types of diabetes, there are a number of related disorders. During pregnancy, some women develop gestational diabetes. Many times it disappears after the baby is born, but about half of these women will later develop non-insulin-dependent diabetes. Secondary diabetes occurs when drugs and other chemicals damage the pancreas. Impaired glucose tolerance, previously known as latent diabetes, refers to a condition in which blood-sugar levels hover between normal and diabetic. Impaired glucose tolerance is treated through diet and weight loss.

The Warning Signs of Diabetes

These are the warning signs of insulin-dependent diabetes.

▼ Frequent urination (may include bed-wetting in children who have been toilet trained)

▼ Excessive thirst

▼ Extreme hunger

▼ Sudden weight loss

▼ Weakness and fatigue

▼ Irritability

▼ Nausea and vomiting

Non-insulin-dependent diabetes is signaled by the following symptoms.

▼ Any of the insulin-dependent symptoms listed above

▼ Blurred vision or any change in sight

▼ Tingling or numbness in legs, feet, or fingers

▼ Slow healing of cuts (especially on the feet)

▼ Frequent skin infections or itchy skin

▼ Drowsiness

What Causes Diabetes?

For now, there is no definitive answer. Researchers believe people with insulin-dependent diabetes are genetically vulnerable to the disease. Perhaps an outside force, such as a virus or pollutants, along with the immune system's mistaken attack on insulin-producing cells, triggers the disease response.

Genetics is also suspected of playing a major role in non-insulin-dependent diabetes. But researchers believe certain diets and long-term obesity deserve part of the blame as well.

Exercise is important for diabetic patients because it helps to both control weight and burn food, thus reducing the demand on the pancreas to produce insulin. People with diabetes should check with a doctor before starting an exercise program.

Where Is Diabetes Most Common?

Below the Mason-Dixon line. According to 1987 figures, the South had a rate of 31.8 per 1,000 persons. The West had the lowest rate—24.2 per 1,000 persons.

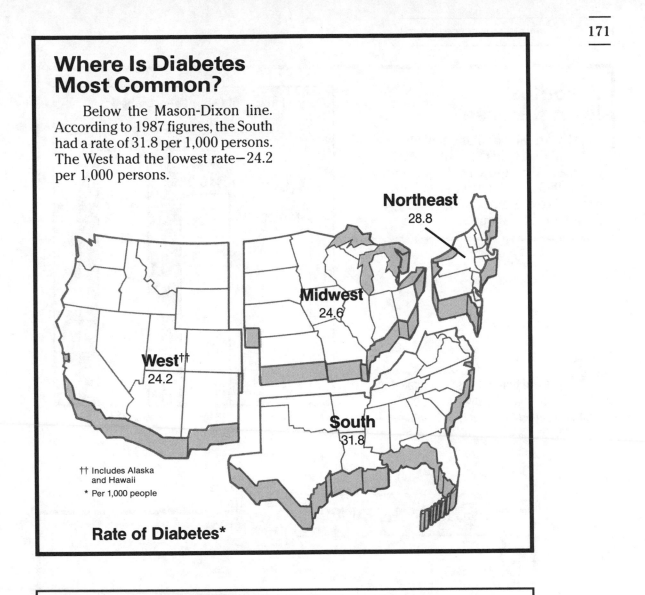

Northeast
28.8

Midwest
24.6

West††
24.2

South
31.8

†† Includes Alaska and Hawaii

* Per 1,000 people

Rate of Diabetes*

Who Is Most Likely to Get Diabetes?

▼ People who are overweight

▼ People with a family history of diabetes

▼ People who are 40 and older

▼ Blacks (they have a 33 percent higher chance of developing non-insulin-dependent diabetes)

▼ Hispanics (they have a more than 300 percent higher chance of developing non-insulin-dependent diabetes)

▼ Native Americans (they have a 33 to 50 percent higher chance of developing non-insulin-dependent diabetes)

Diabetes Is on the Rise

The total population of diagnosed diabetics in the United States is expected to grow by 17 percent from 1990 to 2000. And even more growth is expected among the 45-to-64 age group—about 31 percent.

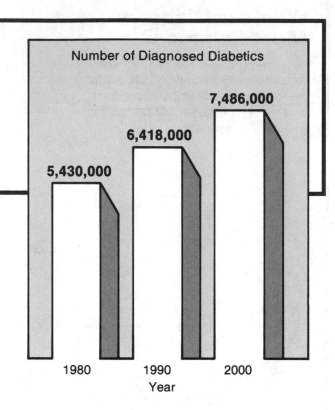

Number of Diagnosed Diabetics

5,430,000

6,418,000

7,486,000

1980   1990   2000

Year

Direct and indirect costs for diabetes reach $20.4 billion annually and account for nearly 5 percent of total U.S. health care costs.

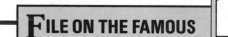

FILE ON THE FAMOUS

Diverse, Distinguished, and Diabetic

Thomas Edison had it. So did Ernest Hemingway, Jackie Gleason, Jackie Robinson, and Elvis Presley. Diabetes didn't prevent them from living successful lives. Here are some more high achievers with diabetes whom you may have heard of:

Wilford Brimley

William Conrad

Ella Fitzgerald

Catfish Hunter

Peggy Lee

Mary Tyler Moore

Thomas P. (Tip) O'Neill

Mario Puzo

Fred Silverman

How to Recognize Diabetic Emergencies

There are two common diabetic emergencies—low blood sugar and high blood sugar. Both require quick action.

Condition	Onset	Signs	Causes	Treatment
Low blood sugar (insulin reaction or hypoglycemia)	Sudden	Staggering; poor coordination; anger, bad temper; pale color; confusion, disorientation; sudden hunger; sweating; eventual stupor or unconsciousness.	Failure to eat before strenuous exercise; delayed or missed meals.	*Provide sugar.* If the person can swallow without choking, offer any food or drink containing sugar, such as soft drinks, fruit juice, candy. *Do not use diet drinks when blood sugar is low.* If the person does not feel better in 10–15 minutes, take him or her to the hospital.
High blood sugar (hyperglycemia with acidosis)	Gradual	Drowsiness; extreme thirst; very frequent urination; flushed skin; fruity or winelike odor on breath; heavy breathing; eventual stupor or unconsciousness.	Undiagnosed diabetes; insulin not taken; stress, illness, injury; too much food or drink or both.	*Take this person to the hospital.* If you are uncertain whether the person is suffering from high blood sugar or low blood sugar, give some sugar-containing food or drink. *If there is no response in 10–15 minutes, this person needs medical attention.* Remember: Do not give food or drink if the person is unable to swallow.

Every year 500,000 more Americans are diagnosed with diabetes.

Help from Soluble Fiber

Soluble fiber helps prevent drastic shifts in blood sugar levels, making it an attractive weapon in the war against diabetes. At the University of Kentucky School of Medicine, diabetes expert James W. Anderson, M.D., has been especially successful in treating diabetic patients with high-fiber diets. Foods high in soluble fiber include fruits, vegetables, oats, and dried beans.

A Higher Rate of Hospitalization

In general, chronic health problems are more likely to put a diabetic in the hospital than a nondiabetic. According to 1987 figures, this held true for cardiovascular, ophthalmic, neurologic, and renal complications. And diabetics were more likely to be hospitalized than nondiabetics in each of the four age groups examined.

Chronic Complications by Age	Rate for Diabetics*	Rate for Nondiabetics*
Cardiovascular complications		
under 25	12.4	0.6
25–44	23.0	4.4
45–64	108.0	31.1
65+	187.7	107.4
Ophthalmic complications		
under 25	5.5	0.1
25–44	6.9	0.2
45–64	5.2	0.6
65+	5.1	3.6
Neurologic complications		
under 25	9.0	0.1
25–44	7.2	0.6
45–64	6.8	0.9
65+	5.8	0.9
Renal complications		
under 25	14.7	1.1
25–44	12.0	1.6
45–64	11.6	2.5
65+	17.3	10.9
Other complications		
under 25	0.0	0.0
25–44	2.3	0.0
45–64	2.5	0.1
65+	3.5	0.8
Total	**162.7**	**72.5**

*per 1,000 patients

Everything Under Control? These Tests Can Tell

Regular self-monitoring is crucial for diabetics. Blood testing, done by pricking the finger for a drop of blood which is then placed on a chemically sensitive strip, is recommended by most doctors because it gives a precise indication of blood sugar level at any given moment. Urine test readings are much less exact because they don't show when blood sugar was high or how high it was. They only show that it was high enough at some point to cause sugar to spill into the urine.

People with insulin-dependent diabetes are often advised to test blood sugar levels two to four times a day, before or after meals. People with non-insulin-dependent diabetes may be able to test less often.

Other tests measure ketones in the urine. Ketones are acids that collect in the blood and urine when the body uses fat—instead of glucose—for energy. Ketones in the urine are a signal that the diabetes is poorly controlled and that prompt medical attention is needed. It's a good idea to test for ketones when you are sick or under stress—times when diabetes is more likely to go out of control.

Finally, a glycohemoglobin test should be administered by a doctor every three to six months. This test measures the average blood-sugar level over the past 30 to 60 days.

Eye Disease—A Likely Complication

The longer a person has had diabetes, the greater the chance of developing diabetic retinopathy—a disease that damages blood vessels in the eye and leads to blindness.

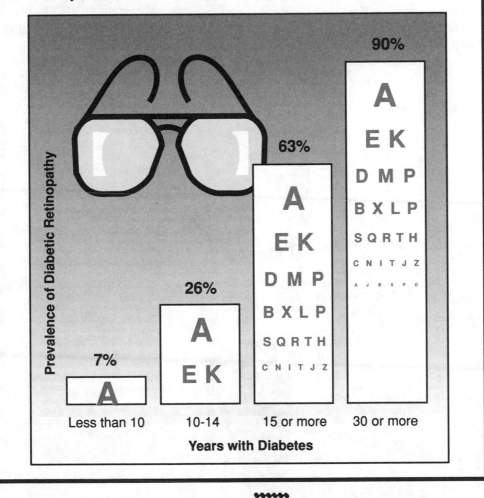

90%

63%

26%

7%

Prevalence of Diabetic Retinopathy

Less than 10   10-14   15 or more   30 or more

Years with Diabetes

~~~~~**P**eople with diabetes should not eat concentrated sugars because insulin cannot be produced fast enough to burn them.

Diet Recommendations Have Changed

In the 1990s, as in the 1950s, the American Diabetes Association and the American Dietetic Association advise diabetics to follow a carefully planned diet. But the suggested makeup of that diet has changed over the years. Today, they recommend more carbohydrates (especially the high-fiber kind) and less fat. And wherever possible, saturated fat should be replaced with unsaturated fat to minimize the cardiovascular complications of the disease. In the case of an 1,800-calorie diet, for example, here's how the guidelines have changed.

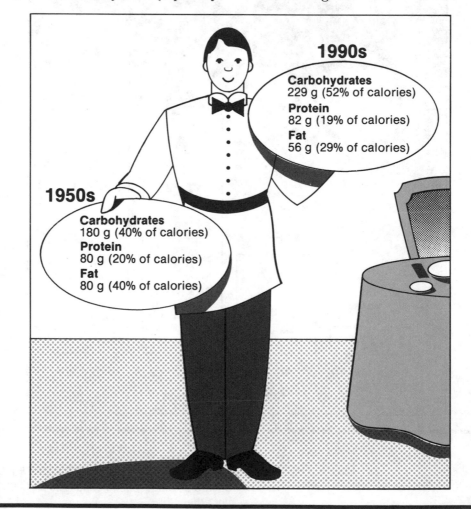

1990s

Carbohydrates
229 g (52% of calories)

Protein
82 g (19% of calories)

Fat
56 g (29% of calories)

1950s

Carbohydrates
180 g (40% of calories)

Protein
80 g (20% of calories)

Fat
80 g (40% of calories)

Life Expectancy for Diabetics

Today people who keep their diabetes under control can expect to live long lives. In fact, as both men and women with diabetes age, the difference between their life expectancy and that of nondiabet- ics narrows. The greatest discrepancy in life expectancy is among those under 40 years of age. Still, even diabetic patients between the ages of 15 and 20 can expect to live more than another 50 years.

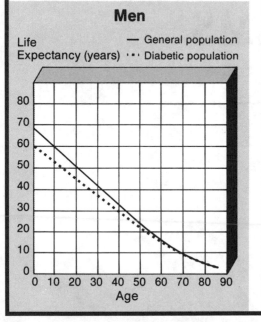

Men

Life Expectancy (years)

— General population
··· Diabetic population

Age

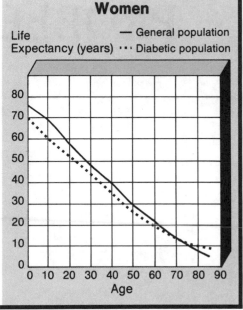

Women

Life Expectancy (years)

— General population
··· Diabetic population

Age

Predicting, and Preventing, Diabetes

Research from the College of Medicine, University of Florida, Gainesville, offers hope for predicting who will develop insulin-dependent diabetes. Analysis of blood test records of 5,000 Florida children uncovered 12 who developed insulin-dependent diabetes. The fascinating part: All 12 carried a particular antibody called 64K. The normal children did not carry the antibody 64K.

The researchers are continuing to follow the children for further evidence of 64K antibodies. They hope it will someday be possible to selectively destroy 64K antibodies, thereby stopping the disease process.

17

DIGESTIVE PROBLEMS

Indigestion is a common enough malady, often caused by overeating or eating the wrong foods. Symptoms may include nausea, regurgitation, vomiting, heartburn, bloating, stomach discomfort, or abdominal fullness. Sometimes you'll feel these symptoms after overeating, other times as an emotional reaction to disturbing events. But sometimes the symptoms warn of peptic ulcer, gallbladder disease, gastritis, or other serious digestive diseases.

Over 34 million Americans have one of the more than 40 gastrointestinal problems collectively called digestive disease. Those conditions range from common indigestion to serious, life-threatening illnesses.

Approximately 2 million Americans are disabled due to digestive disease. Digestive disease is the leading cause of time lost from work for male employees. It accounts for 15 percent of all absences from work among employees aged 17 to 64.

The U.S. Public Health Service estimates that more than $50 billion is spent annually on digestive disease.

Chronic Problems for Many

This table shows the frequency of some commonly reported chronic digestive problems in the United States.

Problem	Rate*
Frequent indigestion	23.6
Abdominal hernia	21.9
Frequent constipation	19.5
Ulcer	17.1
Gastritis	11.8
Colitis	10.1
Diverticulosis	6.7
Spastic colon	4.7

*per 1,000 persons

An after-dinner mint may rid you of more than just the scent of garlic on your breath. Peppermint can be effective medicine for banishing excess stomach gas, according to one gastroenterologist. A mixture of eight drops of spirits of peppermint in 2 ounces of warm water, swallowed, will relax the circular muscle, or sphincter, at the base of the esophagus, allowing stomach gas to escape. Peppermint candy doesn't have enough oil to be effective, although some imported mints do. Peppermint tea, made from leaves, is a good alternative. Warning: Someone with heartburn due to reflux (stomach acid splashing up into the esophagus) should avoid this remedy because it will further relax an already too-loose lower sphincter.

Who's at Greatest Risk?

Of all the doctor's office visits for digestive problems, approximately 59 percent are by women and 41 percent are by men. According to a National Health Interview Survey, chronic digestive diseases reported more commonly by women than men include gallbladder problems (2.8 women for every man), gastritis and duodenitis (1.3 to 1), diverticulosis (3.6 to 1), and frequent constipation (3.2 to 1). The survey showed no sexual division for ulcers of the stomach or duodenum, but male predominance was noted for abdominal hernia (1.1 men for every woman) and upper gastrointestinal disorder (1.3 to 1).

This table shows some chronic digestive problems as reported by age and sex.

Condition	Number of Cases*					
	Men			Women		
	Under 45	45-64	65+	Under 45	45-64	65+
Hernia	9.1	42.3	91.4	7.4	37.1	64.6
Ulcer	10.8	30.9	32.9	11.4	32.3	26.8
Gastritis	4.2	20.7	18.3	8.2	28.1	27.8
Diverticulosis	0.5	10.4	17.4	0.6	17.0	43.5
Frequent constipation	5.7	5.6	44.4	17.0	36.8	79.7

*per 1,000 persons

Off-the-Shelf Digestive Aids

Drugstore shelves are lined with pills, creams, and powders aimed directly at your digestive tract. Their active ingredients vary with the nature and site of the problem. Some of the ingredients you may find in over-the-counter drugs are listed below.

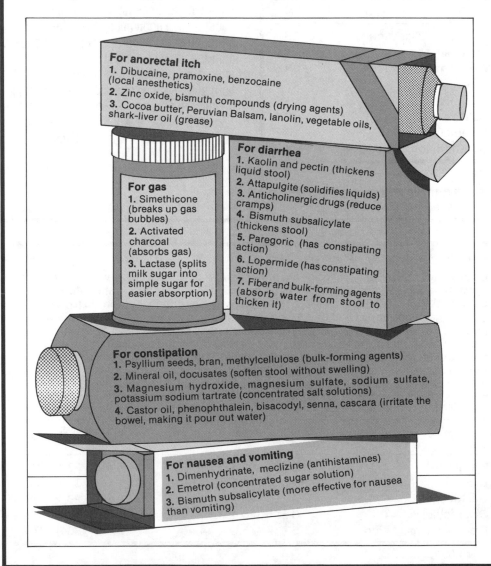

For anorectal itch
1. Dibucaine, pramoxine, benzocaine (local anesthetics)
2. Zinc oxide, bismuth compounds (drying agents)
3. Cocoa butter, Peruvian Balsam, lanolin, vegetable oils, shark-liver oil (grease)

For diarrhea
1. Kaolin and pectin (thickens liquid stool)
2. Attapulgite (solidifies liquids)
3. Anticholinergic drugs (reduce cramps)
4. Bismuth subsalicylate (thickens stool)
5. Paregoric (has constipating action)
6. Lopermide (has constipating action)
7. Fiber and bulk-forming agents (absorb water from stool to thicken it)

For gas
1. Simethicone (breaks up gas bubbles)
2. Activated charcoal (absorbs gas)
3. Lactase (splits milk sugar into simple sugar for easier absorption)

For constipation
1. Psyllium seeds, bran, methylcellulose (bulk-forming agents)
2. Mineral oil, docusates (soften stool without swelling)
3. Magnesium hydroxide, magnesium sulfate, sodium sulfate, potassium sodium tartrate (concentrated salt solutions)
4. Castor oil, phenophthalein, bisacodyl, senna, cascara (irritate the bowel, making it pour out water)

For nausea and vomiting
1. Dimenhydrinate, meclizine (antihistamines)
2. Emetrol (concentrated sugar solution)
3. Bismuth subsalicylate (more effective for nausea than vomiting)

A Guide to Digestive Diseases

This table lists and describes some of the most common digestive disorders that plague more than 34 million Americans.

Condition	Description	Symptoms	Treatment
Anal fissure	Small crack or tear in mucous membrane of rectum or skin around anus	Severe pain, especially during bowel movements	High-fiber diet; stool softeners; local anesthetic ointments; sitz baths; sometimes surgery
Appendicitis	Inflammation of the appendix	Pain, tenderness in abdomen, nausea, vomiting, fever	Surgery
Cirrhosis	Damage in liver is replaced by scar tissue, causing malfunction	Mild cirrhosis—few symptoms; advanced cirrhosis—massive fluid buildup in abdominal cavity, swelling from ribs to groin, red spider marks on face, arms, upper trunk; jaundice; mental confusion	Avoidance of alcohol; well-balanced diet; low salt intake; sometimes steroid therapy
Crohn's disease	Inflammation of the intestinal tract	Diarrhea; abdominal pain; rectal bleeding; fever; decreased appetite, weight loss; stunted growth	Dietary changes; steroid and antibiotic therapy; occasionally surgery
Diverticulitis	Pouches (diverticula) in the weakened muscle walls of intestine trap food residue, which ferments and putrefies, causing inflammation	Pain; tenderness, diarrhea, constipation, fever	Surgery; bed rest; antibiotics; high-fiber diet
Gallbladder disease	Stones formed from cholesterol or bile lodge in the cystic duct	Severe, steady pain in upper abdomen that last from 20 minutes to 4 hours; pain between shoulder blades or in right shoulder; nausea; vomiting	Surgery, change in diet
Gastritis	Inflammation of the stomach lining	Abdominal pain; loss of appetite; nausea; vomiting	No food, small amounts of liquid for 24 hours, then small amounts of bland foods; antacid or anti-emetic

(continued)

A Guide to Digestive Diseases—*Continued*

Condition	Description	Symptoms	Treatment
Hemorrhoids	Small distended veins in the rectum and anus	Pain; possibly bright red blood on toilet tissue or in stool	High-fiber diet; stool softeners; bulk-forming agents; sitz baths; avoidance of straining at stool
Hiatal hernia	Stomach slips through the opening in the diaphragm, presses upward into the chest	Belching; general discomfort	Small, frequent meals; weight reduction; high-fiber diet
Irritable bowel syndrome (IBS)	Believed to be due to abnormalities in gastrointestinal motility	Abdominal pain; bloating; constipation; diarrhea	High-fiber diet for constipation; psychotherapy; antispasmodic drugs; antidepressants
Lactose intolerance	Reduced levels of digestive enzyme lactase in the body	Gas; bloating; pain, diarrhea after consuming milk or milk products	Adding lactase to milk and milk products or avoiding them
Malabsorption syndrome	Group of diseases that interfere with absorption of nutrients	Pale, foul-smelling, bulky stools; painful abdominal bloating; failure to grow; iron deficiency anemia	Eliminate wheat and other gluten-rich grains from diet; nutritional supplements
Pancreatitis	Inflammation, causing pancreatic enzymes to digest pancreatic tissue	Tenderness and severe pain in midabdomen	Hospitalization; painkillers; intravenous fluids
Peritonitis	Inflammation of the two-layered membrane that lines the abdominal cavity and covers stomach, intestines, and other abdominal organs	Abdominal pain; tenderness; rigidity; nausea; fever; vomiting	Antibiotic therapy
Proctitis	Inflammation of the rectum and anus	Pain; discharge; straining at stool	Rest; sitz baths
Ulcerative colitis	Chronic inflammation of the colon	Diarrhea; abdominal pain, rectal bleeding	Low-fiber diet; steroids
Ulcers	Sores thought to be caused by imbalance between stomach acids and gastrointestinal tract's natural defenses	Burning, gnawing pain around the breastbone, lasting between 30 minutes and 3 hours	Antacids; acid-blocking medicines and barrier drugs; avoidance of smoking, coffee, alcohol, and aspirin

Where Gas Comes From

Doctors call it aerophagia—a fancy name for swallowing air. Swallow enough—as many of us do—and you'll swell up, then belch. And since one good swallow deserves another, you'll often belch again.

Occasionally swallowed air winds its way through the system and into the intestines. And that is where the other gas—flatus—comes in. Or out. Most flatus is caused by colonic bacteria, which ferment undigested food and create gas as a by-product. While most of us know that beans cause gas, other foods containing starches and especially high-fiber foods can also cause flatulence.

The average person passes gas about 14 times a day, although doctors documented 70 passages in 4 hours in one person, 141 passages in one day in another.

This chart indicates the gas-generating potential of many common foods.

High Gas	Moderate Gas	Low Gas	Low Gas
Dairy products	Potatoes	Meat, fowl, fish	Grapes
Onions	Pastries	Lettuce	Berries
Beans	Eggplant	Cucumber	Rice
Bagels	Citrus fruits	Broccoli	Potato chips
Pretzels	Apples	Peppers	Popcorn
Prunes	Bread	Avocado	Nuts
Apricots		Tomato	Eggs
Carrots		Zucchini	Gelatin
Celery		Okra	Graham crackers
Bananas		Olives	Nonmilk chocolate
Raisins		Asparagus	Fruit ice
Brussels sprouts		Cauliflower	Cantaloupe
Wheat germ			

Don't turn your bathroom into a library. Restrict your toilet time to 5 minutes per sitting, if you can. Sitting on the toilet can put undue pressure on the blood vessels of the anal area, leading to hemorrhoids. So bowel specialists advise patients not to use the toilet for anything other than strictly business.

Choosing the Right Firefighter

Antacids commonly use one of four active ingredients (or a combination).

Sodium bicarbonate. This is baking soda. Taken once a week or less, it's fine. It's not useful for a chronic condition such as ulcers. It shouldn't be used by anyone on a salt-restricted diet because it's loaded with sodium.

Magnesium hydroxide. Less potent at neutralizing acid than sodium bicarbonate. It shouldn't be used by people with kidney disease because problems with magnesium excretion can result in a potentially serious disorder called hypermagnesemia.

Aluminum hydroxide. The weakest of the acid neutralizers, it's mostly combined with magnesium products or with sodium bicarbonate or with both calcium carbonate and magnesium hydroxide. One side effect is constipation. Another concern is that aluminum absorbed into the blood may cause a loss of phosphate, fluoride, and calcium, possibly weakening the bones.

Calcium carbonate. A fast-acting, inexpensive acid neutralizer in small doses. Large doses can cause constipation.

This table lists some antacid products and their ingredients.

Product (mfr.)	Dosage Form	Ingredient(s)			
		Calcium	Aluminum	Magnesium	Other
Alka-Mints (Miles)	Chewable tablet	1			
Alka-Seltzer Effervescent Antacid (Miles)	Tablet				9
Basaljel (Wyeth-Ayerst)	Capsule, suspension, tablet		6		
Citrocarbonate Antacid (Upjohn)	Granule				9
Di-Gel Advanced Formula (Plough)	Tablet	1		2	11
Di-Gel Advanced Formula (Plough)	Liquid		5	2	
Gaviscon (Marion)	Tablet		5	4	9
Gaviscon (Marion)	Liquid		5	3	
Gelusil (Parke-Davis)	Tablet, liquid		5	2	11
Gelusil-II (Parke-Davis)	Tablet, liquid		5	2	11
Maalox (Rorer Consumer)	Tablet, suspension		5	2	
Maalox Extra Strength Plus (Rorer Consumer)	Tablet, suspension		5	2	11
Mylanta (Stuart)	Tablet, liquid		5	2	11
Mylanta-II (Stuart)	Tablet, liquid		5	2	11
Phosphaljel (Wyeth-Ayerst)	Suspension		7		
Riopan (Whitehall)	Tablet, chewable tablet, suspension		8	8	
Riopan Plus (Whitehall)	Tablet, suspension		8	8	11
Rolaids (Warner-Lambert)	Chewable tablet				10
Tums (Norcliff Thayer)	Chewable tablet	1			

1—Calcium carbonate   5—Aluminum hydroxide   9—Sodium bicarbonate
2—Magnesium hydroxide   6—Aluminum carbonate   10—Dihydroxyaluminum sodium carbonate
3—Magnesium carbonate   7—Aluminum phosphate
4—Magnesium trisilicate   8—Magaldrate   11—Simethicone

Fiber Keeps Things Moving

In the mid-1960s, British surgeon Denis Burkitt, M.D., laid the foundation for our knowledge of the importance of fiber to a healthy digestive system. He was among the first to propose that many disorders of Western civilization, including diverticulitis, hemorrhoids, constipation, and bowel cancer, could be traced to a lack of dietary fiber. In particular, he found that relatively unrefined carbohydrate foods, like whole grains and fresh vegetables, provide the bulk needed to keep stools moving through the intestines in a rapid and trouble-free way. The chart shows differences in stool bulk and transit time (the time needed for a given meal to be digested and eliminated), which he recorded among various population groups.

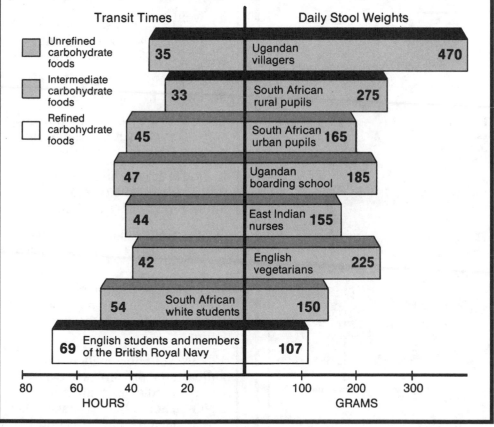

Transit Times — Daily Stool Weights

Unrefined carbohydrate foods
Intermediate carbohydrate foods
Refined carbohydrate foods

Group	Transit Time (Hours)	Daily Stool Weight (Grams)
Ugandan villagers	35	470
South African rural pupils	33	275
South African urban pupils	45	165
Ugandan boarding school	47	185
East Indian nurses	44	155
English vegetarians	42	225
South African white students	54	150
English students and members of the British Royal Navy	69	107

HOURS — GRAMS

Time For Supper

How long will it take tonight's dinner to travel through each portion of your gastrointestinal tract? This chart follows the path. Keep in mind that times will vary depending on the meal's fiber content.

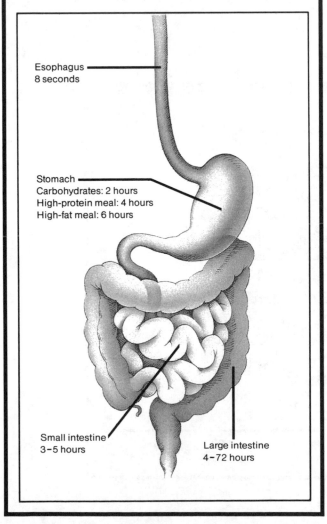

Esophagus
8 seconds

Stomach
Carbohydrates: 2 hours
High-protein meal: 4 hours
High-fat meal: 6 hours

Small intestine
3–5 hours

Large intestine
4–72 hours

Twelve Ways to Aid Digestion

1. Eat a well-balanced diet. Include fresh fruit, vegetables, and whole grain breads and cereals.

2. Eat slowly. Relax for 30 minutes after each meal.

3. Exercise regularly.

4. Be cautious taking over-the-counter medications. Follow your doctor's instructions for prescription medicine.

5. Avoid greasy foods.

6. If you are lactose intolerant, eliminate milk and milk products.

7. Don't skip meals, allowing acid to build up in your stomach.

8. Don't pacify your hunger with coffee, which increases stomach acid.

9. Don't take aspirin for a hangover. It can further irritate a stomach already irritated by alcohol.

10. Avoid smoking, which decreases the stomach's natural bicarbonate, an acid buffer.

11. If you drink, do so only with meals or on a full stomach, so the alcohol won't irritate the stomach lining.

12. Ask your doctor about the antibacterial properties in over-the-counter medicines containing bismuth. Some studies suggest that certain bacteria may be a contributing cause of stomach ulcers.

Cooling the Fire with an Antacid

More than $500 million is spent on antacids in the United States each year. And they do seem to work—neutralizing stomach acid and relieving indigestion.

Here's how to make your antacid work best.

▼ Try a liquid. It works faster because more surface area is exposed to the antacid.

▼ Take your antacid on a full stomach. Taken an hour or two after a meal, an antacid will neutralize acid for up to 3 hours. Taken on an empty stomach, it will work for only 20 to 40 minutes.

▼ Small doses over time are more effective than one large dose. A single large dose can be quickly emptied out of the stomach.

Diverticulosis/ Diverticulitis— Which Is Which?

The colon, or large intestine, is formed by two groups of muscle tissue: an inner, circular layer that surrounds the colon's contents, and an outer, longitudinal layer. Sometimes little grapelike pouches occur in the muscular layers of the colon, forming in weak points in the colon wall. When there is pressure in the colon as the muscles contract to move the contents along, the thin-walled sacs balloon through the outer wall. These are called *diverticula*. Once you have them, they never go away.

Anyone who has diverticula is said to have *diverticulosis*. The pouches are not necessarily inflamed or infected at this point, just present.

Diverticulosis usually affects people in their forties and fifties and occurs in about 10 to 15 percent of the population in Western nations. It is rarer in underdeveloped parts of the world where people eat a high-fiber diet.

Diverticula may lie quietly in the gut, never causing a problem. Sometimes, however, they become infected and inflamed, developing into boils along the colon wall. This is called *diverticulitis*. Symptoms include fever and persistent pain. Treatment of such a flare-up usually includes a liquid diet and antibiotics. Many times a hospital stay is required, and sometimes surgery is necessary.

Understanding Ulcers

Ulcers come in two forms—duodenal and gastric. This table summarizes their differences and their similarities.

Type	Description	Symptoms	Possible Causes and Risk Factors	Self-Treatment	Medications
Duodenal	A duodenal ulcer is a raw area in the lining of the duodenum, the first part of the small intestine. This kind of ulcer is usually less than ½ inch wide. Duodenal ulcers are more common in men than in women. Studies show that there may be a third fewer duodenal ulcers now than in the 1950s, when incidence reached an all-time high.	Gnawing pain, resembling hunger pains, in the middle abdomen, is typical. This pain may occur several hours after a meal and can be quieted temporarily with antacids, milk, or a few crackers.	Heredity. Blood type: People with type O blood have 40% higher risk. Bacterial infection: Doctors have found *Campylobacter pyloridis* bacteria in the stomach of 90% of people with duodenal ulcers. Cigarettes: Smokers have twice the ulcer rate of non-smokers.	50–70% of all ulcers disappear in 6 weeks with no treatment, although proper care can raise that figure. Doctors suggest: 1. Stop smoking. 2. Avoid alcohol and caffeine. 3. Use antacids. 4. Eat frequent small meals. 5. Get plenty of rest.	"H₂" or histamine blockers (these reduce the body's histamine, which in turn reduces acid) such as cimetidine (Tagamet), ranitidine (Zantac), and famotidine (Pepcid); stomach-coating drugs such as sucralfate (Carafate).
Gastric	A gastric ulcer is a raw spot, usually more than an inch wide, in the lining of the stomach. Gastric ulcers occur only a third to a quarter as often as duodenal ulcers. Men and women seem equally affected. Most occur in middle age or later. About 3% turn out to be cancerous.	The primary symptom is burning, gnawing pain in the upper abdomen or lower chest that lasts 30 minutes to 3 hours. Attacks come and go, with painful weeks followed by pain-free periods. Pain may start after eating or not until hours afterward.	Bacterial infection: Doctors have found *Campylobacter* in the stomach of 70–80% of gastric ulcer patients. Faulty valve: A defective sphincter allows bile to back up into the stomach. Aspirin: About a third of gastric ulcer patients take 15 or more aspirin a week.	Same as duodenal	Same as duodenal

The Facts about Gallstones

The gallbladder is a thumb-sized sac tucked into the lobes of the liver just below the right ribcage. It collects bile, a cholesterol-rich digestive fluid secreted by the liver, and then pumps the bile into the small intestine.

Sometimes bile becomes oversaturated with cholesterol. Then particles of cholesterol separate from the fluid and clump together, forming large stones. In many people, gallstones may sit quietly, causing no problems. But for some of the approximately 25 million Americans with the problem, the stones may flow out with the bile and get stuck in the bile duct. Intense pain in the upper right side of the abdomen begins to build and peaks after only a few hours. The stone is either passed into the small intestine or it falls back into the gallbladder.

Who gets them. The most likely candidates for gallstones are women who have been pregnant, overweight people who eat a diet high in animal fat, and people over age 60.

Home care. Doctors suggest a low-cholesterol, low-fat diet may be of some help. Others say a high-fiber diet may help reduce the cholesterol content of the bile. Eating frequent small meals helps maintain the flow of bile through the gallbladder. Some research has shown a link between high-sugar diets and increased risk.

A daily dose of a nonsteroidal anti-inflammatory drug (NSAID) such as ibuprofen or aspirin may also block gallstones in people with recurring gallstones. Researchers from St. Thomas's Hospital in London studied 75 people who had previous gallstone treatment. Twelve of those people took NSAIDs daily and had no recurrence of gallstones. Twenty who never or rarely took NSAIDs had gallstones return. Be sure to check with your doctor before you begin taking any drugs.

High-tech care. Ever since shock waves first pulverized kidney stones, doctors had hoped to apply the same treatment to gallstones. Unfortunately, they found that, while shock waves could break the stones into small fragments, drug treatment was still necessary to dissolve the pieces. And only about 20 percent of patients were good candidates.

A newer, more refined shock-wave procedure, which delivers the jolt directly to the stones (instead of from the outside of the body), now looks more promising. Doctors insert a thin tube with a wire probe into the gallbladder. They locate the stone and send an electrical charge down the wire along with a salt solution to act as a conductor. Then, an electrical spark is converted into a shock wave. The stone breaks and the fragments are scooped up in a tiny basket for removal. The process takes about an hour and recovery time is three to four days—compared with three to six weeks for traditional surgery, which removes the gallbladder.

There is one drawback: Stones can recur. There's a 10 percent chance per year of recurrence.

IS THAT A FACT?

Ulcer disease occurs mostly among high-powered executives.

Ulcers affect people in all walks of life. In fact, studies show that ulcers are most common among people in lower socio-economic groups. Also, studies show a link between smoking cigarettes and ulcers. A smoker is not only more likely to have an ulcer, but his ulcer is less likely than a nonsmoker's to heal.

Another risk group: People who take aspirin four or more days a week for three or more months increase their chances of gastric ulcer. Aspirin also increases the likelihood of bleeding from an ulcer.

Bowel regularity means a bowel movement every day—achieved with laxatives if necessary.

The frequency of bowel movements in normal, healthy individuals varies from three movements a day to three a week.

Laxatives can be a short-term cure for constipation, but long-term use may weaken the natural muscle action of the intestinal walls required for defecation. Overuse of mineral oil, a popular laxative, may inhibit the absorption of vitamins A, D, E, and K.

Your Appendix: Good for Nothing

The appendix is a worm-shaped pouch, 3½ inches long, located in the lower right side of the abdomen just underneath where the small and large intestines come together. In some animals, such as rabbits, it plays a role in the digestive process. But in humans, it seems to have no function, although it can become diseased. About 10 to 20 percent of all people can expect to experience an attack of appendicitis—including pain, fever, and nausea or vomiting. It usually strikes 5- to 30-year-olds.

Got that burning sensation? It could be your workout, say researchers at Bowman Gray School of Medicine at Wake Forest University. Vigorous aerobic exercise can cause gastric reflux. The more agitating the exercise, the more acid that's likely to spill over into the esophagus. Running produced the most and bicycling the least, they found.

Seven Ways to Fix a Hemorrhoid

Eight out of ten people get hemorrhoids, yet preventing them isn't that complicated. Short toilet sessions, plenty of fiber in the diet, and lots of liquids are recommended measures. But if the advice comes too late, medicated pads, salves, suppositories, and sitz baths may relieve some of the symptoms. Here are seven other courses your doctor might take.

Sclerotherapy. Hemorrhoids are injected with a 5 percent solution of phenol in almond oil. The hemorrhoids then wither away. This procedure is used to treat only small hemorrhoids.

Rubber band ligation. In an office procedure, the hemorrhoid is tied at its upper end with an elastic band. Within 7 to 20 days the hemorrhoid "strangles," then falls off with a minimum of pain and risk of bleeding.

Infrared photocoagulation. A doctor can zap a hemorrhoid with infrared heat. The blood inside coagulates and the hemorrhoid collapses.

Cryotherapy. This method destroys hemorrhoids by freezing. Popular during the 1960s, cryotherapy is now thought to be less advisable than surgery.

Laser therapy. Internal hemorrhoids are shot with bolts of electromagnetic radiation through a flexible tube.

Electric current. Hemorrhoids receive low-power DC current for 6 to 9 minutes in one to three treatments. The tissue dies and falls off in three to ten days.

Surgery. Considered a final option. Using a local anesthetic, the doctor removes the offending portion of the blood vessel. Patients can leave the hospital pain-free the next day.

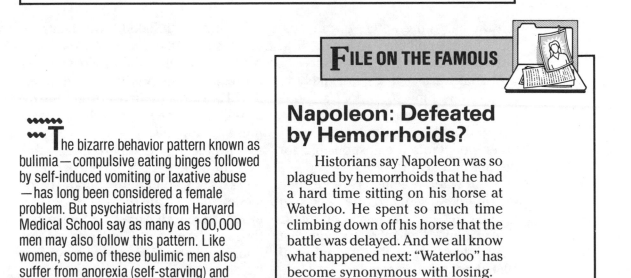

The bizarre behavior pattern known as bulimia—compulsive eating binges followed by self-induced vomiting or laxative abuse —has long been considered a female problem. But psychiatrists from Harvard Medical School say as many as 100,000 men may also follow this pattern. Like women, some of these bulimic men also suffer from anorexia (self-starving) and major depression or manic-depressive illness.

FILE ON THE FAMOUS

Napoleon: Defeated by Hemorrhoids?

Historians say Napoleon was so plagued by hemorrhoids that he had a hard time sitting on his horse at Waterloo. He spent so much time climbing down off his horse that the battle was delayed. And we all know what happened next: "Waterloo" has become synonymous with losing.

18

ENVIRONMENT AND HEALTH

In the air, in the water—even inside our homes—pollution is a hazard to public health.

That's a fact that's not likely to change any time soon. PCB's (polychlorinated biphenyls), asbestos, carbon monoxide, radon, and many, many other pollutants are responsible for disease and death.

But when pollutants are cleaned up, or at least reduced, the effects on health can be positive—and dramatic. One example: Federal regulations that went into effect at the beginning of 1986 drastically decreased the lead content of gasoline.

The result: 5,000 fewer heart attacks and 1,000 fewer strokes each year, according to the Environmental Protection Agency (EPA). In addition, the EPA estimates there are now nearly 2 million fewer cases of high blood pressure annually.

Protecting our environment, and in turn our health, is of course everyone's responsibility. For your own protection, investigate the quality of your drinking water, have your home tested for radon, and try to keep the use of household pesticides and other chemicals to a minimum.

Pollution: Our Most Pressing Problem?

Asked in a survey to name the most critical problem currently facing the United States, most Americans found economic issues and drug abuse to be more troubling than the state of the environment. But environmental pollution was more often a concern than the quality of education or the threat of war.

Public Concerns	Percentage of Vote*
Drug abuse	27
Poverty	10
Economy (general)	8
Other economic problems	8
Other noneconomic problems	8
Federal budget deficit	7
No opinion	7
Crime	6
Unemployment	6
Moral decline	5
Environmental pollution	**4**
International/foreign aid	4
Cost of living/inflation	3
Quality of education	3
Trade deficit	3
Dissatisfaction with government	2
Fear of war	2
AIDS	1

*Answers total more than 100% due to multiple responses

Exercising is good for your health, but not if done in areas of heavy traffic. Accelerated breathing during your workout increases the dose of pollutants inhaled.

The 20 Areas with the Worst Smog

Low-level ozone, a precursor of smog, results from the chemical combination of reactive hydrocarbons with nitrogen oxides in the presence of sunlight. Put more simply, in a city with a lot of traffic and industry, bright summer days can easily turn into smog alert days—days when taking a brisk walk or going for a jog can leave you coughing and rubbing your eyes. This list reflects the average number of days the ozone level exceeded the EPA standard of 0.12 parts per million in 1985–1987.

Location	Number of Violations
1. Los Angeles, Calif.	143.5
2. Bakersfield, Calif.	35.1
3. Fresno, Calif.	30.5
4. Houston, Tex.	19.1
5. Modesto, Calif.	16.2
6. Philadelphia area	13.6
7. San Diego, Calif.	12.5
8. Visalia, Calif.	11.9
9. Sacramento, Calif.	9.7
10. El Paso, Tex.	9.0
11. Stockton, Calif.	8.1
12. Baltimore, Md.	7.9
13. New York City area	7.5
14. Chicago area	7.4
15. Providence, R.I. area	6.5
16. Washington, D.C. area	6.2
17. Dallas-Fort Worth, Tex.	6.1
18. Muskegon, Mich.	6.0
19. St. Louis, Mo.	5.4
20. Central Connecticut	4.8

Toxic Emissions: The Top Ten States

The ten states shown here in blue emitted more than half of the 2.4 billion pounds of toxins released into the air in 1987. The EPA estimates that air toxins are responsible for more than 2,000 cases of cancer annually. Omission from the top ten doesn't mean a state's air gets a clean bill of health. The EPA's inventory found that Kansas air, for example, contained nearly 70,000 pounds of phosgene. This gas was used to kill thousands of soldiers in World War I.

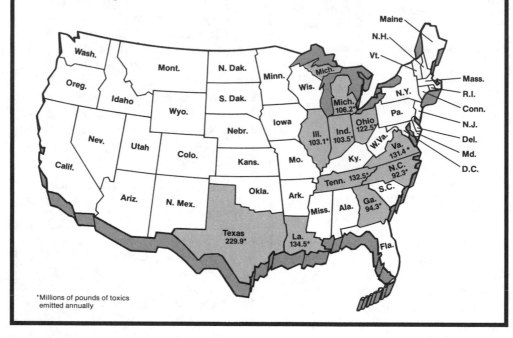

*Millions of pounds of toxics emitted annually

IS THAT A FACT?

Dioxin is the most dangerous chemical pollutant known to man.

Dioxin *is* the most toxic of all cancer-associated substances regulated by the EPA. But in 1987 the EPA drastically reduced its calculations of this chemical pollutant's cancer-causing power.

Dioxins are by-products of combustion processes and the production of pesticides. Very high levels of dioxins were found in the infamous Love Canal toxic waste site in Niagara Falls, New York. But now the EPA says that dioxin is only one-sixteenth as potent as previously thought. Still, dioxin is considered to be a 10,000 times more potent cause of cancer than PCBs (polychlorinated biphenyls).

Using tap water instead of distilled water in ultrasonic humidifiers may increase vulnerability to colds and flu.

Carbon Monoxide—
An Indoor Problem,
Too

You may think of carbon monoxide (CO) as a nasty by-product of motor vehicles, but studies show that indoor levels of CO in homes where natural gas is used often exceed outside CO levels. Even in a city. So adequate ventilation is crucial. This chart shows how one home's CO levels consistently exceeded outdoor readings, with particularly high readings at suppertime when the stove was used.

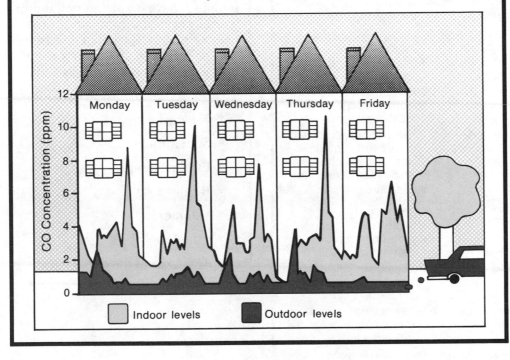

Monday   Tuesday   Wednesday   Thursday   Friday

CO Concentration (ppm)

12
10
8
6
4
2
0

Indoor levels   Outdoor levels

The U.S. government's General Accounting Office says most pesticides used by commercial lawn care companies have never been properly tested.

Where Air Pollutants Come From

Automobiles and smoke-spewing factories aren't the only pollution producers out there, just the most visible. Air pollutants can be found in everything from rocks to particleboard.

Pollutants	Sources
Group I: Predominantly outdoor sources	
Sulfur oxides (gases, particles)	Fuel combustion, nonferrous smelters
Ozone	Photochemical reactions
Pollens	Trees, grasses, weeds, plants
Lead, manganese	Automobiles
Organic substances	Petrochemical solvents, natural sources, vaporization of unburned fuels
Group II: Both indoor and outdoor sources	
Nitric oxide, nitrogen dioxide	Fuel burning
Carbon monoxide	Fuel burning
Carbon dioxide	Metabolic activity, combustion
Particles	Resuspension, condensation of vapors and combustion products
Organic substances	Volatilization, combustion, paint, metabolic action, pesticides, insecticides, fungicides
Spores	Fungi, molds
Group III: Predominantly indoor sources	
Radon	Building construction materials (concrete, stone), water, soil
Formaldehyde	Particleboard, insulation, furnishings, tobacco smoke, gas stoves
Asbestos, mineral and synthetic fibers	Fire-retardant, acoustic, thermal, or electric insulation
Ammonia	Metabolic activity, cleaning products
Mercury	Fungicides in paints, spills in dental care facilities or laboratories, thermometer breakage
Aerosols	Consumer products

Know the Symptoms of "Sick Building Syndrome"

A survey of U.S. government employees found that about 75 percent of them complained of symptoms of indoor air pollution—often referred to as "sick building syndrome." And about half of those surveyed said their symptoms had caused them to miss work. The World Health Organization estimates that 30 percent or more of all modern buildings have indoor air pollution, typically caused by ventilation problems or materials used in construction or furnishing. Here is a list of the most common signs of sick building syndrome.

▼ Headache

▼ Sore throat

▼ Eye irritation

▼ Runny nose

▼ Fatigue

▼ Coughing

▼ Tightness in the chest

An unusually severe smog buildup in London in 1952 is believed responsible—at least in part—for 4,000 deaths.

Now Your Oven's Clean, but . . .

Tests have shown that the use of a commercial oven cleaner containing nonmethane hydrocarbons (which have the potential to cause cancer) can drastically affect indoor air quality in just 90 minutes. And, as the chart shows, it may take several hours after use for indoor air quality to return to its previous level. In addition to making sure your house is well-ventilated, it's a good idea to stay out of the kitchen for a while after using such a product. Cleaning your oven right before leaving for work or going shopping might be the best option.

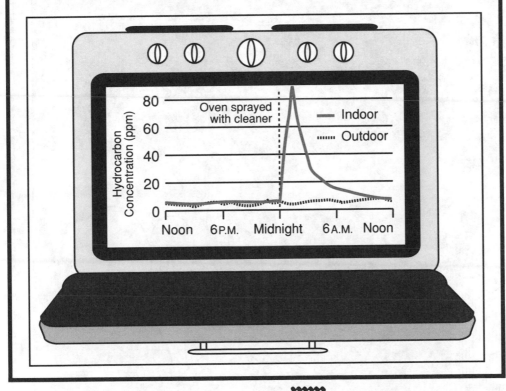

Even low levels of carbon monoxide in the air may impair heart function and significantly limit the exercise capacity of people with heart disease.

What's Going Up in Smoke?

Literally, toxins, carcinogens, and suspected carcinogens. Almost literally, your health if you're a smoker or spend a lot of time around smokers. Here's a partial list of contaminants in cigarette smoke.

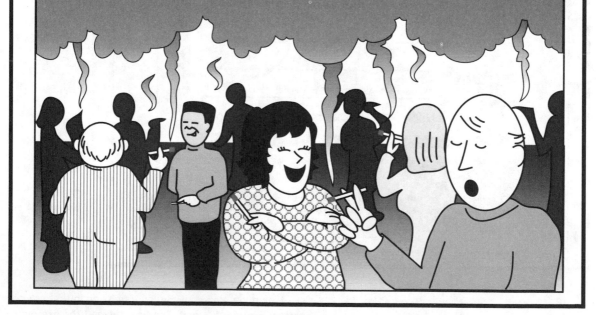

TOXINS

Acetaldehyde   Acetone   Acetonitrile   Ammonia

Argon   Butylamine   Cadmium   Carbon dioxide

Carbon monoxide   Creosol   Endrin   DDT

Hydrogen sulfide   Hydrogen cyanide   Lead

Methane   Methyl alcohol   Nickel compounds

Nicotine   Nitrogen dioxide   Particulate matter

Phenol   Pyridine   Other gases

CARCINOGENS and Suspected Carcinogens

Benzene   Chrysene

Formaldehyde

Lead-210   Polonium-210

Benzo (a) pyrene

Dibenzo (a,h) anthracene

Dibenzo (a,h) pyrene

Other hydrocarbons

Are Neighbors of Nuclear Plants at Risk?

Obviously, an accident at a nuclear power plant, such as occurred in Chernobyl in the Soviet Union, can be a serious threat to health. But what about just living near a normally functioning nuclear plant, as millions of people do? The chart shows cancer death rates per 100,000 people before and after the start-up of the Millstone Nuclear Power Plant in Waterford, Connecticut. In Waterford itself, the cancer death rate increased by 58 percent.

Site	Approx. Dist. from Millstone	Before (1970)	After (1975)	Percentage of Change
Vermont	200 mi. NW	176.1	173.9	− 1
Connecticut	35 mi. NW*	168.1	188.4	+12
New Haven, Conn.	30 mi. W	200.9	255.5	+27
Waterford, Conn.	**0**	**152.6**	**241.8**	**+58**
New London, Conn.	5 mi. E	177.4	255.0	+44
Rhode Island	50 mi. NE	200.1	216.0	+ 8
Massachusetts	70 mi. NE	185.0	198.4	+ 7
New Hampshire	120 mi. NE	180.4	182.4	+ 1
Maine	200 mi. NE	197.7	185.0	− 6

*Population center of Connecticut (Hartford-Waterbury area)

What You Should Know about Radon

Radon is odorless, but far from harmless. The EPA estimates that radon is responsible for 5,000 to 20,000 lung cancer deaths each year.

What exactly is radon? It's one of several naturally occurring radioactive decay products (sometimes called "radioactive daughters") created as uranium in rock and soil gradually breaks down. But unlike other decay products, radon is a gas. So it can escape out of water, the ground, or even building materials. As a result, we may breathe this radioactive gas into our lungs.

Radon is a major health concern across the country; the EPA estimates that 8 to 12 percent of all U.S. homes have dangerous radon levels. The EPA has set as a safety guideline a level of 4 picocuries of radon per liter of indoor air. If tests show your home has more than this level, action should be taken to reduce the problem.

Where Radon Risk Is Greatest

You're most likely to have a radon problem if your house is in one of the states shown here in blue. The EPA says these 14 states have the highest levels of cancer-causing radon.

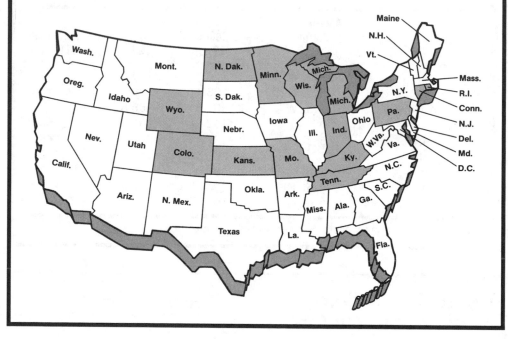

The Right Way to Test for Radon

A quick, one-time test for radon may provide an inaccurate reading of the average level of this contaminent in a house or other building. Radon levels are not consistent over time, and can be affected by a number of factors, including the use of stoves, furnaces, and bathroom exhaust fans. Also, radon levels average about 60 percent higher in the winter, when houses are not as well ventilated. Only long-term monitoring of radon levels can provide accurate information about a potential threat.

Other People's Smoke Can Pollute *Your* Lungs

Being a smoker puts you at the highest risk for lung cancer. But being around a smoker isn't too healthy either. When nonsmoking women with nonsmoking husbands were compared with nonsmoking women who had smoking husbands, the latter had significantly higher rates of lung cancer.

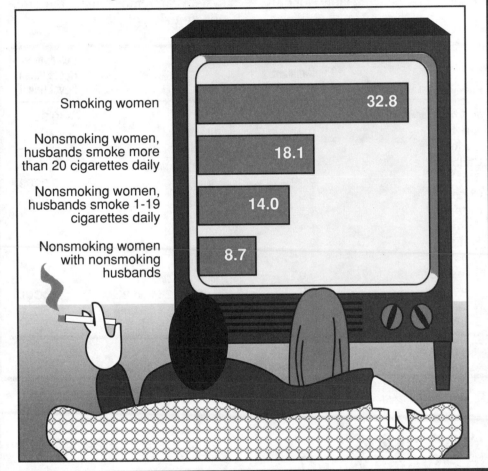

Smoking women — 32.8

Nonsmoking women, husbands smoke more than 20 cigarettes daily — 18.1

Nonsmoking women, husbands smoke 1-19 cigarettes daily — 14.0

Nonsmoking women with nonsmoking husbands — 8.7

An estimated 750 million tons of toxic chemical wastes have been dropped into 30,000 to 50,000 hazardous waste sites in the United States since the late 1950s. Several studies have shown that people living in the vicinity of such sites have more cancers of the rectum, large intestine, bladder, and stomach.

Water: What's Safe to Drink

A glass of water usually looks benign, but it may contain levels of pollutants that can put your health at risk. So far the EPA has determined maximum safe levels (shown in the accompanying table) for only a fraction of the contaminants known to occur in drinking water.

If you're thinking of having your own tap water tested, you might want to compare the results with the figures shown here. A water-filtering system can remove many, but probably not all, pollutants.

Pollutant	Maximum Safe Contaminant Level (mg/l)	Pollutant	Maximum Safe Contaminant Level (mg/l)
Inorganic chemicals		Silver	0.05
Arsenic	0.05	Sulfate	250.0
Barium	1.0	Total dissolved solids	500.0
Cadmium	0.01	*Organic chemicals*	
Chromium	0.05	Endrin	0.0002
Copper	10.0	Lindane	0.004
Detergents	0.5	Methoxychlor	0.1
Fluoride	1.4	Toxaphene	0.005
Iron	0.3	Total trihalomethanes (THM)	0.1*
Lead	0.025	*Radioactive substances*	
Manganese	0.05	Radium 226 and 228	5 pCi/l
Mercury	0.002	Gross alpha particle activity	15 pCi/l
Nitrites and nitrates	10.0		
Selenium	0.045		

*The EPA has stated a future goal of 0.01–0.025 mg/l for THM.

Windsurfing in Polluted Water? Be Careful Not to Fall

You don't have to drink polluted water by the glass to get sick. A study of competitive windsurfers found that the more times they fell in polluted water, the more likely they were to experience symptoms of gastroenteritis, skin infections, and other illnesses. *All* the windsurfers who fell more than 30 times suffered some symptoms.

What We're Doing to Make the Environment Healthier

According to a national survey, most Americans are taking concrete steps to help the environment. Only 2 percent of respondents said they had done nothing in the last year.

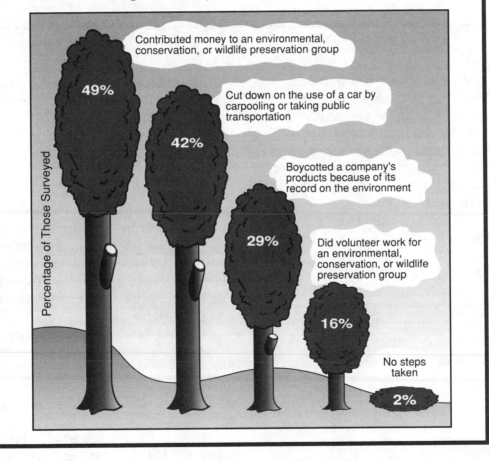

Air pollution poses a greater risk to children than adults. According to a study in California, children breathing the same polluted air as adults may receive more than six times the amount of airborne pollutants.

19

FITNESS

Over the past two decades, there has been a dramatic trend toward greater fitness. People everywhere are running more, swimming more, bicycling more, walking more. Tennis, volleyball, racquetball, and other leisure-time competitive sports are immensely popular.

All this attention to physical activity has its rewards. A more fit lifestyle brings with it a slimmer and more robust appearance, stronger bones, less depression and anxiety, better self-image and more self-confidence, greater energy throughout the day, sharper concentration, and more restful sleep. In addition:

▼ Exercise protects the heart. Studies have shown that lack of regular physical activity may be an even more important heart-disease risk factor than smoking or high blood pressure.

▼ The fit live longer. A 20-year study showed that physically active men live an average of 2.1 years longer than men who love to loaf.

▼ Vigorous exercise can help older people maintain a high level of sexual interest and activity, as well as improve their memory, reasoning, and reaction time.

Perhaps the best news of all is that fitness can be fun in many ways. You can get fit by swimming. Participation by about 66 percent of all Americans makes this the nation's most popular recreational sport. Many experts rate swimming the best all-around exercise you can find.

Or you can try fitness walking, America's second-most popular sport. Fifty-eight percent of Americans walk for fitness, and the number is growing fast, particularly among the over-40 crowd.

Or you can ride a bicycle. Fifty-three percent of Americans bike. It's great exercise and can save you money on transportation.

Fitness can also come from physical activity that isn't sport at all. Gardening, for instance, can burn an impressive 400 to 450 calories an hour.

The Best Fitness Activities

What is fitness really all about? Undoubtedly, the most important component of a fitness program is aerobic exercise. That's what keeps your heart and lungs in top working order. But different forms of exercise can also burn up calories (fat loss), build muscular strength, and improve flexibility. If your aim is total fitness, pick one or two activities from this list that have good ratings in all categories, such as swimming and cross-country skiing, or try alternating between activities that are complementary, such as weight lifting and running.

Activity	Aerobic Power (Endurance)	Fat Loss	Strength	Flexibility
Aerobic dance	High	High	Moderate	High
Baseball	Low	Low	Low	Low
Basketball	High	Moderate	Moderate	Moderate
Biking	High	High	Moderate	Low
Bowling	Low	Low	Moderate	Low
Brisk walking	Moderate	Moderate	Low	Low
Golf	Low	Low	Low	Moderate
Jogging	High	Moderate	Low	Low
Rowing	High	High	High	Moderate
Running	High	High	Moderate	Low
Skating	High	Moderate	Moderate	Moderate
Skiing				
Cross-country	High	High	Moderate	Moderate
Downhill	Low	Low	Moderate	Low
Soccer	High	Moderate	Moderate	Moderate
Swimming	High	Moderate	Moderate	High
Tennis				
Singles	Moderate	Moderate	Low	Moderate
Doubles	Low	Low	Low	Moderate
Weight lifting	Low	Low	High	Moderate

From *THE ATHLETE WITHIN: A Personal Guide to Total Fitness* by Harvey B. Simon, M.D. and Steven R. Levisohn, M.D. Copyright © 1987 by Charter Oak Trust and Harvey B. Simon Family Trust. By permission of Little, Brown and Company.

Exercise to your heart's content. A study of 3,100 men conducted at the University of North Carolina at Chapel Hill found that cardiovascular (aerobic) exercise offers more heart protection than pushing back the clock 19 years.

Where You'll Find the Fit

Southerners are more likely to be serious about fitness than easterners, but not as serious as westerners. That's the conclusion of a *Prevention* magazine survey that asked people all around the United States how often they exercise. Here are the percentages of respondents who said they exercise strenuously three or more days per week.

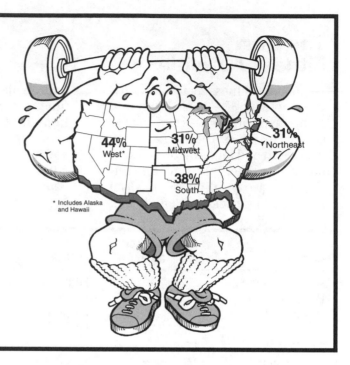

44% West*

31% Midwest

31% Northeast

38% South

* Includes Alaska and Hawaii

Where Do Couch Potatoes Grow?

These five states have higher than average percentages of sedentary adults:

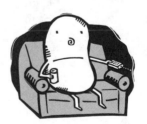

Tennessee—67.8 percent

Rhode Island—65.1 percent

South Carolina—64.5 percent

Indiana—64.5 percent

Georgia—63.8 percent

These five states boast lower than average percentages of sedentary adults:

Idaho—44.2 percent

Montana—45.0 percent

Arizona—46.1 percent

Utah—47.5 percent

Florida—51.5 percent

The More Degrees, the More Activities

Forget any stereotypes you once had about dumb jocks. The fact is that people with more education tend to be more physically active. That's the conclusion of researchers at the University of Maryland, whose fig-ures are shown here. The numbers represent the percentage of Americans aged 25 and older who participated in each activity during the previous 12 months.

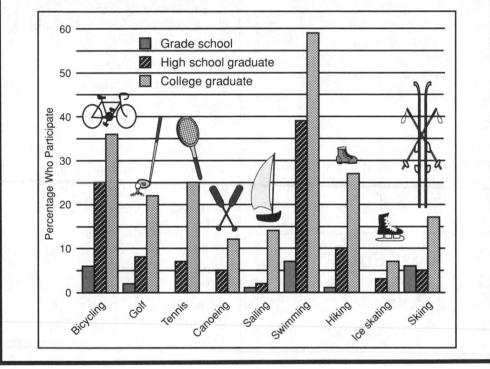

Playing baseball is good for your health. A follow-up look at former major-league players reveals that their overall death rate is 6 percent lower than that of the general population. And those with the best records tend to live longest. Statistics show that infielders have the lowest death rate, followed by pitchers and outfielders. Death tends to catch up with catchers the earliest.

FILE ON THE FAMOUS

Patriot, Scientist, and Swimmer

Benjamin Franklin was more than a leader of America's fight for independence and a man who liked to fly kites in thunderstorms. He was also an excellent swimmer who often urged others to learn and personally taught many to swim.

Stronger abdominal muscles can improve posture and lower the chance of back injury, an increasing problem in middle age. Best bet: bent-knee sit-ups.

The Best Spot for Taking Your Pulse

To find your pulse, you could either reach for the side of your neck or your wrist. Following heavy exercise, however, your choice becomes clear: Go for the wrist. Pressure on the carotid artery in your neck can slow your heart rate, giving you a false reading on the intensity of your workout. That could create a possible health hazard, especially if you're a heart patient. Taking your pulse at the wrist, however, does not affect heart rate.

Eight Signs of Exercise Excess

While most people don't get enough exercise, there are a few overzealous types who overtrain. Here's how to recognize whether you fall into this extra-sweaty group.

1. You crawl out of today's exercise session and loathe the thought of tomorrow's.

2. You have trouble sleeping.

3. You have no energy to enjoy doing other things.

4. Your morning pulse rate is high.

5. Your appetite is out of control, or you have no appetite at all.

6. You begin to develop aches and pains you never had before.

7. You need orthopedic devices, ice bags, and massage to keep up your exercise routine.

8. Your spouse occasionally comments that it's nice to have you around the house for a change.

Your basic metabolic rate (the rate at which calories are burned to fuel the body's basic biological functions) does slow down with age—but only 2 to 3 percent every decade after age 19. The bigger problem is that as those decades roll by, we tend to eat more and exercise less.

~~~**P**umping iron can pump up your image. A study of young and middle-aged women found that in addition to boosting physical strength, lifting weights lifted the women's self-esteem.

Take Your Pulse . . . Fast!

To find your heart rate, check your pulse. But take a shortcut. There's no need to count to 60 to find the number of heartbeats per minute. Simply take your pulse for 10 seconds and multiply by six.

Active People Live Longer

Active life, long life: The two are practically synonymous. Those who regularly expend energy—either by walking, climbing stairs, or participating in sports and exercise programs—can expect to live longer than those who pass their hours lounging. Here are some examples of how the death risk drops as the number of calories burned a week (in this case by walking) steadily increases.

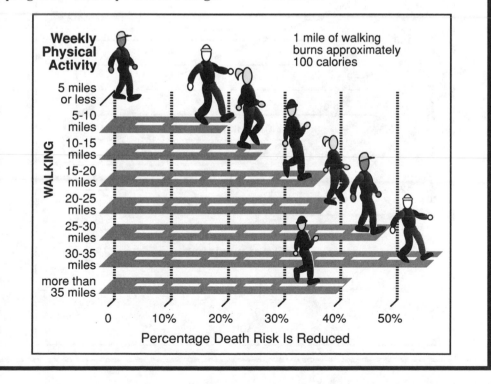

Weekly Physical Activity

1 mile of walking burns approximately 100 calories

WALKING

- 5 miles or less
- 5-10 miles
- 10-15 miles
- 15-20 miles
- 20-25 miles
- 25-30 miles
- 30-35 miles
- more than 35 miles

0   10%   20%   30%   40%   50%

Percentage Death Risk Is Reduced

Train at the Rate That's Right for Your Heart

Airplanes need to reach a certain speed before they can leave the ground, water must reach a certain temperature before it boils, and your heart must beat at a certain rate before it (and your lungs) get the kind of aerobic conditioning best suited to building endurance and health. This target rate, according to the American Heart Association, is between 60 and 75 percent of your maximum heart rate. And *that*

rate is determined by subtracting your age from 220. So if you're 30 years old, for example, you would have a maximum heart rate of 190 ($220 - 30 = 190$), and a target heart rate of between 114 ($0.60 \times 190 = 114$) and 142 ($0.75 \times 190 = 142$). If your heart rate rises above 142, you're probably exercising too vigorously. And if it falls below 114 during exercise, you'd do yourself a favor by working a little harder.

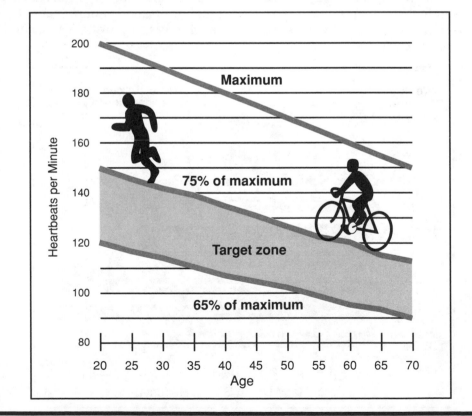

How Hot Is Too Hot?

If you exercise when it's terribly hot outside, you run the risk of collapsing from heat exhaustion or heat stroke. But it's not heat alone that puts you at risk. Humidity also plays a critical role. Here's a chart from the doctors at Duke University to help you decide if it's too hot and humid to exercise outside today. If the temperature and humidity readings indicate that you're in the danger zone, do yourself a favor—wait for the heat wave to pass, or find yourself an air-conditioned gym.

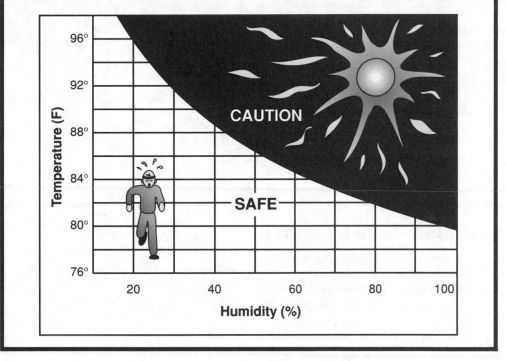

The Tarahumara Indian tribe of Mexico boasts some of the world's greatest long-distance runners. Tarahumara hunters have been known to run 200 miles over a period of three days and nights, chasing a deer until it drops from exhaustion. Two Tarahumara were entered in the 1928 Olympics in Amsterdam. They ran the marathon (26 miles) but lost. "Too short," was their explanation. Apparently prepared to run a much longer race, they mistook the marathon for a mere warm-up!

How Fit Are Kids Today?

Chances are that Beaver Cleaver and Dennis the Menace were a lot fitter than kids today. Skinfold measurements on the upper arms and shoulders show a marked increase in body fat for boys and girls in the 1980s compared with the 1960s. (The chart summarizes data for the eight-year-old groups. Keep in mind that the *lower* the score, the better.) Researchers say children in the decade of hula hoops and hopscotch were substantially slimmer—and probably fitter—than kids in the decade of video games and MTV.

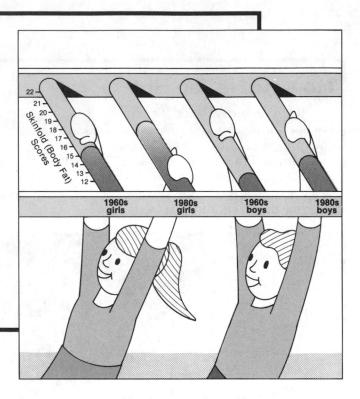

Fitness for Mr. Fix-It

Some doctors today think that you can maintain your heart in good working order without ever putting on a pair of running shoes or saddling a bicycle. But you won't do it by lounging around the house watching TV. Instead, pick up a hammer, an ax, or a paintbrush and get to work on that project in the yard or garage that you've been putting off for years. Here's a list of around-the-house chores, that—if done vigorously for more than half an hour a day, every day—may substitute for more strenuous exercise at the gym.

Activity	Calories Burned per Hour*
Bricklaying	235
Carpentry	
light	200–270
heavy	415
Chopping wood	
by hand	525
with power saw	260
Cleaning windows	295
Gardening (weeding, hoeing, digging)	400–450
House painting	245
Lawn mowing (pushing a power mower)	310
Scrubbing floors	295
Shoveling snow	710
Stacking wood	400–440
Washing and polishing car	270

*Based on body weight of 180–200 lb.

Walking on the Job: Who Does the Most?

Back in the days when most folks tilled the land from sunrise to sunset, people got the exercise they needed while they worked. These days, things are different. For many of us, the only thing we may exercise on the job is a little caution when the boss walks by. But there are still some jobs in this age of computers that do offer the chance for beneficial exercise, especially in the form of walking. Check this list to see if yours is one of them.

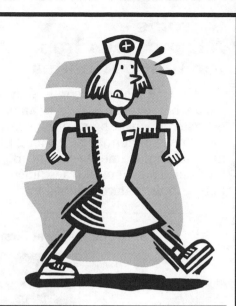

Job	Miles Walked per Day	Job	Miles Walked per Day
Hospital nurse	5.3	Newspaper reporter	2.1
Security officer	4.2	Banker	2.0
City messenger	4.0	Accountant	1.8
Retail salesperson	3.5	Teacher	1.7
Waiter/waitress	3.3	Lawyer	1.5
Hotel employee	3.2	Housewife	1.3
Doctor	2.5	Magazine editor	1.3
Advertising rep.	2.4	Radio announcer	1.1
Architect	2.3	Dentist	0.8
Secretary	2.2		

If you're having trouble sticking with your walking program, finding a partner may help you stay motivated. Fifty-one men enrolled in a hospital-based exercise program at St. Francis Medical Center in Peoria, Illinois, were twice as likely to continue their walking program for a year if their wives exercised with them.

Steroids— A Dangerous Trap for Young Athletes

Olympic athletes aren't the only ones who sometimes turn to anabolic steroids in the hopes of improving athletic performance. Although they can damage the liver and heart, raise blood pressure, and cause infertility and premature balding, these body-building drugs also appeal to many high school athletes looking for a competitive edge or simply hoping to look more like the Hulk. Here are the results of a survey that appeared in the *Journal of the American Medical Association.*

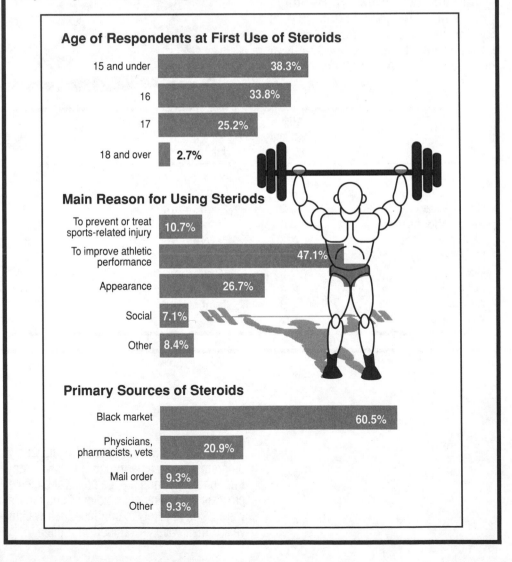

Age of Respondents at First Use of Steroids

15 and under	38.3%
16	33.8%
17	25.2%
18 and over	2.7%

Main Reason for Using Steriods

To prevent or treat sports-related injury	10.7%
To improve athletic performance	47.1%
Appearance	26.7%
Social	7.1%
Other	8.4%

Primary Sources of Steroids

Black market	60.5%
Physicians, pharmacists, vets	20.9%
Mail order	9.3%
Other	9.3%

The Sports with the Most Injuries

More Americans hurt themselves playing football than any other sport, according to a University of Rochester study. Doctors there say that football fields are home to more than 12 times the number of injuries seen on basketball courts, the next most common site of sports injuries.

And what is the most common kind of injury? In all of the five major sports studied, knee problems were the most prevalent, accounting for more than a third of all football injuries, and almost two-thirds of all basketball injuries.

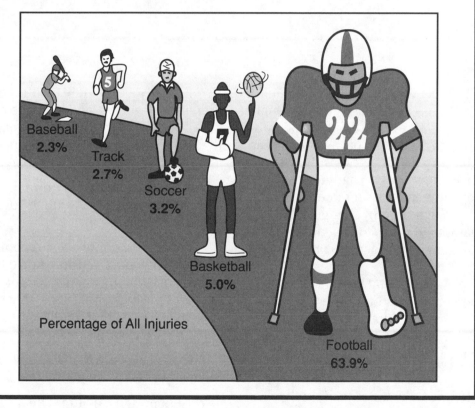

Baseball
2.3%

Track
2.7%

Soccer
3.2%

Basketball
5.0%

Football
63.9%

Percentage of All Injuries

You're never too old. Men in their sixties and seventies were able to increase their muscle size by an average of 11 percent and their strength by a staggering 170 percent after just 12 weeks in a weight-training program.

20

FOOD AND HEALTH

The National Academy of Sciences (NAS) has linked faulty diet to a higher risk of heart disease, high blood pressure, cancer, tooth decay, liver disease, obesity, and diabetes. And there's lots of evidence that changing your diet for the better can reduce your risk.

What kind of changes? The NAS has issued the following dietary guidelines aimed at reducing chronic disease.

▼ Reduce total fat intake to 30 percent or less of calories. Reduce saturated fat intake to less than 10 percent of calories, and daily cholesterol intake to less than 300 milligrams.

▼ Increase consumption of complex carbohydrates to more than 55 percent of total calories. Every day eat five or more servings of vegetables and fruits, especially green and yellow vegetables and citrus fruits. Also eat six or more servings of complex carbohydrates—breads, cereals, and legumes. Whole-grain products are especially good.

▼ Eat only a moderate amount of protein—no more than 1.6 grams per kilogram (2.2 pounds) of body weight. Even that level is twice the Recommended Dietary Allowance (RDA).

▼ Keep your weight at normal levels by balancing how much you eat with exercise.

▼ Drinking alcohol is not recommended. If you must drink, don't drink more than the equivalent of 1 ounce of pure alcohol a day—that's two cans of beer, two small glasses of wine, or two average cocktails.

▼ Don't eat more than 6 grams of salt a day.

▼ Get enough calcium. The best sources are low-fat or nonfat dairy products and dark-green vegetables.

▼ Don't exceed the RDA for dietary supplements.

▼ Maintain an optimal intake of fluoride, especially during childhood.

What Concerns Shoppers Most

Shoppers interviewed in supermarkets seem to be most concerned about excess sodium and fat in the foods they buy.

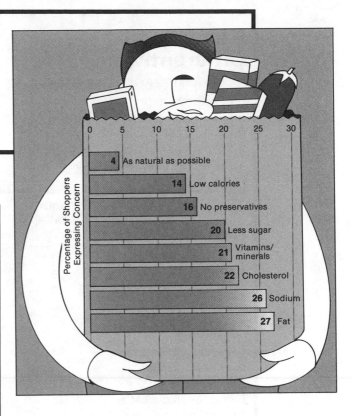

Percentage of Shoppers Expressing Concern

4	As natural as possible
14	Low calories
16	No preservatives
20	Less sugar
21	Vitamins/minerals
22	Cholesterol
26	Sodium
27	Fat

The Story of a Peanutaholic

A 48-year-old woman went to see Neil Scheier, M.D., a New York physician, with a cholesterol count of more than 300 and a high triglyceride count as well. Both are potent risks for heart disease and stroke. Yet she wasn't fat, there was no history of high cholesterol in her family, and she had no other risk factors for heart disease. Except for the cholesterol and triglycerides, her diagnostic tests were normal.

Dr. Scheier decided the woman needed to go on a diet to bring her cholesterol and triglycerides under control. Going over the packet of information, the woman noticed that peanuts are loaded with triglycerides. It was then she told Dr. Scheier that while at work she snacked on more than two pounds of peanuts a week, following that up with peanut butter at every meal!

Ten days after she stopped eating peanuts and peanut butter, her cholesterol and triglyceride counts had dropped dramatically to normal levels.

IS THAT A FACT?

Americans eat more fat now than in "the good old days."

Yes. In 1909 the average American consumed about 121 grams of fat daily—about 4.3 ounces. By 1985, that figure had risen to 169 grams—almost 6 ounces. But the news is not all bad: Saturated fat consumption has hung around the 55- to 60-gram level for the last 80 years, while the consumption of healthier monounsaturated fat has risen from 48 to 68 grams and polyunsaturated fat from 13 to 33 grams.

Fixing Food Differently

Two-thirds of shoppers surveyed report they are preparing their food differently than they did three to five years previously. More women than men have changed their habits, and people in the 50-to-64 age group lead the way—nearly 75 percent have changed. This table shows the myriad ways people are putting into practice the lessons they're learning about food and health.

Change Made	Percentage Reporting Change	Change Made	Percentage Reporting Change
Using less salt	40	Eating more fruit	4
Frying less	35	Using more margarine	3
Using less added fat	29	Eating less/smaller quantities	3
Broiling more	20	Changing length of cooking time	3
Eating more vegetables/fresh foods	20	Eating more chicken	3
Lowering cholesterol	18	Eating more fish	2
Microwaving more	17	Eating a more nutritionally balanced diet	2
Eating less sugar	17	Eating fewer or more healthful desserts	2
Eating less red meat	15	Using a barbecue or outdoor grill	1
Baking/roasting more	13	Using fewer sauces	*
Steaming more	10	Other	23
Eating fewer calories	7	Not sure	1
Using a wider variety/more recipes	5		
Using fast foods/prepared foods	5		
Changing spices or seasoning	4		

*Less than 0.5 %

San Francisco Giants president and general manager Al Rosen had a heart attack after the 1988 season. And baseball fans at Candlestick Park reaped the benefits. At Rosen's request, the stadium began offering healthy snacks like yogurt, tofu dogs, pasta salad, fresh fruit, and bottled water.

The Fat Finder

We love the rich taste of fat-marbled meat, fried chicken skin, and ice cream. Yet fatty foods have been implicated in heart disease and cancer, and so major health organizations recommend that fat should account for no more than 30 percent of your total daily calories. Since Americans typically get 40 percent of their calories from fat, we need to begin monitoring our diets for excess fat. This extensive list of foods showing percentages of calories from fat is a good beginning. But numbers don't tell the whole story. While keeping your total fat intake down, try to replace artery-clogging saturated fat (signified by S next to the number when this type of fat predominates) with protective polyunsaturated (P) and monounsaturated (M) fats.

Food	Portion	Total Calories	Fat (g)	Fat Calories (%)
Breakfast foods				
Bacon, fried or broiled	1 slice	36	3.1	77 S,M
Bagel, egg or water	1 (2 oz.)	163	1.4	8
Breakfast strips	3 strips	80	6.0	68
Canadian bacon, grilled	1 slice	43	2.0	41 M
Cereals				
corn bran	1 cup	124	1.3	9
cornflakes	1 cup	98	0.1	1
Cream of Wheat	1 cup	144	0.6	3
granola, homemade	½ cup	298	16.6	50 P,M
granola, purchased	½ cup	252	9.8	35 S
grits	1 cup	146	0.5	3
oat flakes	1 cup	177	0.7	4
oatmeal	1 cup	145	2.4	15
"O-shaped" oats	1 cup	91	1.1	11
crispy rice	1 cup	109	11.9	11
puffed rice	1 cup	56	0.1	2
shredded wheat	1 cup	83–169	0.6	5
wheat bran flakes	1 cup	146	0.7	5
wheat bran flakes with raisins	1 cup	169	0.8	4
Croissant, frozen	1	109	6.1	50
Danish pastry, plain	1	250	13.6	49 S
Doughnut, yeast, glazed	1	205	11.2	49 M
Eggs				
raw or poached	1	79	5.6	63 S
scrambled with milk and butter	1	95	7.1	67 S
substitute*	¼ cup	25	0.0	0
white	1	16	0.0	0
Eggs, sausage, hash browns, frozen	5¼ oz. pkg.	360	28.0	70
French toast				
frozen	1 slice	85–135	2.5–7.0	27–48
homemade	1 slice	153	6.7	40
Instant breakfast drink	1 cup	280	8.0	26

*Read labels carefully. Some foods in this category may be surprisingly high in fat.

(continued)

The Fat Finder — *Continued*

Food	Portion	Total Calories	Fat (g)	Fat Calories (%)
Breakfast foods — continued				
Pancakes				
from mix	1	58	2.1	32
frozen	1	80	3.5	39
Pastry, toaster	1	196	5.8	26
Sausage links, low-fat	2–3	160	11.5	66
Scrambled eggs, home fries, frozen	4⅝ oz. pkg.	280	21.0	68
Waffles				
from mix	1	205	8.0	35
frozen	1	106	4.8	31
homemade	1	245	12.6	46
Wheat germ, toasted	1 Tbsp.	27	0.8	25 P
Combination foods: dinners				
Beef cannelloni, light, frozen	9.6 oz.	260	10.0	35
Beef dinner, frozen	12 oz.	320	9.0	25
Beef teriyaki, light, frozen	8 oz.	240	3.0	11
Cheese cannelloni, light, frozen	9.1 oz.	270	10.0	33
Chicken with broccoli, light, frozen	9.5 oz.	290	11.0	34
Chicken cacciatore, frozen	11.2 oz.	310	11.0	32
Chicken chow mein, light, frozen	11.2 oz.	250	5.0	18
Chicken dinner, frozen	11.5 oz.	660	33.0	45
Chicken divan, frozen	8.5 oz.	335	22.0	59
Chicken parmigiana, frozen	11.5 oz.	400	20.0	45
Chicken with vegetables and rice, light	8.5 oz.	270	8.0	27
Fish and chips, frozen	7.9 oz.	500	30.0	54
Lasagna Florentine, light	11.2 oz.	280	5.0	16
Lasagna, frozen	10.5 oz.	385	14.0	33
Lobster Newburg, frozen	6.5 oz.	350	29.0	75
Manicotti, with cheese, frozen	8.5 oz.	310	13.0	38
Meatballs with noodles, frozen	11 oz.	475	27.0	51
Meat loaf dinner, frozen	11 oz.	412	23.7	52
Salisbury steak, frozen	11 oz.	390	24.6	57
Shells with beef, frozen	9 oz.	290	11.0	34
Shells with cheese, frozen	9 oz.	320	14.0	39
Shells with chicken, frozen	9 oz.	400	22.0	50
Shrimp creole, light, frozen	10 oz.	200	2.0	9
Sirloin tips, frozen	11.5 oz.	390	18.0	42
Sweet and sour chicken, frozen	11.2 oz.	460	22.0	43
Tuna with noodles, frozen	5.7 oz.	200	9.0	41

Food	Portion	Total Calories	Fat (g)	Fat Calories (%)
Turkey breast, premium dinner, frozen	11.2 oz.	470	24.0	45
Turkey dinner, with potatoes, frozen	11.5 oz.	340	10.0	27
Vegetable lasagna	11 oz.	400	24.0	54
Yankee pot roast, frozen	11 oz.	360	15.0	38
Zucchini lasagna, light	11 oz.	260	7.0	24
Dairy products				
Buttermilk	1 cup	99	2.2	20 S
Cheese				
American, process	1 oz.	106	8.9	75 S
American, singles	1 oz.	45	2.0	40
blue	1 oz.	60	4.9	73 S
Brie	1 oz.	95	7.9	74 S
Cheddar	1 oz.	114	9.4	74 S
Colby	1 oz.	112	9.1	73 S
feta	1 oz.	75	6.0	72 S
Monterey Jack	1 oz.	106	8.6	73 S
Monterey Jack, light	1 oz.	80	6.0	68 S
mozzarella, whole-milk	1 oz.	80	6.1	69 S
mozzarella, part-skim	1 oz.	72	4.5	56 S
Parmesan, grated	1 Tbsp.	29	1.9	59 S
ricotta, whole-milk	¼ cup	107	8.0	67 S
ricotta, part-skim	¼ cup	85	4.9	52 S
Swiss	1 oz.	107	7.8	65 S
Swiss, diet	1 slice (1 oz.)	50	2.0	36
Cottage cheese	¼ cup	58	2.5	39 S
low-fat (1%)	¼ cup	41	0.5	13
Cream cheese	1 oz.	99	9.9	90 S
Cream				
heavy, whipping	1 Tbsp.	51	5.5	97 S
light	1 Tbsp.	29	2.9	89 S
Half-and-half	1 Tbsp.	20	1.7	79 S
Milk				
chocolate	1 cup	208	8.5	37 S
evaporated	1 Tbsp.	21	1.2	51 S
evaporated skim	1 Tbsp.	12	0.1	2
low-fat (1%)	1 cup	102	2.6	23 S
skim	1 cup	86	0.4	5 S
whole	1 cup	150	8.2	49 S
Nondairy creamer	1 Tbsp.	10	1.0	80 S

(continued)

The Fat Finder—*Continued*

Food	Portion	Total Calories	Fat (g)	Fat Calories (%)
Dairy products—continued				
Nondairy whipped topping, frozen	1 Tbsp.	15	1.2	72 S
Sour cream				
cultured	1 Tbsp.	31	3.0	88 S
imitation	1 Tbsp.	28	2.6	84 S
Yogurt				
low-fat	1 cup	144	3.5	22 S
nonfat	1 cup	127	0.4	3
whole-milk	1 cup	139	7.4	48 S
Delicatessen foods				
Bagel				
with cream cheese	2 oz. bagel	361	21.1	53
with lox and onion	2 oz. bagel	243	3.9	15
Salads				
chef's	average	722	56.1	70
chef's, no dressing	average	344	20.1	53
chicken	average	509	39.0	69
cucumber	average	43	2.2	47
egg	average	425	41.0	86
Greek, with feta cheese	average	377	21.5	51
macaroni	average	286	25.1	79
potato, German	average	164	3.3	18
Sandwiches				
grilled cheese	1	440	31.0	63
ham and cheese on rye with mustard and mayonnaise	1	615	37.7	55
hero	4.75-oz. roll	1,154	62.2	49
pastrami, beef, on rye	1	541	36.0	60
pastrami, turkey, on whole-wheat	1	297	11.6	35
Reuben, grilled, on rye	1	835	59.5	64
roast beef with horseradish on rye	1	444	18.8	38
roast beef with mayonnaise, tomato, lettuce on rye	1	576	35.1	55
tuna/cheese melt	1	640	48.2	68
turkey club	1	626	33.5	48
turkey club on whole-wheat	1	357	14.3	36
Desserts and sweets				
Brownies				
fudge, microwave	1	180	9.0	45

Food	Portion	Total Calories	Fat (g)	Fat Calories (%)
iced	1 oz.	105	5.0	43 M,S
with nuts, no icing, homemade	1 oz.	135	8.5	57 S
with nuts, no icing, mix	1 oz.	121	5.7	42 S
Candy				
caramel, plain and chocolate	1 oz.	115	3.0	23 S
milk chocolate bar	1 oz.	145	9.0	56 S
chocolate bar with peanuts	1 oz.	154	10.8	63
semisweet chocolate bar	1 oz.	144	10.2	64 S
fudge	1 oz.	115	3.0	23 S
gumdrops	1 oz.	100	0	0
chocolate-covered peanuts	1 oz.	160	12.0	68 S
Cakes				
angel-food, mix	2 oz.	142	0.1	1
coffeecake, mix	2.5 oz.	230	7.0	27 S
cheesecake	3 oz.	257	16.3	57
devil's-food, iced, mix	2.5 oz.	235	8.0	31 S
pound, homemade	2 oz.	275	17.2	56 S
sponge, homemade	2.3 oz.	188	3.1	15 S
pineapple upside-down, homemade	2.5 oz.	221	8.5	35
Cookies				
chocolate chip, homemade	1 small	46	2.7	52 P,M
chocolate chip, mix	1 small	50	2.4	44 S,M
fig bar	1 average	53	1.0	16 S
fudge	1 small	25	1.0	36
gingersnap, homemade	1 small	34	1.6	42 S
macaroon	1 average	90	4.5	45
peanut butter, homemade	1 average	59	3.3	50
peanut butter, mix	1 small	50	2.6	48
vanilla wafer	1 small	19	0.6	29 M
Custard, baked	1 cup	305	15.0	44 S
Eclair, custard-filled, iced	3.5 oz.	239	13.6	51
Gelatin, fruit-flavored	1 cup	161	3.1	17
Ice cream				
hot fudge sundae	6 oz.	312	10.9	31
vanilla, soft	1 cup	377	22.5	54 S
vanilla, regular	1 cup	349	23.7	61 S
Ice milk				
vanilla, soft	1 cup	223	4.6	19 S
vanilla, regular	1 cup	184	5.6	28 S

(continued)

The Fat Finder—*Continued*

Food	Portion	Total Calories	Fat (g)	Fat Calories (%)
Desserts and sweets—continued				
Marshmallows	1 oz.	90	0	0
Mousse, chocolate, homemade	⅔ cup	445	35.7	72 S
Pies				
apple, homemade	5 oz.	323	13.6	38 S
banana cream, homemade	4.5 oz.	285	12.0	38 S
blueberry, homemade	5 oz.	325	15.0	42 S
cherry, homemade	5 oz.	350	15.0	39 S
chocolate cream, homemade	3.5 oz.	264	15.1	52
lemon meringue, homemade	4 oz.	300	11.2	34 S
pumpkin, homemade	4.5 oz.	275	15.0	49 S
Pudding				
chocolate, homemade	1 cup	385	12.0	28 S
rice, with raisins, homemade	1 cup	387	8.2	19
tapioca, homemade	1 cup	220	8.0	33 S
vanilla, homemade	1 cup	285	10.0	32 S
Sherbet, orange	1 cup	270	3.8	13 S
Tofutti	1 cup	210	12.0	51
Turnovers				
apple	1 oz.	85	4.7	50
lemon	1 oz.	93	5.0	49
Yogurt, frozen, fruit-flavor	1 cup	216	2.0	8
Meats				
Beef				
chicken-fried steak	3½ oz.	389	30.0	69
chipped, dried	2½ oz.	117	2.8	21 S,M
corned beef, canned	3 oz.	213	12.7	54 S,M
corned beef hash	¼ cup	100	6.3	56 S
eye round roast	3 oz.	155	5.5	32 S,M
ground, up to 30% fat, fried	3 oz.	260	19.2	66 S,M
ground, up to 30% fat, baked or broiled	3 oz.	244	17.8	66 S,M
ground, 21% fat	3 oz.	231	15.7	61 S,M
ground, 10% fat	3 oz.	217	13.9	58 S,M
liver, fried	3 oz.	184	6.8	33 S
London broil (top round)	3 oz.	162	5.3	29 S,M
pot roast	3½ oz.	231	10.0	39 S,M
rib roast, trimmed	3 oz.	203	11.7	52 S,M
rib steak	3½ oz.	225	11.6	46 S,M
roast beef, lean, trimmed	3 oz.	189	8.7	41 S,M

Food	Portion	Total Calories	Fat (g)	Fat Calories (%)
sirloin steak, trimmed, broiled	3 oz.	202	10.1	45 S,M
tenderloin, broiled	3 oz.	174	7.9	41 S,M
Frankfurters				
beef/pork	1	183	16.6	82 S,M
beef/pork with cheese	1	141	12.5	80 S,M
Lamb				
leg, roasted, trimmed	3 oz.	156	6.0	35 S
chop, broiled	3 oz.	360	32.0	80 S
shoulder, lean	3 oz.	173	8.0	42 S
Pork				
canned ham, roasted	3 oz.	193	12.9	60 S,M
ham, extra-lean	3 oz.	116	4.1	32 M
ham, roasted, with bone	3 oz.	151	7.7	46 S,M
pork chop, trimmed, broiled	3 oz.	218	13.0	54 S,M
pork loin, trimmed, roasted	3 oz.	213	11.6	49 S,M
pork shoulder, lean, roasted	3 oz.	207	12.8	55 S,M
spareribs, braised	3 oz.	338	25.7	68 S,M
pork tenderloin, roasted	3 oz.	141	4.1	26 S,M
Rabbit, stewed	3 oz.	183	8.6	42
Sausage				
bratwurst	3 oz.	256	22.0	77 S,M
Italian, pork	3 oz.	275	21.8	71 S,M
kielbasa	3 oz.	265	23.1	78 S,M
knockwurst, pork/beef	1 (2.4 oz.)	209	18.9	81 S,M
Vienna, canned, pork/beef	1 link	45	4.0	81 S,M
Veal				
cutlet, broiled	3 oz.	185	9.0	44 S,M
rib, roasted	3 oz.	230	14.0	55 S
Venison, roasted	3½ oz.	146	2.2	14
Poultry				
Chicken				
capon, roasted	3 oz.	194	9.9	46 M
breast, batter-fried	½	364	18.5	46 M
breast, roasted	½	193	7.7	36 M
breast, roasted without skin	½	142	3.0	19 S,M
leg, roasted	1 (4 oz.)	265	15.4	52 M
leg, roasted without skin	1 (4 oz.)	218	9.6	40 M
liver, simmered	3 oz.	133	4.6	31 S
liver pâté	1 Tbsp.	26	1.7	59

(continued)

The Fat Finder—*Continued*

Food	Portion	Total Calories	Fat (g)	Fat Calories (%)
Poultry—continued				
Duck				
roasted	3 oz.	286	24.1	76 S,M
roasted without skin	3 oz.	171	9.5	50 S,M
Turkey				
breast, roasted without skin	3 oz.	115	0.6	5 S,P
leg, roasted without skin	3 oz.	135	3.2	21 S,P
Nuts and seeds				
Almonds, dry roasted, whole	1 cup	810	71.3	79 M
Brazil nuts	1 cup	919	92.7	91 P,M
Cashews, dry roasted	1 cup	787	63.5	73 M
Chestnuts, roasted	1 oz.	68	0.3	5 M
Coconut				
dry, flaked	1 cup	341	24.4	64 S
raw, shredded	1 cup	283	26.8	85
Filberts (hazelnuts)	1 cup	727	72.0	89 M
Macadamia nuts	1 cup	940	98.8	95 M
Peanuts, dry roasted, without salt	1 cup	867	76.5	79 M
Pecans	1 cup	721	73.1	91 P,M
Pistachios, dry roasted	1 cup	776	67.6	78 M
Sesame seeds, dried	1 cup	825	71.5	78 P
Sunflower seeds				
dried	1 cup	821	71.4	78 P
oil roasted	1 cup	830	77.6	84 P
Walnuts, English	1 cup	770	74.2	87 P
Snacks				
Corn chips	1 oz.	155	9.1	53 P,M
Crackers				
animal	1	9	0.2	21
cheese	1	5	0.3	55 S
graham, plain	1	28	0.5	16 M
rye	1	9	0.4	37
wheat	1	9	0.4	35
Hummus	1 Tbsp.	26	1.3	45
Popcorn				
microwave, plain	1.3 cups	110	7.0	57

Food	Portion	Total Calories	Fat (g)	Fat Calories (%)
homemade, plain	1 cup	25	0	0
with oil and salt	1 cup	40	2.0	45
Potato chip	1	11	0.7	61 P
Pretzel	1	60	1.0	15
Rice cake	1	35	0.3	7
Tortilla chips	1 oz.	139	6.6	43 M
Soups				
Bean with bacon, canned	1 cup	173	5.9	31
Beef noodle, canned	1 cup	84	3.1	33
Beef stock, canned	1 cup	16	0.5	30 S
Celery, canned, with milk	1 cup	165	9.7	53 S
Chicken noodle, homemade	1 cup	184	2.7	13
Chicken stock				
canned	1 cup	39	1.4	32 M
homemade	1 cup	166	10.3	56 S,M
Clam chowder				
New England	1 cup	163	6.6	36 S,M
Manhattan	1 cup	78	2.3	27 P
Cream of chicken, canned	1 cup	191	11.5	54 S,M
Cream of mushroom	1 cup	203	13.6	60 S,P
Minestrone	1 cup	83	2.5	27 P
Onion, canned	1 cup	57	1.7	27 M,P
Oyster stew, canned with milk	1 cup	134	7.9	53 S
Pea, green				
canned	1 cup	239	7.0	26 S
homemade	1 cup	296	7.0	21
Tomato, canned				
with milk	1 cup	160	6.0	34 S
with water	1 cup	86	1.9	20 P
Vegetable, canned	1 cup	72	1.9	24 P,M
Vegetable beef, canned	1 cup	79	1.9	22 S,M
Vegetable stock, homemade	1 cup	83	0.4	4
Vegetable with barley	1 cup	99	4.4	40 P,M

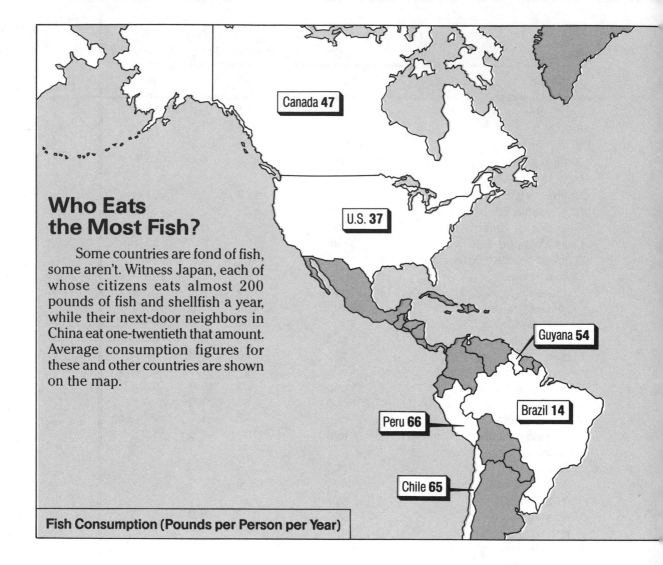

Who Eats the Most Fish?

Some countries are fond of fish, some aren't. Witness Japan, each of whose citizens eats almost 200 pounds of fish and shellfish a year, while their next-door neighbors in China eat one-twentieth that amount. Average consumption figures for these and other countries are shown on the map.

Canada **47**

U.S. **37**

Guyana **54**

Brazil **14**

Peru **66**

Chile **65**

Fish Consumption (Pounds per Person per Year)

The more fermented milk products you consume, the lower your risk of breast cancer, according to a 1989 study from the Netherlands. For those who included more than 1.5 glasses of fermented milk products like yogurt or buttermilk in their diet daily, the odds of getting breast cancer were about half as great as for those who ate no fermented milk products.

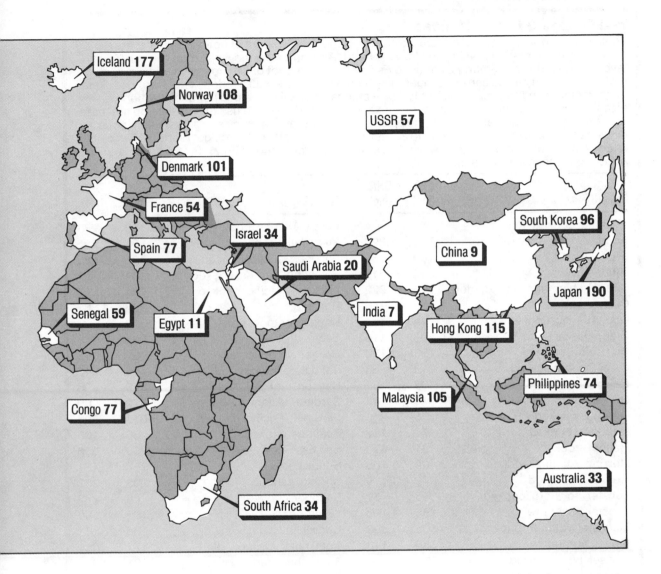

Iceland **177**

Norway **108**

USSR **57**

Denmark **101**

France **54**

South Korea **96**

Israel **34**

China **9**

Spain **77**

Saudi Arabia **20**

Japan **190**

India **7**

Senegal **59**

Egypt **11**

Hong Kong **115**

Congo **77**

Philippines **74**

Malaysia **105**

Australia **33**

South Africa **34**

By 1997, Americans will be buying $7.5 billion worth of frozen dinners each year, analysts say. About $3 billion of that will be low-calorie dinners.

The Omega-3 Fish Oil Finder

While excess dietary fats and oils are implicated in the development of heart disease, there's a type of fat in fish that's actually good for your heart. Applying what they leaned about very low levels of heart disease among Greenland Eskimos, who eat a lot of fish, researchers have shown that omega-3 fatty acids can cut dangerously high blood levels of LDL cholesterol (the "bad" kind of cholesterol) and triglycerides. Two types of omega-3 fish oils have this beneficial action: eicosapentaenoic acid (EPA) and docosahexaenoic acid (DHA). The fish themselves do not make these fats; they are actually made by sea plants. The plants are eaten by small fish, which are eaten by bigger fish, and the oils accumulate as they ascend the food chain. You get plenty of fish oil by eating 4 or 5 servings of EPA/DHA-rich fish a week. This table shows how much of these fatty acids are found in various seafoods.

Food (3½ oz.)	EPA (mg)	DHA (mg)	Food (3½ oz.)	EPA (mg)	DHA (mg)
Abalone, cooked	54	—	Perch, Atlantic, cooked	103	271
Anchovy, canned in oil	763	1,292	Pike, walleye, raw	86	225
Bass, striped, raw	169	585	Pollock, walleye, cooked	185	283
Bluefish, raw	252	519	Pompano, Florida, cooked	131	28
Catfish, channel, breaded, fried	119	222	Rockfish, Pacific, cooked	181	262
Clam, canned	138	146	Roe, raw	983	1,363
Cod, Atlantic, cooked	4	154	Roughy, orange, raw	10	—
Crab, Alaskan king, cooked	295	118	Sablefish, smoked	891	945
Crab, blue, canned	193	170	Salmon, Atlantic, raw	321	1,115
Crab, Dungeness, raw	219	88	Salmon, coho, cooked	414	616
Eel, cooked	108	81	Salmon, pink, canned	845	806
Gefilte fish, sweet	75	45	Sardines, Atlantic, canned	473	509
Grouper, cooked	35	213	Sardines, Pacific, canned	611	993
Haddock, cooked	76	162	Scallops, cooked	86	103
Halibut, cooked	91	374	Sea bass, cooked	206	556
Herring, Atlantic, cooked	909	1,105	Shark, cooked	258	431
Herring, kippered	970	1,179	Shrimp, canned	293	252
Lobster, northern, cooked	53	31	Snapper, cooked	48	273
Lobster, spiny, raw	265	108	Squid, cooked	162	380
Mackerel, Atlantic, cooked	504	699	Swordfish	138	681
Mullet, striped, raw	180	148	Trout, rainbow, cooked	177	551
Mussel, blue, cooked	276	506	Tuna, white, canned in water	191	515
Octopus, common, raw	76	81	Tuna, bluefin, cooked	363	1,141
Oyster, eastern, raw	211	228	Tuna, yellowfin, raw	37	181
Oyster, eastern, steamed	422	456	Whitefish, raw	317	941

Of the 560 million pounds of pesticides used annually by American farmers, 375 million pounds are thought to be carcinogenic.

Salty Facts

In her book *Lot's Wife: Salt and the Human Condition,* Sallie Tisdale has come up with myriad facts about salt. Among them:

▼ The ocean, blood, and amniotic fluid have roughly equal percentages of salt content.

▼ The oceans have enough salt to cover the continents in a 500-foot-thick blanket.

▼ Planet Earth has 120 trillion tons of salt in ocean and rock.

▼ The word "salary" stems from the Roman custom of paying soldiers part of their pay in salt.

▼ Cities named for salt: Salina, Kansas; Salamis, Cyprus; Salinae, Italy; Salins, France.

The fastest-growing beverage in popularity is . . . water. Bottled water, that is. The market grew by almost 15 percent in 1988 alone. Americans guzzled 1.5 billion gallons of it, enough to fill 14,000 Olympic-size swimming pools. West Coast residents lead the trend, accounting for more than one-third of the total.

The Two Kinds of Fiber

Fiber is divided into two basic types, soluble and insoluble. Although fiber-containing foods usually have some of each type, most have more insoluble fiber. Also known as roughage or bulk, this fiber is poorly digested by the body. It's concentrated in the peels, skins, stalks, and husks of fruits, vegetables, and whole grains. Insoluble fiber helps relieve constipation and may help prevent colorectal cancer by speeding cancer-causing agents through the digestive system before they have time to do damage. It may also prevent hemorrhoids and diverticular disease.

Soluble fiber works its beneficial action higher up in the digestive system, forming bulk in the stomach. More digestible than insoluble fiber, it's found in fruits, vegetables, legumes, and whole grains. Carrots, potatoes, oat bran, cantaloupes, oranges, and strawberries all have amounts of soluble fiber equaling or surpassing the amount of insoluble fiber. Soluble fiber's bulk creates a sensation of fullness in the stomach, making it ideal for weight control. It also slows the rate at which the body absorbs glucose, thus helping control diabetes. For many people, oat bran can help keep cholesterol counts within normal ranges as well as most drugs can, but with fewer side effects.

The Fiber Finder

Experts recommend that we include more fiber-rich foods in our daily diet. Approximately 20–35 grams of fiber a day are considered an optimum range. This list of more than 100 fiber-rich foods can help you meet that goal.

Food	Portion	Dietary Fiber (g)
Bread		
Country oat	2 slices	6.0
Whole-wheat, stone-ground	2 slices	4.5
Wheat, reduced-calorie	2 slices	4.0
Mixed grain	2 slices	3.2
Rye	2 slices	3.1
English muffin, wheat	1	3.0
Pita, whole-wheat	1 pocket	2.8
Cornbread, whole-ground	1 piece	2.7
Cracked wheat	2 slices	2.6
Bran muffin	1	2.5
Bran oat cakes	2	2.0
Breakfast cereals, cold		
100% bran-type with added fiber	½ cup	14.0
100% bran-type	⅓ cup	10.0
100% bran-type with oat bran	½ cup	8.0
Multibran	⅓ cup	6.5
Oatmeal flakes	1 cup	6.0
Corn bran, ready-to-eat	⅔ cup	5.4
40% bran-type flakes	⅔ cup	5.3
Bran-type flakes with raisins	1 oz.	5.0
Oat bran, crunchy types	1 oz.	5.0
Bran squares	⅔ cup	4.6
Breakfast cereals, hot		
Multibran, cream, instant, dry	¼ cup	8.0
Oat bran	⅓ cup	5.0
Oatmeal, cooked	¾ cup	1.6
Fruit		
Figs, dried	5	8.7
Pear	1	6.2
Blackberries	½ cup	4.5

Food	Portion	Dietary Fiber (g)
Dates	5	3.2
Orange	1	3.1
Raspberries	½ cup	3.1
Prunes	5	3.0
Apple, with skin	1	3.0
Strawberries	¾ cup	2.9
Apricots, dried	10 halves	2.7
Kiwifruit	1	2.6
Nectarine	1	2.2
Cantaloupe	½	2.0
Applesauce, unsweetened	½ cup	1.9
Raisins	¼ cup	1.9
Banana	1	1.8
Plums	3 small	1.8
Blueberries	½ cup	1.7
Rhubarb	½ cup	1.6
Apricots, fresh	2	1.5
Grapefruit	½	1.5
Peach	1	1.4
Grains		
Corn bran, raw	1 oz.	23.0
Wheat bran, toasted	1 oz.	14.1
Rice bran, raw	1 oz.	6.2–9.5
Bulgur, raw	1 oz.	5.2
Barley, raw	1 oz.	4.9
Oat bran, raw	1 oz.	4.5
Wheat flour, whole grain	1 oz.	3.6
Cornmeal, whole grain	1 oz.	3.1
Wheat germ	1 oz.	3.0
Oats, rolled, dry	1 oz.	2.9
Millet, hulled, raw	1 oz.	2.4
Legumes and peas		
Baked beans, vegetarian, canned	½ cup	9.8
Kidney beans, cooked	½ cup	9.0

Food	Portion	Dietary Fiber (g)
Pinto beans, cooked	½ cup	8.9
Black-eyed peas, cooked	½ cup	8.3
Miso (soybeans)	½ cup	7.5
Chick-peas	½ cup	7.0
Lima beans, cooked	½ cup	6.8
Navy beans, cooked	½ cup	6.8
Lentils, cooked	½ cup	5.2
White beans, cooked	½ cup	5.0
Green peas, cooked	½ cup	2.4
Nuts and seeds		
Almonds, oil-roasted	¼ cup	4.4
Pistachio nuts	¼ cup	3.5
Mixed nuts, oil-roasted	¼ cup	3.2
Peanuts	¼ cup	3.2
Pecans	¼ cup	2.3
Sunflower seeds, oil-roasted	¼ cup	2.3
Cashews, oil-roasted	¼ cup	2.0
Rice, pasta, and tortillas		
Pasta, multigrain with quinoa, dry	2 oz.	8.0
Pasta, multigrain with triticale, dry	2 oz.	6.5
Pasta, whole-wheat ribbon, dry	2 oz.	6.0
Pasta, multigrain with oat bran	2 oz.	6.0
Rice, wild, cooked	½ cup	5.3
Tortilla, corn	2	3.1
Rice, brown, long-grain, cooked	½ cup	1.7
Snacks		
Crackers, stone-ground wheat	1 oz.	3.9
Crisps, thin oat	½ oz.	3.2
Cookies, oat plus fruit	2	3.0
Crackers, hearty wheat	4	3.0

Food	Portion	Dietary Fiber (g)
Crisps, thin rye	½ oz.	3.0
Graham crackers, oat bran	7 (1.2 oz.)	3.0
Cookies, oat bran	2	2.8
Graham crackers, honey	1 oz.	2.4
Popcorn, gourmet	½ oz.	2.0
Fig bars	2	1.3
Saltines, whole-wheat	5	1.0
Vegetables		
Artichoke, raw	1 medium	6.7
Brussels sprouts, boiled	5	4.5
Mixed vegetables, frozen, cooked	½ cup	3.5
Sweet potato, baked	1	3.4
Corn, cooked	1 cob	2.8
Parsley, chopped	1 cup	2.8
Parsnips, cooked	½ cup	2.7
Broccoli, raw, chopped	1 cup	2.5
Kale, frozen	½ cup	2.5
Potato, with skin	1 medium	2.5
Carrot, raw	1	2.3
Beets, canned	½ cup	2.2
Spinach, boiled	½ cup	2.1
Asparagus, cut	1 cup	2.0
Cauliflower, cooked	5 florets	2.0
Zucchini, cooked	½ cup	1.8
Cabbage, raw, shredded	1 cup	1.7
Olives, green	10 large	1.7
Bean sprouts, raw	½ cup	1.6
Green beans, string, cooked	½ cup	1.6
Leeks, raw	½ cup	1.6
Turnips, boiled, cubed	½ cup	1.6
Winter squash, cooked	½ cup	1.6
Mushrooms, raw, sliced	½ cup	1.5
Tomato, raw	1 medium	1.5

More Vegetables, Less Lung Cancer

Beta-carotene, a substance found in red, orange, yellow, and dark-green vegetables like squash and carrots, has consistently been linked to a low risk of lung cancer. In a study of more than 1,000 people, scientists at the University of Hawaii Cancer Research Center found a strong link between lowered lung cancer risk and high consumption of dark-green vegetables, cruciferous vegetables (the cabbage family), tomatoes, and *all* vegetables in general. Apparently more was at work than just beta-carotene. The researchers report that substances known as lutein (in dark-green vegetables),

lycopene (tomatoes) and indoles and phenols (cruciferous vegetables) may be the additional responsible agents. In general, as the charts show, the protective effect was even more dramatic for women than for men. The researchers theorize that the combination of protective factors gained by eating a *variety* of vegetables is the key. The vegetables included in the study were tomatoes (including juice), watercress, spinach, bok choy, Swiss chard, taro leaves, Romaine lettuce, mustard cabbage, broccoli, green peppers, Chinese cabbage, head cabbage, green beans, peas, zucchini, asparagus, and head lettuce.

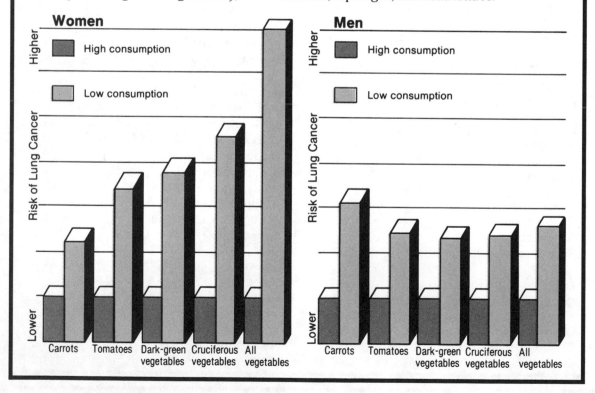

People Prefer Organic

Organic food retailers are reporting growing demand for pesticide-free produce. A 1988 Louis Harris poll conducted for *Organic Gardening* magazine dug up these facts:

▼ Eighty-four percent of those surveyed would buy organic produce if it cost the same as regular produce.

▼ Fifty percent would buy organic even if it cost more.

▼ Of the 48 percent who had eaten organic produce, 56 percent did so for its healthfulness, 21 percent for nutritional value, and 18 percent for taste.

A Berry Good Cancer Fighter?

A substance found in strawberries seems to reduce the risk of cancer. Thought to act as a scavenger of cancer-causing substances, ellagic acid combats nitrosamines found in tobacco smoke and some foods; aflatoxin, the mold that often contaminates peanuts; and hydrocarbons in polluted air and tobacco smoke. The only problem so far: It's not easily absorbed by the body.

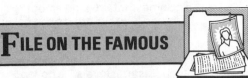

FILE ON THE FAMOUS

Dining with the King

He may have been the king of rock and roll, but when it came to food, Elvis Presley had down-home tastes. Mary Jenkins, one of Presley's cooks at Graceland for 14 years, writes in her book, *Memories beyond Graceland Gates,* that Elvis loved such things as collard greens, string beans and greens, well-done meat, creamed potatoes, and hamburgers. He was partial to bananas, especially peanut butter-and-banana sandwiches, and banana pudding topped with meringue.

Jenkins says Presley served guests turkey for holidays while sticking with ham steaks himself. And he refused to eat fish. In his later years, Elvis got pretty heavy—up to 250 pounds—but rejected his doctor's orders to reform his eating habits, Jenkins says. Before going on tour, he would crash diet on a regimen of crackers, milk, and Gatorade.

Some experts estimate that the pesticide Alar will cause 323 cases of cancer for every 1 million people who ate Alar-contaminated apples.

The 100 Healthiest Foods

Some contain good amounts of available iron, making them beneficial for the blood. Others are high in calcium, a mineral that is essential for strong bones and teeth. Calcium, as well as magnesium and potassium, may help control blood pressure. The fiber, beta-carotene, and vitamins C and E in many of the listed foods have been linked to lower risk of cancer. Low-fat foods protect the heart and control cholesterol levels, as do foods containing soluble fiber. The omega-3 fatty acids found in fish reduce levels of triglyceride fats in the blood, and lower the risk of dangerous clots. Foods that are low-fat, low to moderate in calories, and high in nutrients can help maintain normal weight. The foods listed here as helpful to weight control contain no more than 30% of their calories in the form of fat.

Food	May Be Beneficial for	Why It's Good
Fish 1. Flounder 2. Haddock 3. Tuna 4. Bluefish 5. Mackerel 6. Trout 7. Herring 8. Salmon	Blood, heart, blood pressure, weight loss	Good source of easily absorbed iron; high in magnesium, potassium, phosphorus, zinc, B vitamins; flounder and haddock are low in fat; the others contain moderate-to-high levels of omega-3 fatty acids
Poultry 9. Duck 10. Goose 11. Turkey 12. Chicken	Blood, cancer prevention, heart, weight loss	Duck and goose are high in absorbable iron; goose is rich in vitamin E; turkey and chicken (without skin) are low in fat
Red meats 13. Extra-lean pork 14. Extra-lean beef 15. Extra-lean lamb 16. Venison	Blood, heart, weight loss	Good source of iron; extra-lean cuts are low in fat; venison is also low in cholesterol
Shellfish 17. Clams 18. Mussels 19. Oysters	Blood, heart, weight loss	All are low-fat, mineral-rich; clams and oysters are very high in iron
Dairy foods 20. Skim milk 21. Low-fat milk (1% fat) 22. Low-fat cottage cheese (1% fat) 23. Low-fat cheese 24. Nonfat yogurt	Bones, cancer prevention, heart, blood pressure, weight loss	All are rich in calcium, some are fortified with vitamin D to increase absorption; 1% milk contains only 20% of calories from fat, skim milk only 2%
Cruciferous vegetables 25. Cabbage 26. Bok choy (Chinese cabbage)	Cancer prevention, heart, blood pressure, weight loss, blood, bones	High in insoluble fiber, vitamin C, and folate; brussels sprouts and broccoli also have good levels of calcium, iron, and beta-carotene

Food	May Be Beneficial for	Why It's Good
27. Cauliflower		
28. Brussels sprouts		
29. Broccoli		
Orange-yellow fruits and vegetables	Cancer prevention, heart, blood pressure, weight loss, blood	All are rich in beta-carotene; last four are also good vegetable sources of iron
30. Winter squash		
31. Cantaloupe		
32. Apricots		
33. Mangoes		
34. Papaya		
35. Carrots		
36. Sweet potatoes		
37. Acorn squash		
38. Butternut squash		
39. Pumpkin		
Dark green, leafy vegetables	Cancer prevention, heart, blood pressure, weight loss	High in beta-carotene and vitamin C
40. Romaine lettuce		
41. Chicory		
42. Endive		
43. Watercress		
44. Spinach		
45. Kale		
46. Swiss chard		
47. Arugula		
48. Dandelion greens		
49. Turnip greens		
High-carbohydrate vegetables	Cancer prevention, heart, weight loss, blood, blood pressure	Both are rich in complex carbohydrates; potatoes are high in vitamins C and B_6, copper, magnesium, phosphorus, potassium, iron, and fiber; corn is high in B_6, folate, and fiber
50. Potatoes		
51. Corn		
Grains	Blood, cancer prevention, heart, blood pressure, weight loss, bones	Good sources of fiber and trace minerals, including iron; oatmeal lowers cholesterol; amaranth is high in calcium; high-fiber cereals and whole-grain bread are fortified with calcium, iron, and vitamins
52. Whole-wheat pasta		
53. Buckwheat		
54. Barley		
55. Wheat germ		
56. Brown rice		
57. Oatmeal		
58. Amaranth		
59. High-fiber cereals		

(continued)

The 100 Healthiest Foods—*Continued*

Food	May Be Beneficial for	Why It's Good
Grains—*continued*		
60. Whole-grain bread		
Beans	Blood, heart, blood pressure, weight loss	High in soluble fiber, iron, and other minerals; anasazi beans cause less gas
61. Pinto beans		
62. Navy beans		
63. Lima beans		
64. Lentils		
65. Kidney beans		
66. Peas		
67. Garbanzo beans (chick-peas)		
68. Adzuki beans		
69. Anasazi beans		
Vitamin C-rich fruits	Cancer prevention, heart, blood pressure, weight loss	Rich sources of vitamin C; most are good sources of potassium
70. Kiwifruit		
71. Acerola		
72. Pineapples		
73. Honeydew melons		
74. Pomegranates		
75. Persimmons		
Citrus fruits	Cancer prevention, heart, blood pressure, weight loss	Rich in vitamin C; stringy sections and inner peels are good sources of fiber (pectin, for cholesterol control); tangerines and pink grapefruit have small amounts of beta-carotene
76. Oranges		
77. Grapefruit		
78. Tangerines		
79. Lemons		
80. Limes		
Peppers	Cancer prevention, heart, blood pressure, weight loss	Very high in vitamin C
81. Sweet or bell peppers		

What's high in fiber, even higher in protein, low in fat, and has no cholesterol? Myco-protein, a chemical compound made from fungus. It's been available in the United Kingdom since 1985. Once it's approved in the United States, promoters expect it to be used as imitation beef, poultry, or ham.

Food	May Be Beneficial for	Why It's Good
82. Chili peppers		
Berries 83. Blueberries 84. Raspberries 85. Blackberries	Cancer prevention, heart, blood pressure, weight loss	High in vitamin C; seeds are very high in fiber
Nuts and seeds 86. Dried sunflower seeds 87. Dried pumpkin/ squash seeds	Blood, bones	Contain vitamin E and minerals: calcium, copper, iron, magnesium, phosphorus, potassium, zinc
Dried fruits 88. Raisins 89. Peaches 90. Prunes 91. Figs	Blood, cancer prevention, heart, blood pressure	High in fiber, low in fat; contain copper, iron, magnesium, phosphorus, potassium, zinc
High-fiber fruits 92. Apples 93. Bananas 94. Pears 95. Cherries	Cancer prevention, heart, blood pressure, weight loss	Rich sources of fiber, especially pectin
Garlic group 96. Garlic 97. Onions 98. Leeks	Heart, weight loss	Reduce cholesterol levels
Oils 99. Olive oil 100. Canola oil	Heart	High proportion of monounsaturated fat, which lowers total cholesterol and raises levels of HDL ("good") cholesterol

A garden in space—that's what NASA's planning for its space station. Under development now, the self-sustaining garden will produce food, recycle carbon dioxide and waste, and grow plants for fiber and medicines. Planned installation of the first unit: 1997.

Dumpty Takes Plunge

The yolk's on you, Humpty. So many people have decided to cut back on cholesterol by reducing egg consumption, they've given you a little nudge off that wall you've been perched on for so long.

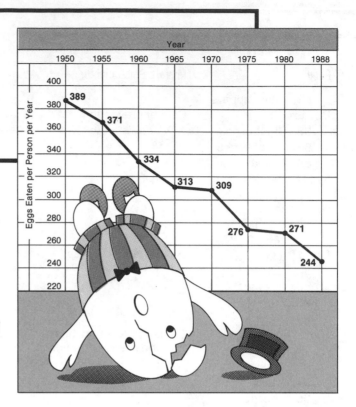

Americans are tossing away their brown bags, according to Campbell Soup Company. The "soup is good food" folks say fewer people than five years ago are taking their lunch to work. And when they do brown-bag it, they're favoring chips, fruit, and yogurt over salads and sandwiches.

Space Shuttle Cuisine

Astronauts on shuttle missions aren't exactly dining at Maxim's, but they do have some options. Many of their dishes are dehydrated and packed in plastic containers: The astronauts just inject water produced by the shuttle's fuel cell system.

For breakfast, they can wake up to thermostabilized peaches, rehydratable beef patty, rehydratable scrambled eggs, rehydratable bran flakes, rehydratable cocoa mix, and rehydratable orange drink.

Lunch might consist of thermostabilized hot dogs, rehydratable tur-key tetrazzini, irradiated bread, freeze-dried bananas, a totally natural almond crunch bar, and rehydratable apple drink.

The big meal of the day starts off with rehydratable shrimp cocktail, thermostabilized irradiated beef steak, rehydratable rice pilaf, rehydratable broccoli au gratin, thermostabilized fruit cocktail, thermostabilized butterscotch pudding, and rehydratable grape drink.

There's no provision for before- or after-dinner martinis.

Trends in Healthy Eating

Just as Americans are passing up meat and eggs for poultry and fish, so are they turning away from processed fruits in favor of fresh. Grain consumption is also up, along with fresh vegetables.

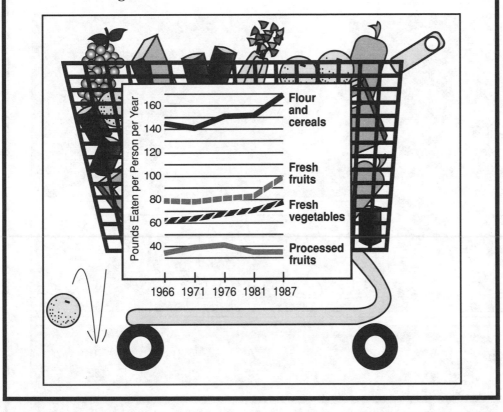

Eating Less May Prolong Life

Reducing daily calories has been shown to extend the life span of laboratory animals. It also delays age-related diseases and decreases their symptoms. How can this happen? Studies indicate that many of the characteristics of aging are associated with a declining ability of the liver to process protein. Researchers have found that the livers of animals on food-restricted regimens retain more of their protein-processing capabilities.

Our Favorite Salad Fixings

In 1989 researchers asked American salad munchers to pick their favorite 7 ingredients from a list of 20. This was the result.

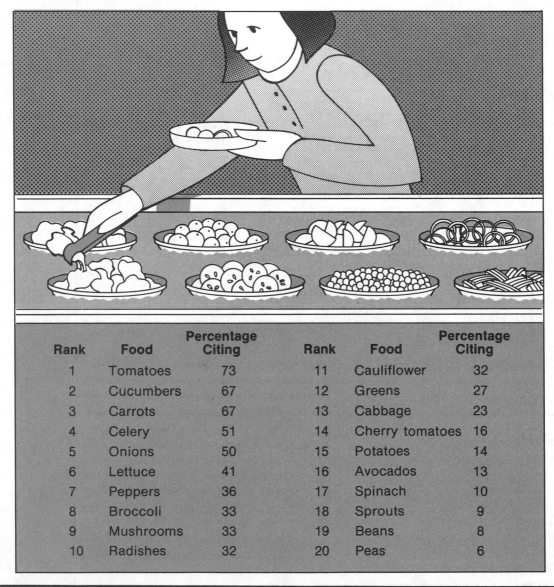

Rank	Food	Percentage Citing	Rank	Food	Percentage Citing
1	Tomatoes	73	11	Cauliflower	32
2	Cucumbers	67	12	Greens	27
3	Carrots	67	13	Cabbage	23
4	Celery	51	14	Cherry tomatoes	16
5	Onions	50	15	Potatoes	14
6	Lettuce	41	16	Avocados	13
7	Peppers	36	17	Spinach	10
8	Broccoli	33	18	Sprouts	9
9	Mushrooms	33	19	Beans	8
10	Radishes	32	20	Peas	6

Heads above Iceberg: The Best Leafy Greens

There's lettuce, and then there's lettuce. A look at this table tells you that America's favorite lettuce, iceberg, isn't the healthiest, not by a long shot. And lettuce in general pales by comparison with darker greens.

Greens	Characteristics	Vitamin A (I.U.)	Vitamin C (mg)	Calcium (mg)	Iron (mg)	Potassium (mg)
Amaranth greens	Bland, mild taste that combines well with other flavors.	2,917	43.3	215.0*	2.3	611
Arugula	Sharp, spicy, mustard flavor. An interesting change from spinach.	7,422	91.0	309.0	9.5	145
Beet greens	Earthy, beety, chardlike taste. Best when leaves are young and tiny.	6,100	30.0	119.0*	3.3	547
Butterhead lettuce (buttercrunch, Boston)	Sweet, succulent lettuces with distinctive flavor and smooth, buttery texture.	970	8.0	35.0	0.3	257
Crisphead lettuce (iceberg, Great Lakes)	A mild-flavored, crunchy, lettuce with brittle leaf texture.	330	3.9	19.0	0.5	158
Dandelion	Pungent. Very nutritious. Use young leaves in salads; sauté tough leaves.	13,720	34.4	182.0	3.0	388
Endive (also includes escarole)	An agreeably bitter taste with chewy crispness and a strong texture. Inner leaves are sweet and mild.	2,050	6.5	52.0*	0.8	314
Kale	A strong-flavored green. Tender young leaves are more delicate in flavor than older leaves.	8,900	120.0	135.0	1.7	447
Loose-leaf lettuce (oak-leaf, ruby, black-seeded Simpson)	Tender lettuces with exceptionally good texture. Leaves range from smooth to wrinkly and are green or red in color.	1,900	18.0	68.0	1.4	264
Parsley, curly	Tangy and sweet. Helps to bring out flavor of other herbs and seasonings.	5,200	90.0	130.0*	6.2	536
Radicchio	Appealingly bitter. Vivid red with a snappy flavor.	462	26.4	9.8	2.5	N/A
Romaine	Strong taste. Used in Caesar salads.	2,548	23.5	39.2	1.1	284
Spinach	Bright and leafy; sports a grassy flavor. Thick leaves supported by tough stems.	6,715	28.1	99.0*	2.7	558
Turnip greens	Strong flavor. More nutritious than the root vegetable. Eat raw or cooked.	7,448	58.8	185.5	1.1	290

NOTE: All nutrient values are based on 3½-oz. servings.

*These greens contain oxalic acid, which inhibits absorption of calcium, so not all the calcium in the greens is bioavailable.

Food, Guilt, and Self-Indulgence

People seem to know what foods are good for them. Witness the results of this first survey, in which people confess that they need to eat more of the healthiest foods. But a second survey shows that people also know which foods make them feel better when they need to indulge themselves. When it comes to indulgence, note that women favor desserts and treats, while men favor entrées.

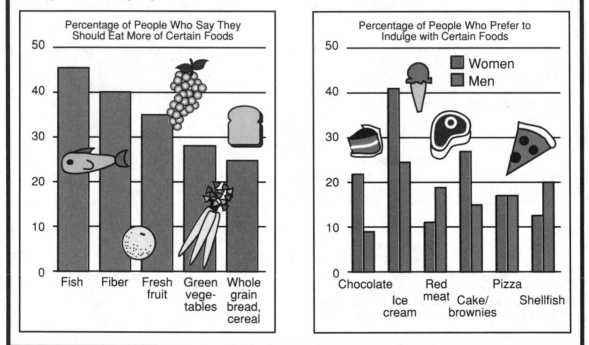

Is That a Fact?

Chocolate in milk interferes with your body's ability to absorb calcium.

Apparently not. Creighton University School of Medicine researchers gave a small number of women calcium from a variety of sources, including milk, chocolate milk, yogurt, cheese, and calcium supplements. Tests of blood calcium levels indicated the same degree of absorption, no matter where the calcium came from—including chocolate milk.

Comparing Diets: Soviets and Americans

Political systems notwithstanding, Soviets and Americans have at least one thing in common—a diet high in fat, cholesterol, and calories. Here's how the two superpowers match up in terms of overall nutrition.

Nutrient*	U.S.S.R.	U.S.
Food energy	3,200 calories	3,400 calories
Protein	100 g	100 g
Fat	100 g	160 g
Cholesterol	400 mg	490 mg
Carbohydrate	490 g	390 g
Minerals		
Calcium	760 mg	870 mg
Zinc	12 mg	12 mg
Iron	15 mg	17 mg
Magnesium	420 mg	330 mg
Vitamins		
Thiamine	1.8 mg	2.1 mg
Riboflavin	1.8 mg	2.3 mg
Vitamin C	120 mg	120 mg
Vitamin A	5,800 I.U.	7,700 I.U.
Vitamin B_6	2 mg	2 mg
Vitamin B_{12}	6.6 mcg	9.1 mcg

*Per capita per day. U.S. data include iron, thiamine, vitamin C, vitamin A, vitamin B_6, and vitamin B_{12} added by enrichment and fortification.

When Do People Eat Fresh Fruit?

Fresh fruit is one of America's favorite between-meal treats. To be truly superior, a snack should be healthy, convenient, fresh, and above all, good tasting. Fresh fruit fills the bill for many.

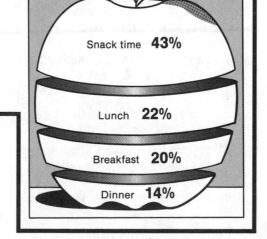

Snack time **43%**

Lunch **22%**

Breakfast **20%**

Dinner **14%**

Almost 50 percent of American lunches are eaten away from home.

America's Favorite Ethnic Cuisines

When it comes to ethnic eating, Chinese cuisine rules in America, with the most restaurants in northern California, the South, the Midwest, the Pacific Northwest, and eastern New England. But Italian dominates most of the East Coast, while Mexican prevails in the plains, mountains, and Southwest.

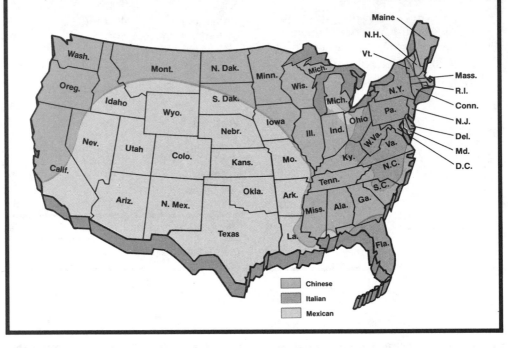

Chinese

Italian

Mexican

Food Facts

Rank of white bread, rolls, and crackers as calorie sources in the American diet: 1. Rank of doughnuts, cookies, and cake: 2. Rank of alcohol: 3.

Equivalent in M&M's of the daily amount of glucose the human brain needs: 250.

Rank of snails, brains, squid, shark, and tripe in list of foods Americans hate the most: 1, 2, 3, 4, 5.

Percentage of Americans who nibble corn-on-the-cob from side to side like a typewriter: 20.

Guinness Book of World Records' record for number of baked beans eaten one by one with a cocktail stick in 30 minutes: 2,780.

Record number of bananas eaten in 2 minutes: 17.

Pounds of chocolate eaten by the average American in 1986: 8.6.

Quarts of popcorn eaten by the average American per year: 42.

21

FOOT PROBLEMS

Your feet ache? Three out of four Americans echo your complaint, and little wonder. Every workday, most of us spend a quarter of our time standing on our feet. Every year, we walk the distance between Chicago and California's Yosemite National Park, about 2,000 miles. In a lifetime, we rack up enough mileage to have circled the globe not once, not twice, not thrice, but *four* times.

That's a big feat for a couple of little feet, but they're built to handle it. Simple as they may seem down there in the shadow of our big bodies, our feet are actually quite smartly constructed. A single foot has 18 muscles, 31 tendons, 107 ligaments, 30 joints, and 28 bones—all working together to take us where we want to go with efficiency and grace.

No two feet are alike, not even your own—one is usually larger than the other, for instance. And they're always changing. If you gain weight, they'll get wider. If you lose weight, they'll slim down. As you age, your muscles lose their tone, causing your foot to lengthen. Age also brings a thinning of the layers of protective padding along your foot's bottom and between the skin and bones, leaving you more susceptible to foot injuries and other maladies.

About 85 percent of Americans have a foot problem some time during their lives—mostly after the age of 50. More women develop blisters, corns, painful bunions, calluses, and ingrown toenails. More men suffer from athlete's foot, foot injuries, and foot odor.

An estimated 60 to 70 percent of foot problems are inherited. Your genes dictate a characteristic foot shape which may then be aggravated by poor care or ill-fitting shoes. The 1 billion people in the world who go shoeless have fewer foot problems than anybody else. In more "civilized" cultures, shoes may contribute to as many as 80 percent of all foot problems. Nevertheless, 20 percent of men and 45 percent of women in the United States admit that in order to be fashionable they're willing to wear shoes that hurt.

247

Why Your Tootsies Are Tired Tonight

Your feet are under an incredible amount of pressure. The sensitive soles, heels, and toes of a person who weighs just 135 pounds absorb a cumulative pressure of more than 2.5 million pounds while stepping through a typical day. If you're heavier, you're piling on even greater pressure.

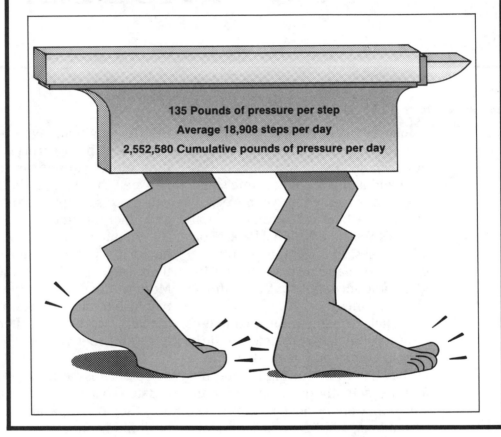

135 Pounds of pressure per step

Average 18,908 steps per day

2,552,580 Cumulative pounds of pressure per day

Is That A Fact?

Cutting a "V" in the center of an ingrown toenail will encourage the nail to grow toward the center and away from the ingrown edge.

Not true. The fact is, all nails grow straight forward only, from back to front. Cutting out a section won't make any difference.

The Top Five Foot Complaints

Doctors nationwide reported that 39 percent of their patients complained about sore feet, according to a survey conducted by Scholl's. The chart shows the five most frequently reported foot problems.

Complaint	Percentage of Patients Affected
1. Sore, aching feet	39
2. Ingrown toenails	28
3. Corns	24
4. Warts/Plantar Warts	21
5. Calluses	18

Pronation vs. Supination: Which Side Are You On?

Your feet naturally lean slightly to one side or the other when they strike the ground during a step. *Pronation* is your foot's tendency to roll inward when it strikes the ground. The movement absorbs shock and helps you balance by getting a maximum amount of your foot onto the ground. But too much of a good thing, *overpronation* in this case, can cause your foot to roll inward excessively and your knee to twist inward, putting you at risk for injuries. Overpronation is a common cause for concern among runners. You can compensate for overpronation by wearing well-reinforced shoes that help control and stabilize your foot's motion.

In *supination,* your foot leans outward and the outside of your foot strikes the ground first. Wearing shoes with strong ankle and heel support can help compensate.

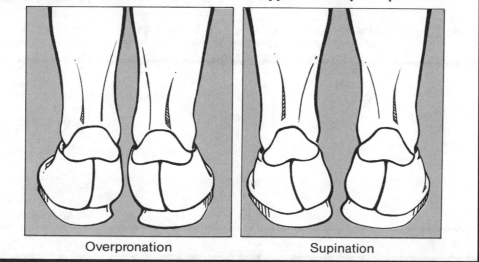

Overpronation   Supination

A Guide to Everyday Foot Problems

Foot problems are just about as common as feet. Who among us hasn't hobbled around with a callused sole or a blistered heel? Fortunately, many foot problems lend themselves to self-treatment. A few don't. This chart will help you tell the difference. Be sure to consult a foot specialist for a major foot problem or if a minor one persists.

Problem	Description	Cause	Prevention	Treatment
Corn	Small area of thickened dead skin, generally on top of a toe or on the sole of the foot.	Usually results from shoe friction.	Wear well-fitted shoes that don't rub against toes or push toes together. Avoid tight hosiery.	Soften a hard corn by soaking the foot in warm, soapy water, then applying a drop of oil to the corn. Gently rub off the top layer with an emery board or pumice. Do not remove too much at once. Wash and cover with a corn pad. Protect a hard corn with moleskin or with petroleum jelly under a bandage. Do not try to cut a corn or remove it with over-the-counter products.
Callus	Thick, flat pad of dead, hard skin, usually on the heel or ball of the foot.	The foot's structure or the way you walk.	Wear properly fitted shoes. Use cushioned insoles. Keep feet well lubricated with cream or lotion.	As with a corn, soak in warm, soapy water and rub callus gently with moistened pumice to remove the top layer of dead skin. At night before bed, apply cream or petroleum jelly. Protect with moleskin while wearing shoes.

Problem	Description	Cause	Prevention	Treatment
Blister	Fluid-filled cushion that forms when the top layer of skin is damaged.	Excessive friction on the skin from shoes or socks. Also due to skin that is too dry or sweaty.	Wear well-fitted shoes and socks. If the shape of your feet causes them to rub against every pair of shoes you buy, apply moleskin padding to the problem areas. If feet are too dry, apply a thin coat of petroleum jelly before activity. If feet are too sweaty, sprinkle cornstarch in socks and shoes.	Cover a small blister with a sterile dressing and let it heal by itself. For a large blister, sterilize a needle with 70% isopropyl alcohol, clean the blister with an antiseptic, then make small holes in it with the needle to release the fluid. Blot the fluid with sterile gauze, apply antibiotic cream, and cover with protective pad.
Bunion	Gradual enlargement and dislocation of the big toe joint, often accompanied by an inward tilt of the big toe and inflammation. (Bunionettes are bunions on the sides of the little toes.)	An inherited tendency, aggravated by shoes that are not wide or roomy enough.	None, but good shoes may keep it from worsening.	Wear low-heeled shoes with rounded toes. Apply ice to painful bunions, elevate feet for 20 minutes, and follow with a soak in warm water. A foot specialist may recommend special pads, physical therapy, or surgery.

(continued)

A Guide to Everyday Foot Problems—*Continued*

Problem	Description	Cause	Prevention	Treatment
Hammertoes	Permanently bent toes, sometimes accompanying painful corns on the joints or under the tips of the toes.	Possibly an inherited tendency irritated by tight shoes.	Wear shoes with wide toes.	If the problem is very painful or persistent, see a physician, who may recommend surgery.
Ingrown toenail	Painful condition in which the side of a nail grows and digs into the skin, sometimes leading to inflammation and infection.	Improper nail cutting, toe injury, or fungal infection.	Avoid pointed or tight shoes that press on toenails. Keep nails cut but not too short. Use clean nail clippers made to cut straight across.	Soak foot in lukewarm water to soften nail, then tuck a small wisp of cotton between the nail edge and skin to hold nail away from flesh. Do this daily until nail grows out beyond the corner.
Athlete's foot	Itching, burning, cracking, and blistering skin, usually between the toes.	Fungal infection.	Keep feet clean and dry. Wear absorbent socks and shoes made of a breathable material like leather or canvas.	Wash feet twice a day and apply an over-the-counter antifungal preparation. Sprinkle shoes with medicated powder every day and spray them once or twice a week with disinfectant.
Plantar warts	Spongy, flat warts on the soles of the feet.	Highly contagious virus.	Don't go barefoot at places like the beach or health club, where virus may be lurking. Keep feet dry.	See a foot specialist for treatment with chemicals, dry ice, surgery, or lasers. Avoid over-the-counter treatments.

A Quick and Easy Foot Massage

Treat your feet to a good massage to help prevent foot soreness, relieve tiredness, and keep your muscles loose and flexible.

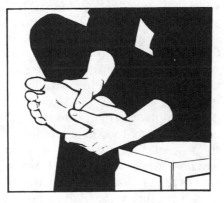

1. Sit on a chair and place one foot on the opposite thigh. Rub some massage oil or lotion on your foot. Apply pressure with your thumbs to the sole of your foot, working from the bottom of the arch to the top near your big toe. Repeat five times.

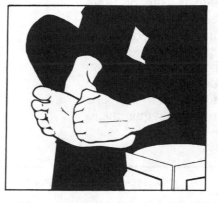

2. Make a fist and use your knuckles to move from your heel to your toes. Repeat five times.

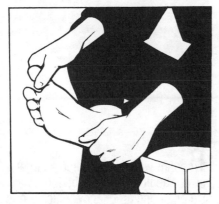

3. Massage each toe by holding it firmly and moving it from side to side. Apply pressure to the areas between the toes.

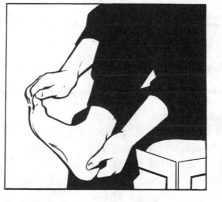

4. Hold all your toes with one hand and bend them backward, holding for 5 to 10 seconds. Bend them in the opposite direction and hold. Repeat three times.

Big Shoes for Bigfoot

If there really is a gigantic ape-like man called Bigfoot out there stomping around the American wilderness, he is going to have a hard time finding shoes that fit. Based on 16-inch-long footprints attributed to the semimythical creature, experts calculate Bigfoot's shoe requirements at an awesome size 25. (Extra wide, we presume.)

A Brief History of Shoe Misery

The first shoes, sandals woven from papyrus, were worn about 5,000 years ago by the Egyptians. Shoe styles since haven't always been so simple, let alone so comfortable. In China, women who could squeeze small feet into tiny shoes were considered more sexually desirable, so girls' feet were painfully bound to prevent growth. In the fourteenth century, pointy-toed shoes, believed to protect their wearers against witches, were popular in Europe. Aristocratic Italian women in the fifteenth century wore platform heels as high as 30 inches tall, shoes considered so dangerous that a law was passed to prohibit their use by pregnant women, who put their unborn children's lives at risk by wearing them.

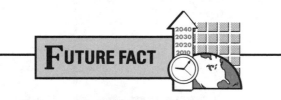

FUTURE FACT

High-Tech Foot Analysis

That's what you may soon be stepping into, via a computerized insole that measures pressure distribution under the foot. The computer displays color-coded images that enable physicians to analyze gait, detect diseases, and prescribe corrections. Called EMED, the system also shows promise for showing athletes the best shoe design for a particular activity, and helping ski boot makers to create designs that minimize injuries.

Pregnant women may need a larger shoe size. The ligaments of the foot relax and stretch during pregnancy, which tends to flatten and spread the foot. Pregnancy may also cause swelling in feet and legs. Sturdy, roomy shoes with good support and wide heels (no higher than 1½ inches) may feel best.

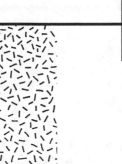

22

GENDER DIFFERENCES

Your sex is determined at the moment of conception. Your mother gives you an X chromosome. Your father gives you either an X or a Y. If he contributes an X, you are female. If his sperm carries a Y, you are male. About seven to ten weeks later, the genitals of the embryo begin to form, becoming either ovaries or testes. And that's when the two sexes begin to branch apart.

Gender differences in health are real. Biologically, females have distinct advantages over males. In the United States, while 125 males are conceived for every 100 females, and 106 live males are born for every 100 females, almost 33 percent more boys than girls die within the first year. Later in life, as well, females enjoy an edge. They are less vulnerable to many of the major life-threatening ailments, and generally outlive their male counterparts.

Scientists once assumed that women would lose their health and life-expectancy advantage as increasing numbers of females entered the job market and were subjected to the same pressures as men. But several studies prove this untrue. Women in executive jobs, for instance, do not show a higher incidence of heart disease than other women. More flexible female roles notwithstanding, women still enjoy a healthy edge.

Seeing the Not-So-Obvious Differences

Just as scientists can see gender differences in chromosomes, they've discovered other minute variations between the sexes, beyond the obvious genital differences. Some of these characteristics, according to anthropologists, were developed in response to special environmental needs. Here are some highlights.

His

Hair—By age 60, 80 percent of white men will have some hair loss. Blame male sex hormones (androgens) and heredity.

Eyebrows—Bushiness is female attraction signal.

Nose—Usually larger than a woman's.

Beard—An average man can grow a foot-long beard in just over two years. It is a natural scent-carrier for man's hormone-induced scents.

Chin—Protuberant chin and heavy jaw.

Chest—Broader, longer.

Fat—More lean body tissue.

Hand—About twice the gripping power of the average woman's hand—up to 120 pounds of pressure.

Belly—More likely to have a pot-belly.

Navel—Less recessed than that of a woman (if both are of average build).

Buttocks—Dimples that show up on women are visible in only 18 to 25 percent of men.

Hers

Hair—No balding, but when she gets old, there may be an overall thinning of hair.

Eyebrows—Naturally less bushy than a man's, but often exaggerated by plucking or shaving.

Belly—More rounded than that of men. Proportionally longer, with greater distance between the navel and genitals.

Upper arms—Usually more fat at this site than in men.

Hand—Lighter, thinner fingers with more flexible finger joints.

Thigh—Usually more fat at this site than in men.

Pelvis—Broader than a man's, with larger space in the middle to accommodate baby during childbirth.

Buttocks—Two dimples, appearing at either side of the base of the spine, are more distinct on a woman because of fat deposits.

Fat—May have up to twice the fatty tissue of a man the same height.

Women Have
More Chronic Illness

Although men are more likely to be injured or impaired, women are much more likely to suffer from chronic health complaints. Here are some selected comparisons.

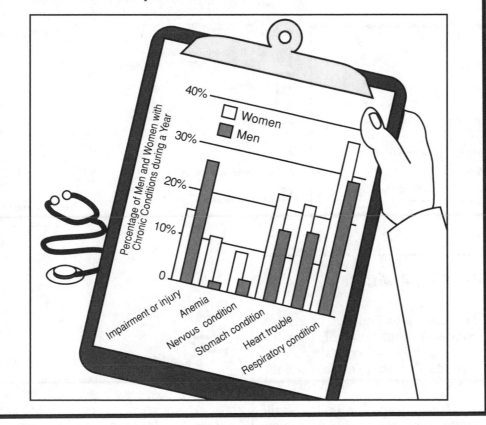

Women are more "coachable" in athletics than men, according to a sports psychologist at Pennsylvania State University. She believes that's because men are accustomed to using their bodies to please themselves, while women are taught to use their bodies to attract and please others.

Different Ways of Dying

Men are more likely than women to die from the two major killers, heart disease and cancer. The chart summarizes death rate differences by sex for the ten leading causes of death.

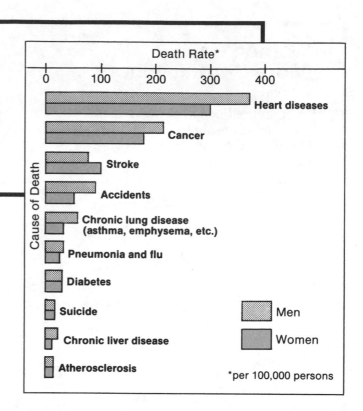

Death Rate*

Cause of Death:
- Heart diseases
- Cancer
- Stroke
- Accidents
- Chronic lung disease (asthma, emphysema, etc.)
- Pneumonia and flu
- Diabetes
- Suicide
- Chronic liver disease
- Atherosclerosis

Men / Women

*per 100,000 persons

While women get sick more often than men, men aren't necessarily more healthy. Men may avoid expressing their pain or asking for help—both feminine characteristics—and by so doing, shorten their lives.

IS THAT A FACT?

Men have an advantage when it comes to weight control. They can eat more and not gain extra pounds. And they can lose weight more easily than women can.

It's all true. The daily calorie intake recommended for women aged 23 to 50 is only 1,600 to 2,000 calories—compared with 2,300 to 2,700 calories for men. And because women have up to twice as much fatty tissue as men of the same height do, the average male has fewer fat cells to fight when he's trying to lose weight.

Women can remember better than men as they grow older, according to research at Johns Hopkins Medical Institutions in Baltimore. Two hundred healthy men and women between ages 40 and 89 were given a 15-noun word list to memorize. Men generally lagged slightly behind women of comparable age throughout the testing. However, men in their late sixties scored a full 20 percent lower than women. It's not that men have more trouble learning, says neurologist Margit Bleecker, M.D., Ph.D. Women appear to be more adept at information *retrieval*.

Life Expectancy at Birth: Girls Have the Edge

Throughout this century, gender has played a part in life expectancy. A baby boy born in 1900 could expect to live 47.9 years. A girl, 50.7 years. A baby boy born today can expect to live 71.3 years. A baby girl can look forward to 78.3 years. By the year 2000, a newborn boy's projected life span will be 73.5 years. A girl's, 80.4.

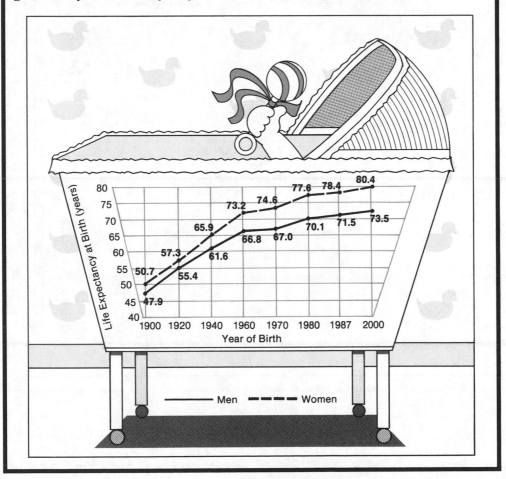

Life Expectancy at Birth (years) vs. Year of Birth

Women: 50.7, 57.3, 65.9, 73.2, 74.6, 77.6, 78.4, 80.4
Men: 47.9, 55.4, 61.6, 66.8, 67.0, 70.1, 71.5, 73.5

Years: 1900, 1920, 1940, 1960, 1970, 1980, 1987, 2000

— Men   - - - Women

A man spending 10 minutes a day shaving will use up 106 days removing his beard by age 60.

How Many Years Are Still Ahead?

At any given age, gender plays a part in determining how many years we have left to live. Here's a chart that demonstrates the ongoing differences in life expectancy between the sexes.

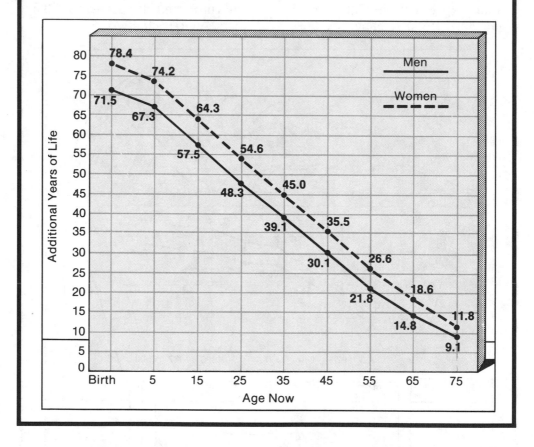

~~~W~~~omen are usually paid only 70 percent of a man's salary for the same work, according to a survey by Significance, a Ridgewood, New Jersey, company.

~~~M~~~en are more skilled than women at using humor to create a relaxed atmosphere. Boys feel freer to tell jokes and do funny things. One study showed girls check the reactions of others before laughing at cartoons.

FILE ON THE FAMOUS

Man, Woman, or a Little Bit of Both?

Sometimes a biologically normal male or female believes that he or she is meant to be of the other gender—and resolves to do something about it. One of the first such persons to have "gender reassignment surgery," or surgery to become the other gender, was George Jorgensen.

At an early age Jorgensen identified with female characteristics: He wished for a doll with long golden hair; he avoided rough-and-tumble games; he described himself as being frail and introverted. Jorgensen was drafted into the service at the end of World War II, when he was 19. He weighed 98 pounds, had underdeveloped genitals and almost no beard.

He felt emotionally attached to several men and said he wished he could relate to them and to the rest of the world as a woman.

In 1950, Jorgensen moved to Copenhagen, Denmark, where gender reassignment surgery was being done. In 1952, he had three operations. Then, at age 26, he returned to the United States as a she—Christine Jorgensen.

Thirty years after her sex reassignment made the headlines, Jorgensen described her life in positive terms, saying she didn't regret the surgery and that she might not have survived without it.

Caffeine causes men, but not women, to eat less. In a study at Laval University in Quebec, men consumed 22 percent fewer calories after ingesting 300 milligrams of caffeine. Women ate the same amount of food as they would normally. Caffeine—in this case an amount equal to about three cups of coffee or four and a half cans of cola—activates the sympathetic nervous system and increases energy expenditure. Women tend to conserve energy when their systems are triggered; men don't.

Men are more likely to abuse illegal drugs than women. Male heroin addicts, for example, outnumber women three to one. But women are more likely to use legal prescription drugs and more likely to have drugs prescribed for them. Two-thirds of the prescriptions for the mind-affecting drugs Valium and Librium are for women.

Answering Nature's Call

You've seen the lines at the ladies' restroom. And, you've seen the way men whoosh in and out of their restroom. Is it your imagination, or do women really need more time? Cornell University engineering students analyzed toilet-use patterns at highway rest stops for the Washington State Department of Transportation. The results show just how unequal the sexes are.

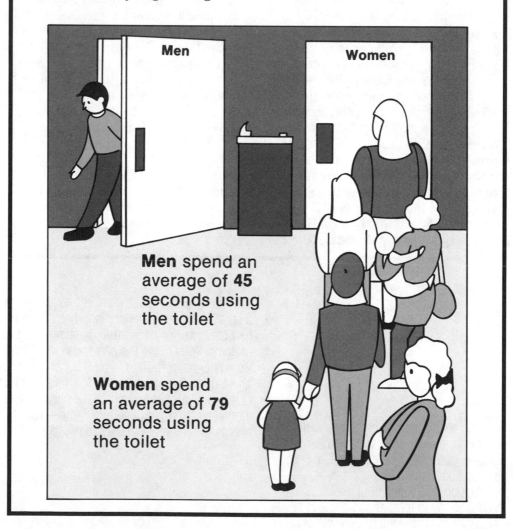

Men

Women

Men spend an average of **45** seconds using the toilet

Women spend an average of **79** seconds using the toilet

The Creativity Connection

Some experts think there is a link between creativity and the ability to draw upon both the male and female aspects of our personalities. Studies in California comparing creative male architects to their less creative colleagues found that the former scored higher in measures of femininity. Another study (illustrated here), of 10- and 11-year-old school children, showed that those with versatile use of both sides of their sexual makeup were more creative than their gender-regimented schoolmates, with top honors going to the masculine girls.

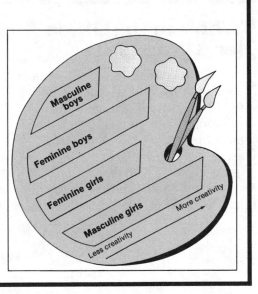

Vital Statistics

Percentage of men happy with their weight: 67
Percentage of women: 50

Percentage of women who change their diet to reduce cholesterol intake: 50
Percentage of men: 33

Average number of days per year missed in the office by working mothers: 9
By fathers: 4

Average number of days spent in the hospital by men: 7.0
By women: 6.3

Percentage of working mothers who stay home with a sick child: 66
Percentage of working fathers: 21

Percentage of men who are color blind: 8
Percentage of women: 0.5

Percentage of men who say they can eat pretty much what they want without gaining weight: 61
Percentage of women: 42

Percentage of wives who mention their housework when describing a typical day: 97
Percentage of husbands: 54

Percentage of women who mention children as part of their typical day: 97
Percentage of men: 69

Percentage of weight that fat accounts for in adult men: 10 to 20
Percentage in women: 25

Percentage of women who have cried in the office: 80
Percentage of men: 50

Percentage of women who say they avoid the sun: 67
Percentage of men: 46

Who's in the Office (and Who Isn't)

Who will call in sick on Monday morning? One study shows female office workers aged 17 to 24 are more likely to call in sick than any other group. Men aged 25 to 44 are the most likely to be at their desks on any given day.

Accidental injuries were the leading cause of lost workdays among male office personnel. Next were respiratory system problems and diseases of the digestive system. For women, pregnancy and maternity-related conditions were the most cited excuses. Respiratory diseases and accidental injuries followed.

Here's how the genders' attendance records compared.

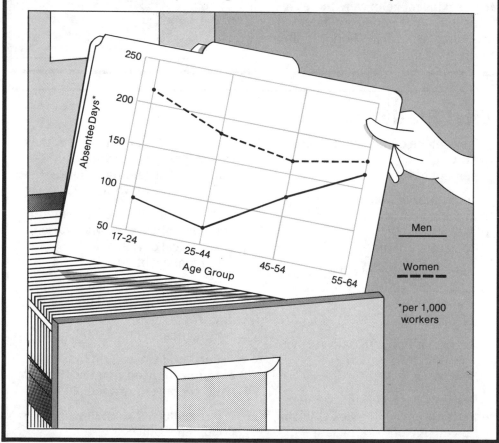

Men

Women

*per 1,000 workers

Women with Alzheimer's disease outnumber men by more than two to one.

Gender at the Gym

While women are only slightly more inclined to exercise regularly than men (22 percent versus 18 percent), they do dominate five of seven popular fitness activities. The illustration compares levels of participation.

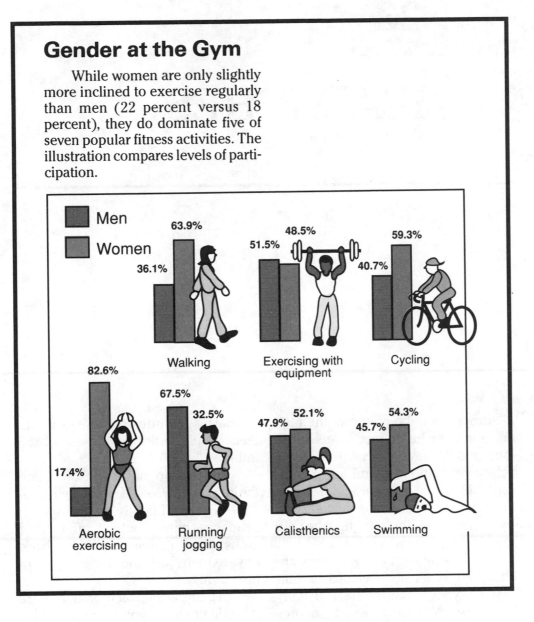

Men and women both use hand gestures when speaking, but men tend to gesture more slowly.

23

HEADACHES

Almost everybody knows the misery of headache. In fact, three out of four people have at least one headache a year. And for 45 million Americans, headaches are a chronic problem. Fortunately, most headaches are not signs of serious illness, though the pain may be very annoying.

Ninety percent of headaches are classified as tension headaches, and that everyday villain, stress, is usually the cause. Migraines, which involve the cerebral arteries, bring even more severe pain and affect 16 to 18 million people, the majority of them women.

The sum of all this head pain is more than $4 million a year spent on over-the-counter remedies and an annual loss to industry—due to absenteeism and medical expenses—of $55 million.

Those who suffer the most and the longest may look beyond their medicine chest and family doctor. Special headache clinics, which offer other forms of treatment such as biofeedback, now exist in just about every part of the country.

In general, headache sufferers are more likely to be younger than older. Asked if they had had at least one headache in the preceding 12 months, more than 80 percent of those aged 18 to 34 said yes. But only 50 percent of those 65 and older reported at least one headache in the last year.

How Long Do Headaches Last?

Headaches tend to last at least 5 hours. In the following study of males and females 12 to 29 years of age, the average length of the most recent headache was 5.9 hours for males and 8.2 hours for females.

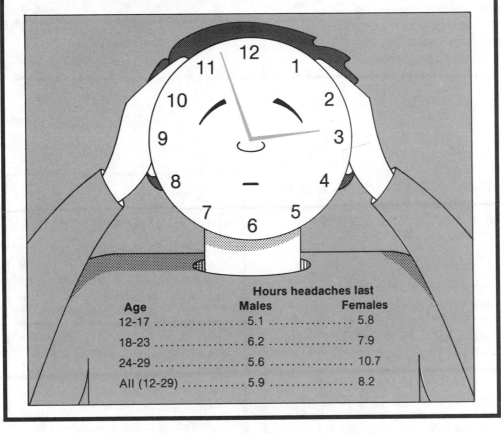

Age	Hours headaches last	
---	Males	Females
12-17	5.1	5.8
18-23	6.2	7.9
24-29	5.6	10.7
All (12-29)	5.9	8.2

What's good for an ailing marriage may also be good for a headache. According to a Canadian study, several headache sufferers attending marital counseling sessions reported marked improvement in their headaches.

Frequency of Headaches

Seventy percent of males who were surveyed reported no more than one headache in the month preceding the study. And while only 6 percent of males reported four headaches or more in the preceding month, more than twice as many females (14 percent) said they had suffered four or more headaches.

Number of Headaches in Past Month	Percentage of Men	Percentage of Women
0	43.0	23.6
1	27.1	28.1
2	18.8	25.4
3	5.0	8.9
4	6.1	14.0

More than half of the new patients at a headache clinic chose not to follow recommendations, leading researchers to speculate that many chronic headache sufferers never take their doctors' advice.

The Cold Facts about "Ice Cream" Headaches

Sudden headaches after eating something very cold, such as ice cream, are fairly common. But this reaction is especially likely in people with a history of migraine, who are three times more likely than non-migraine sufferers to report "ice cream" headaches. Eating ice cream very slowly will help decrease the shock of cold and help head off a headache.

The Top Ten Headache Triggers

Chronic headache sufferers were asked to name two or three regular contributing causes of their headaches. Here are the top ten.

Causes	Percentage of People Surveyed
Stress (unspecified)	50
Other	21
Sinus problems	18
Job stress	14
Fatigue	9
Eye problems/conditions	8
Weather	8
Allergies	7
Dietary conditions/foods	7
Friends/family problems	3

A Guide to Common Headaches

Type	Symptoms	Precipitating Factors	Treatment	Prevention
Tension headaches	Dull, nonthrobbing pain, frequently bilateral, associated with tightness of scalp or neck. Degree of severity remains constant.	Emotional stress, hidden depression.	Rest, aspirin, acetaminophen, ice packs, muscle relaxants; antidepressants if appropriate; biofeedback, psychotherapy; if necessary, *temporary* use of stronger analgesics.	Avoidance of stress; use of biofeedback, relaxation techniques, or antidepressant medication.
Common migraine	Severe, one-sided throbbing pain, often accompanied by nausea, vomiting, cold hands, tremor, dizziness, sensitivity to sound and light.	Certain foods; use of the Pill or menopausal hormones; excessive hunger, change in altitude or weather; bright or flashing lights; excessive smoking, emotional stress; hereditary component.	Ice packs; analgesics such as Darvon or codeine; medications known as vasoconstrictors, such as ergotamine, which constrict the blood vessels; for prolonged attacks, steriods may be helpful.	Avoidance of precipitating factors; biofeedback; Propranolol.
Classic migraine	Same as for common migraine, except victim develops warning symptoms, which may include visual disturbances, numbness in arm or leg, the smelling of strange odors, hallucinations.	Same as for common migraine.	At earliest onset of symptoms use of biofeedback or vasoconstrictors can ward off attack; once pain has begun, treatment is the same as for common migraine.	Same as for common migraine.
Cluster headaches	Excruciating pain around or behind one eye. Tearing of eye, congestion of nose, flushing of face. Pain frequently develops during sleep and may last for several hours. Attacks occur every day for weeks or months, then disappear for up to a year.	Alcoholic beverages, excessive smoking.	Ergotamine or oxygen inhalation.	Steriods, ergotamine, methysergide; small regular doses of lithium carbonate for chronic cluster headaches.

(continued)

269

A Guide to Common Headaches—*Continued*

Type	Symptoms	Precipitating Factors	Treatment	Prevention
Menstrual headaches	Migraine-type pain that occurs shortly before, during, or after menstruation or midcycle, at time of ovulation.	Variance in estrogen levels.	Same as for migraine.	Small doses of vasoconstrictors before and during menstrual period; anti-inflammatory drugs during menstruation may also help. Hysterectomy does not cure menstrual headaches.
Hypertension headaches	Generalized or "hatband" type pain, most severe in morning. Diminishes as day goes on.	Severe high blood pressure over 200 systolic and 110 diastolic.	Appropriate blood pressure medication.	Keep blood pressure under control.
Aneurysm	Early symptoms may mimic frequent migraine or cluster headaches. Cause is balloonlike weakness or bulge in blood-vessel wall. May rupture or allow blood to leak slowly. A ruptured aneurysm (stroke) results in sudden, unbearable headache, double vision, rigid neck. Victim rapidly becomes unconscious.	Congenital tendency; extremely high blood pressure.	If detected early, surgery.	Keep blood pressure under control; if aneurysm is severe, surgery may be indicated.
Sinus headaches	A gnawing pain over nasal area, often increasing in severity as day goes on. Caused by acute infection, usually with fever, producing blockage of sinus ducts and preventing normal drainage. Sinus headaches are rare—migraine and cluster headaches are often misdiagnosed as sinus in origin.	Infection, nasal polyps, anatomical deformities, such as deviated septum that block the sinus ducts.	Antibiotics, decongestants, surgical drainage, if necessary.	None.

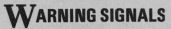 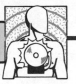

WARNING SIGNALS

Heed These Danger Signs

Usually headaches are not nearly as serious as they are painful. One study of 1,000 chronic headache sufferers found only one brain tumor. But occasionally headaches are symptoms of serious disease. So be alert for the following:

▼ Recurring headaches that appear for the first time after the age of 40

▼ Headaches that are getting stronger

▼ Headaches that are occurring more frequently

▼ Headaches that have changed locations

▼ Headaches that do not fit a pattern (there seems to be nothing in particular that triggers them)

▼ Headaches that have begun to disrupt life and interfere with work and regular activities

▼ Headaches that are accompanied by numbness, dizziness, blurred vision, or memory loss

▼ Headaches that coincide with other pain or medical problems

IS THAT A FACT?

Sex can give you a headache. So can too much sleep.

Unfortunately, both statements are true. Some people develop headaches during sex (it's more common in people with a history of migraine). Sleep most often brings on a headache when the body gets too much of it, like when you sleep late on the weekend or take a nap.

But guess what else is a fact? In some instances, sex and sleep can also bring *relief* from headaches. Many people have great success "sleeping off" a headache. And, in a study of migraine sufferers, several people reported moderate to complete relief from migraine after having sex.

Facts about Migraine

▼ Migraines most often strike women; in fact, 70 percent of migraine sufferers are female.

▼ A nap or the aroma of strong perfume can trigger a migraine attack.

▼ Migraine headaches tend to run in families.

▼ Though many "triggers" for migraine have been identified, the root cause of migraine remains a mystery.

Pain Patterns in Headaches

In comparing headache occurrence over time, migraines tend to strike in waves (see dark spikes on chart) with periods of relative freedom between attacks, while tension headaches tend to follow a continuous pattern. Cluster headaches are so named because they tend to recur in clusters. Each cluster may last several weeks or months and be separated by months or even years of freedom from pain.

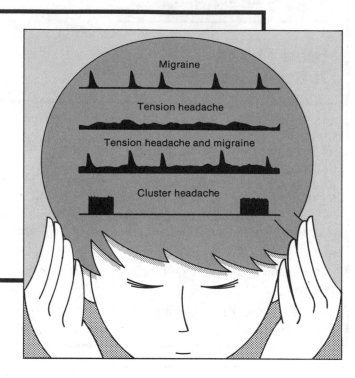

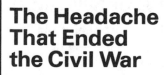 **F**ILE ON THE FAMOUS

The Headache That Ended the Civil War

Just when Ulysses S. Grant was trying to end the Civil War—the Union general had asked his Confederate counterpart, Robert E. Lee, to surrender but Lee had refused—Grant was hit with a horrible headache. He suffered through the night of April 8, 1865, bathing his feet in hot water and mustard and putting mustard plasters on his wrists and neck. None of that helped.

Grant started the next day still feeling awful. Then a message arrived from General Lee. Upon reading the note in which Lee said he would surrender, Grant's pain and nausea vanished. He rode off to accept Lee's surrender and end the Civil War.

Foods That Bring Pain

Many headache sufferers have reported a cause and effect relationship between the foods they eat and the headaches they get. Foods containing the amino acid tyramine are frequently cited. Here is a list of diet components most often linked to headache.

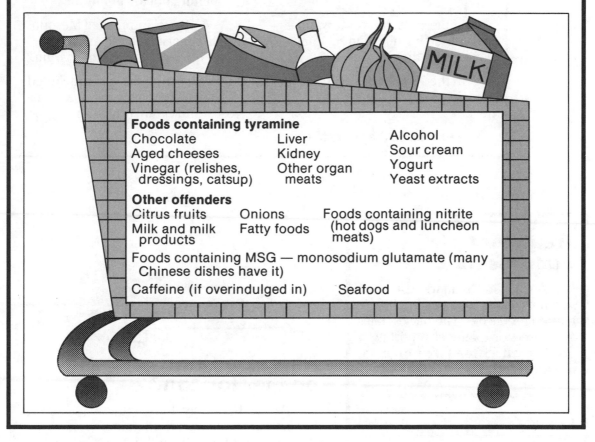

Foods containing tyramine

Chocolate
Aged cheeses
Vinegar (relishes, dressings, catsup)
Liver
Kidney
Other organ meats
Alcohol
Sour cream
Yogurt
Yeast extracts

Other offenders

Citrus fruits
Milk and milk products
Onions
Fatty foods
Foods containing nitrite (hot dogs and luncheon meats)

Foods containing MSG — monosodium glutamate (many Chinese dishes have it)

Caffeine (if overindulged in)   Seafood

People making $50,000 or more a year and people making less than $7,500 a year have about the same amount of headaches.

Desperate "Cures" from the Past

Long before treating headaches became a true medical specialty, people tried just about everything imaginable to relieve the pain. Here are a few methods from the past.

▼ In the sixteenth century, surgeons tried burning and scraping bone under the sliced scalp.

▼ In the 1800s, doctors tried applying a pair of tongs to the neck.

▼ Mexicans in the Sierra Madres believed in stroking the head with a live toad.

▼ The Romans and Europeans used to tie on a hangman's noose (hopefully, not *too* tightly).

▼ A physician-priest of Mesopotamia advocated tying on a headband woven of the hair of a virgin.

▼ "Prescriptions" have included dill blossoms boiled in oil, marijuana, roses, and candied sugar.

Treatment Success Rates

A study in Denmark examined seven methods for treating chronic tension headaches. The success rates are based on patients reporting a positive effect for three or more months.

Treatment	Success Rate (%)
Dental splint	13
Acupuncture	12
Chiropractic	7
Physical therapy	7
Plantar (foot) acupressure	6
Herbal remedies	4
Nerve block	3

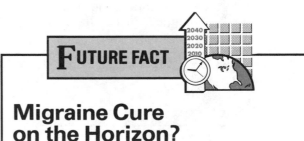

FUTURE FACT

Migraine Cure on the Horizon?

Researchers may have found tomorrow's cure for acute migraine. Preliminary test results of the drug known only as GR43175 are encouraging. Researchers in England and West Germany found that it brought rapid and complete relief in 17 of 24 cases, perhaps by constricting certain arteries believed to open up during migraine attacks.

24

A HEALTH HISTORY OF THE WORLD

In earliest times, the main health concerns centered around getting enough to eat and staying one step ahead of whatever was stalking you for dinner. Primitive people did manage to discover which plants were useful as food and medicine and which were poisonous.

By 3000 B.C. in Egypt, people had turned to their priests for more advanced health advice. Much was learned about the body while preparing mummies. Sanitation became a concern: Egyptian ruins show elaborate bathroom facilities and sewerage systems. Herbs, massage, special diets, and baths were prescribed as medicines in ancient Greece. Ancient Romans devised the first respirators to protect workers from dust.

With the disintegration of the Roman Empire, large cities disappeared, along with roads, aqueducts, and the benefits of organized sanitation. For hundreds of years scientists believed disease was caused by "bad air."

In the mid-1400s, the invention of the printing press led to books on health and medicine. Scientists discovered how the blood circulates and described the functions of the brain and the ear. New tools, such as the thermometer—first employed for fever detection in 1815—brought still more health discoveries. The microscope opened a whole new world.

In 1882, scientists identified germs as the causes of various diseases. Public sanitation systems were perfected. New vaccines were developed. By the mid-1900s antibiotics became another way to protect against disease. And vitamins became an important element in the health-care puzzle.

Ancient Ailments

Anthropologists can chart the health of our earliest ancestors by examining bones, mummies, and other excavated remains. They've discovered that many of the diseases that afflict us today also affected our forebears thousands of years ago. Here are some examples.

Neolithic Europeans

Arthritis

Sinusitis

Tumors

Spina bifida

Congenital dislocation of the hip

Tuberculosis of the vertebral column

Poliomyelitis

Rickets

Ancient Peruvians

Arthritis

Sinusitis

Osteosarcoma

Multiple myeloma (bone marrow cancer)

Osteoporosis

Ancient Egyptians

Arthritis

Poliomyelitis

Tuberculosis of the hip joint

Tuberculosis of the vertebral column

Mastoiditis

Osteoma (bone tumor)

Osteosarcoma (bone cancer)

Club foot

Dwarfism

Osteoporosis of the skull

Arteriosclerosis

Pneumonia

Pleurisy

Kidney stones

Gallstones

Appendicitis

Smallpox

Prolapse of uterus and intestines

Milestones of Health

When were germs discovered? When was the first contact lens worn? When was the first coronary bypass performed? Follow this timeline of the world's health history and find out.

3000 B.C. Teeth are filled in ancient Egypt.

2900 B.C. Imhotep, first recorded doctor, receives medical degree in Egypt. Code of Hammurabi

rules Babylon's doctors. It specifies fees (between two and ten shekels for successful surgery) and malpractice consequences (an unsuccessful surgeon will have his hands cut off).

The First Brain Surgeons

Skulls 8,000 to 10,000 years old from France, northern Africa, Asia, New Guinea, Tahiti, New Zealand, Kodiak Island in Alaska, and Peru carry marks of trephination, believed to be the earliest brain surgery performed.

Our ancestors opened skulls to liberate the evil spirits that might be causing headaches or epilepsy or mental illness, as well as to relieve pressure in head wounds and remove bone fragments left after combat.

Evidence from the ancient Peruvians shows the operation was survivable. At least one skull bears five trephination holes with evidence of postoperative healing. Peruvians used knives of obsidian, stone, and bronze to trim, scrape, saw, and cut openings. Dressings of gourd, bone, shell, and beaten silver covered the holes.

The first degreed medical doctor, Egypt's Imhotep, used spells and incantations, bloodletting, and herbal medicines to treat disease.

Egyptian remedies, circa 3000 B.C.: Moldy bread applied to wounds; castor oil used as a purgative; poppy juice to relieve pain; radishes, garlic, and onions to prevent epidemic disease. Medicines were often mixed into wine or beer to contribute to the patient's feeling of well-being.

Pharmacopoeia, 2100 B.C.

The first drug catalog, or pharmacopoeia, was a collection of prescriptions written by a Sumerian physician on clay tablets in cuneiform script.

The remedies described included one in which the leaves of cassia, myrtle, asafetida, and thyme were collected, dried, and crushed, then added to salves concocted from kushumma wine, cedar oil, pulverized snakeskins, turtle shells, and dried milk. In another, the barks of willow, pear, and fir trees were boiled for potions. Sodium chloride (salt) was used as an antiseptic. And potassium nitrate, made from the urine flowing in sewer drains, made a handy astringent.

1500 B.C.	Edwin Smith Surgical Papyrus (Egyptian medicine) written. Describes the pumping function of the heart, and notes that the pulse can be used to determine how the heart is working.	1000 B.C.	Etruscans use a form of false teeth for cosmetic reasons.		optic nerves, Eustachian tubes, and brain as center of intellect.
		600 B.C.	Massage and acupuncture used by Japanese.	525 B.C.	Asclepius named god of medicine in Greece.
		535 B.C.	Greek physician dissects cadavers, noting	522 B.C.	First medical school founded in Athens.

Cro-Magnon Man Ate Only the Leanest Meat

A third of the diet of Cro-Magnon man, who lived about 25,000 years ago, was meat. Yet he had little hypertension or cardiovascular disease. So why has meat gotten such a bad health reputation today?

The difference is in the fat. Meat from the wild is higher in protein, lower in calories, and lower in saturated fat than what you purchase at the grocery store.

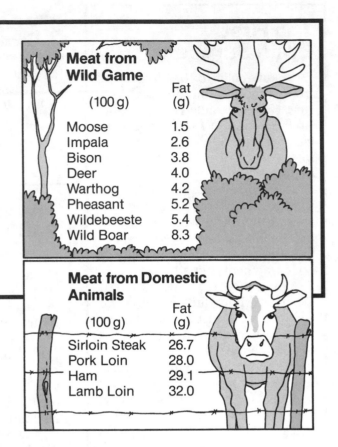

Meat from Wild Game

(100 g)	Fat (g)
Moose	1.5
Impala	2.6
Bison	3.8
Deer	4.0
Warthog	4.2
Pheasant	5.2
Wildebeeste	5.4
Wild Boar	8.3

Meat from Domestic Animals

(100 g)	Fat (g)
Sirloin Steak	26.7
Pork Loin	28.0
Ham	29.1
Lamb Loin	32.0

The Ebers Papyrus, written about 1553 B.C., contains several prescriptions for constipation, a condition that has plagued people for thousands of years. Here's one: "Take thou: Onions. Cook in sweet beer and drink the third part thereof for three days."

500 B.C.	First cataract operations in India.	**A.D. 400**	First hospital founded in western Europe.	**1140**	Norman King Roger II says only licensed physicians may practice medicine.
400 B.C.	Hippocrates notes relationship between diet and health.	**A.D. 541**	Bubonic plague kills 10,000 people a day in Constantinople.	**1270**	First spectacles developed by Venetians.
300 B.C.	Greek physician claims organs develop with exercise and weaken when not used.	**A.D. 643**	Chinese note symptoms of diabetes mellitus, including thirst and sweet urine.	**1320**	French surgeon urges cleansing of wounds and sutures.
				1377	First quarantine set up in

Stone-Age Health Prescription

Many modern experts believe we'd all be healthier if we took some lifestyle cues from the caveman—particularly in the area of diet. Here are some of the things our earliest ancestors were doing right.

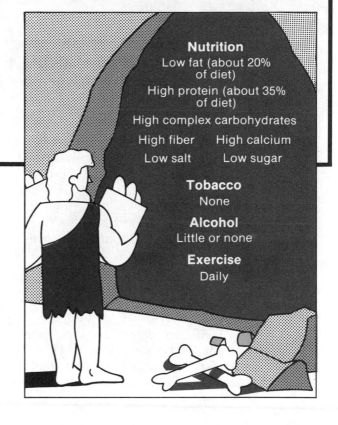

Nutrition
Low fat (about 20% of diet)
High protein (about 35% of diet)
High complex carbohydrates
High fiber   High calcium
Low salt   Low sugar

Tobacco
None

Alcohol
Little or none

Exercise
Daily

Pestilence: The Chain of Transmission

Like a not-so-humorous version of the children's song, "The Farmer in the Dell," plague has been passed along between animals and people throughout history. And it spreads the same way today. Fleas carrying the disease crawl onto rodents such as squirrels, mice, and rats or onto domestic pets such as cats and dogs, then leap onto humans. Or, humans may contract the disease through direct contact with rodents or with rodent-eating cats.

Ships were quarantined in the late 1700s to control yellow fever, a disease carried by mosquitoes. Those ships carrying the fever were forced to fly a yellow flag, thus giving the disease the nickname "yellow jack."

Yugoslavian seaport. Those thought to have plague must stay there 40 days.

1497   Scurvy aboard Vasco da Gama's ships.

1520   Smallpox epidemic among the Aztecs allows Hernando Cortés to take over their empire.

1590   Compound microscope invented providing first view of germs, although connection between germs and diseases wasn't discovered until 1800s.

1667   Animal kept alive by artificial respiration.

1701   Three small children are inoculated against smallpox in Constantinople, Turkey.

1707   English doctor takes pulse during medical exam.

1717   England's Lady Mary Wortley Montagu has her children inoculated against smallpox, following the example she saw while in Turkey.

FILE ON THE FAMOUS

Louis Pasteur

Louis Pasteur was a French chemist, bacteriologist, and consultant to the wine industry. He proved the existence of airborne bacteria and laid the groundwork for vaccines that improved health a hundredfold. His work touches our lives even today. Here's a short chronology of his life and work.

1822 Born the son of a tanner.

1865 Discovers that heating wine in a limited amount of air will kill bacteria that would normally spoil the alcohol. Process is called *pasteurization*.

1879 Discovers that weakened cholera bacteria won't infect chickens but will cause immunity to the bacteria. Paves the way for development of vaccines.

1881 Develops successful anthrax vaccine.

1885 Invents successful rabies vaccine.

1895 Dies at age 73 after a series of strokes.

Who Was Typhoid Mary?

The legendary disease carrier's real name was Mary Mallon, but she was dubbed Typhoid Mary because her body was loaded with typhoid. She became a walking epidemic, spreading the salmonella bacillus, or typhoid germ. As a cook in New York City in the early twentieth century, she infected 53 people. Later she moved to Ithaca, New York, where 1,300 more people got typhoid.

1736 First successful appendectomy.	**1800** Chlorine used to purify water in England.	English commission establishes connection between dirt and epidemic disease.
1774 German Franz Mesmer uses hypnosis to cure disease.	**1834** Amalgam (a mercury alloy) used to fill teeth.	**1865** Joseph Lister uses phenol as disinfectant in surgery.
1796 Citrus fruit juice keeps British Navy men from developing scurvy. Sailors now called "limeys."	**1842** First surgery using anesthesia.	**1869** Paul Langerhans discovers the cells in the pancreas that produce insulin.
	1844 First childbirth using anesthesia.	

Pox, Plague, and Famine: A Grim Scorecard

Throughout history, infection and disease have swept continents, sending hundreds of thousands to their death as populations scrambled for prevention and a cure. Here are a few of the most notable scourges.

When	What	Where	Deaths
A.D. 527–565	Bubonic plague	Egypt, Mediterranean, Constantinople	25% of population
A.D. 762	Bubonic plague	China, Shandong province	More than 50% of population
1346–1351	Black Death (bubonic, pneumonic, and septicaemic plagues)	Eurasia	25–30% of population
1624	Typhoid	Jamestown, Va.	6,454 of 7,549 colonists
1793	Yellow fever	Philadelphia	10% of population
1817	Cholera	India, East Africa, Asia, Japan, Philippines	Massive losses; exact toll unknown
1823–1826	Cholera	Russia	2,140,558 of approximately 30 million people
1831–1832	Cholera	Europe, Russia, Asia	Massive losses; exact toll unknown
1856–1866	Bubonic plague	China	Massive losses; exact toll unknown
1898	Bubonic plague	Bombay, India	Massive losses; exact toll unkown
1918–1919	Influenza	Worldwide	21,640,000
1959–1961	Famine	Northern China	30,000,000

Year	Event
1887	First contact lens developed.
1890	Surgeons begin wearing rubber gloves in surgery.
1892	Water filtration used to control cholera epidemic in Hamburg, Germany.
1900	Sigmund Freud says dreams reveal the unconscious mind.
	Austrian doctor shows there are three types of blood, A, B, and O.
1902	A fourth blood type, AB, found.
1905	First human blood transfusion.
1921	Hermann Rorschach uses inkblots to chart personality.
1928	Alexander Fleming discovers penicillin in mold.
1932	German chemist develops first sulfa drug.
1937	First antihistamine.

"A Shave, a Haircut . . . and a Hemorrhoidectomy"

In medieval society, university-trained doctors considered themselves careful observers, not healers. Surgery was regarded as a menial task. One university in Paris made medical students swear they wouldn't perform surgery. So barbers took up the task.

Barbers clipped and shaved clients, but they also pulled teeth, gave enemas, and performed minor surgery. Eventually doctors reclaimed the surgical duties, but the red-and-white stripes of the barber pole still symbolize arterial blood and the bandages used by the barber-surgeons.

Plague Prevention Tips, Circa A.D. 1345

Worries about Black Death got you down? Here's what your doctor would have prescribed if you had lived in the mid-1300s.

▼ Keep streets cleared of refuse.

▼ Maintain personal cleanliness.

▼ Avoid overeating, drunkenness, and sexual indulgence.

▼ Suck on pomegranates or sour plums. Eat lentils and pumpkin seeds. Drink lemon and onion juices. Pickled onions are healthful for breakfast.

▼ Glaze or cover windows; the safest houses are those that face North.

▼ Bury the dead promptly in graves at least 5 feet deep.

▼ Special prescription: Mix ten-year-old treacle with chopped-up snakes, wine, and 50 other ingredients including powdered emeralds and gold dust.

The Hippocratic Oath, the blueprint for medical ethics over the past 2,000 years, was probably not written by Hippocrates. Scholars think it may have been written by a contemporary or student of Hippocrates, based on principles he taught.

1945 Grand Rapids, Michigan, is first city in the world to fluoridate drinking water to prevent tooth decay.

1952 Jonas Edward Salk uses killed polio virus to make vaccine that will be used in 1954.

1953 Scientists show that tars from tobacco smoke cause cancer in mice.

1956 Birth control pills tested in Puerto Rico.

1957 First high-speed dental drills. Discovery of interferons, natural substances produced by the body to fight viruses.

Albert Sabin develops polio vaccine based on live, weakened viruses.

1967 Mammography used to detect breast cancer.

20-year study in Evanston, Illinois, shows fluorides in water supply reduce cavities by 58 percent.

Microbe Hunting

In 1546 Girolamo Fracastoro proposed that diseases were seed-like things that were passed from person to person. In 1673, Anton van Leeuwenhoek discovered tiny "animals" with the aid of a simple microscope, setting the stage for modern bacteriology. In 1840, one scientist suggested germs might be the cause of communicable disease. Once the first germ was seen under a microscope, the discovery of others followed quickly.

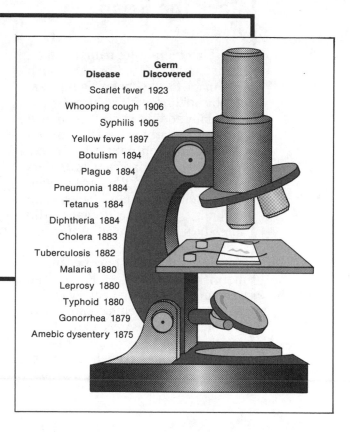

Disease	Germ Discovered
Scarlet fever	1923
Whooping cough	1906
Syphilis	1905
Yellow fever	1897
Botulism	1894
Plague	1894
Pneumonia	1884
Tetanus	1884
Diphtheria	1884
Cholera	1883
Tuberculosis	1882
Malaria	1880
Leprosy	1880
Typhoid	1880
Gonorrhea	1879
Amebic dysentery	1875

Quinine, from the bark of the Peruvian cinchona tree, was the best and only remedy for malaria for 300 years beginning in 1630. The active alkaloid in this remedy suppresses the malaria parasites and acts as a preventive. Today, synthetic drugs have mostly replaced natural quinine.

In 1718, German physician Friedrich Hoffman suggested that muscle tone can be used as a measure of good health. Today doctors know that regular exercise will help protect you from heart disease and aging.

First human heart transplant; recipient lives 18 days.
First coronary bypass surgery.

1977 Two homosexual New York City men are diagnosed with Kaposi's sarcoma, but acquired immune deficiency syndrome (AIDS) is not yet recognized.

1978 First test-tube baby, Lesley Brown, born in United Kingdom.

1981 Centers for Disease Control officially recognize AIDS.

1982 First Jarvik-7 artificial heart implanted; recipient lives 112 days.

1983 Team at University of California at Torrance makes first successful human embryo transfer.

1984 In Denver, Colorado, first successful surgery on baby before birth.

1985 Lasers used to clean out clogged arteries.

Pass the Soap, Please

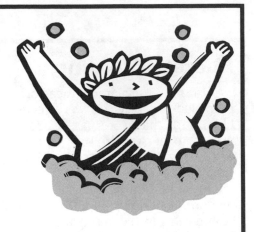

First there were baths . . . then came the soap. The first bar of soap was made by the Phoenicians in 600 B.C. by boiling goat's fat in water and gradually adding wood ashes rich in potassium carbonate. They stirred their concoction until it hardened. Then these Mediterranean traders sold their soap to the Greeks, who saw medicinal value in cleansing wounds, and to the Romans, who already had baths waiting for this bubbly creation.

Even though soap became a flourishing business in France and Italy in the eleventh century and in England in the twelfth century, people of the Middle Ages feared bathing the whole body more than once a month. Some even hesitated to bathe more than once a year. They thought bathing could be fatal, or at least dangerous to health.

By the nineteenth century more people wanted to take more baths, but the tax on imported soap was so high in France and England during the Napoleonic Wars that people secretly made their own soap at night.

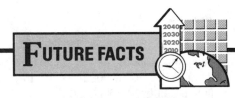

Future Health: 2001

What will your medical care be like in the future? Here are some expert predictions.

▼ Doctors will be more protective of their practices, referring patients to specialists less often and striving to enhance doctor-patient relationships.

▼ Hospitals will be neighborhood clinics connected by computer information networks and served by ground and air transportation.

▼ Medical malls will conveniently group doctors' offices, health food stores, fitness centers, and pharmacies.

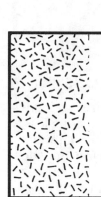

25

HEARING

Hearing impairment is among the nation's leading chronic physical disabilities, and its impact on sufferers has few equals. At least 18 million Americans have some kind of hearing impairment. About 2 million are nearly or totally deaf, a condition Helen Keller said was "a worse misfortune" than being blind. Hearing problems in children can be mistaken for mental retardation or hyperactivity, and by impeding language they can interfere with a child's progress at school. Anyone who can't hear well becomes socially isolated.

This vital ability is based on a stunningly designed miniaturized sensory system. Sound waves entering the ear travel down the ear canal to strike the eardrum, a membrane ½ inch across and less than 1/50 inch thick. The drum's vibrations start the ossicles moving. These three tiniest bones in the body—the malleus, incus, and stapes—amplify the vibrations so they produce waves in the fluid of the inner ear, the cochlea. Inside the cochlea, microscopic hairs growing from cells literally sway in the waves, causing nearby nerve cells to send electrical impulses along the auditory nerve to the brain's hearing centers.

The entire system is exquisitely sensitive to sound. The system is also sensitive to noise, injury, infection, and an array of other hazards. Most people who lose their hearing lose it gradually, beginning in their youth, and in ways that are largely preventable.

Hearing Problems Increase with Age

The percentage of Americans with chronic hearing impairment increases with age, but men are worse off than women because they lead noisier lives. By age 75, one-third of women and almost 40 percent of men have chronic hearing loss.

Number of Hearing-Impaired People*

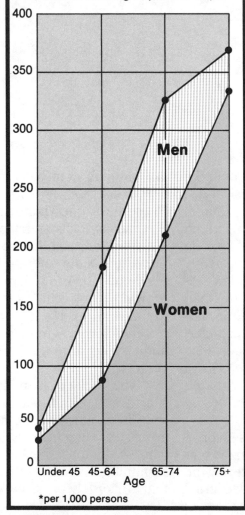

Age

*per 1,000 persons

Equation for Hearing Loss

High blood pressure + a high-fat diet + loud noise = hearing loss, researchers say. Because a fatty diet and high blood pressure impede blood flow to the inner ear, the ear can't recover from the impact of noise as well as a normal ear can.

The High Notes and Low Notes

A sound generates a force that pushes out against air molecules, squeezing them together to form "waves." The number of waves that pass a given point every second is the frequency of the sound, measured in cycles per second, called Hertz (Hz).

Humans interpret frequency as pitch; the greater the frequency, the higher the pitch. A healthy young adult picks up frequencies ranging from 20 Hertz to 20,000 Hertz. By comparison, the lowest note on a piano is 27 Hertz and the highest is about 3,900 Hertz, a range encompassing the human voice and other instruments. Vampire bats can hear frequencies up to 210,000 Hertz, dolphins up to 280,000 Hertz. Humans can hear sounds as high as 200,000 Hertz, but only if the sound source is pressed up against the skull.

How Loud Is That Sound?

A decibel, abbreviated dB, is a measure of the force of sound waves breaking against our ears. The greater the intensity, the louder the sound and the farther it can be heard. A sound 10 times louder than another at the same frequency is 10 decibels higher. Our ears respond to an enormous range of intensity, so the scale has to be enormous. The slightest sound a healthy young adult can hear is arbitrarily set at 0 decibels. The sound of a gentle breeze (50 decibels) is *100,000 times* louder, a jet plane flying 1,000 feet overhead (100 decibels) is *10 billion* times louder, and the noise of a rocket launch, at 160 decibels, is *10 quadrillion* times louder. The table below compares some common sound sources.

Sound Source	Intensity (dB)	Sound Source	Intensity (dB)
Lowest sound audible to human ear	0	Shouted conversation	90
Leaves rustling	20	Motorcycle at 25 ft.	90
Watch ticking	20	Inside subway car	95
Soft whisper	30	Power mower	96
Quiet library	30	Newspaper press	97
Quiet office	40	Farm tractor	98
Living room	40	Jet flyover at 1,000 ft.	103
Normal conversation	50	Stereo headphones	105
Refrigerator	50	Chain saw	110
Gentle breeze	50	Jet engine at 800 ft.	110
Air conditioner	60	Live rock and roll band	114
Sewing machine	60	Screaming baby	115
Auto traffic near freeway	64	Jet plane takeoff	120
Busy traffic	70	Jackhammer	120
Noisy restaurant	70	Sandblaster	120
Vacuum cleaner	70	Thunderclap overhead	120
TV	70	Oxygen torch	121
Dishwasher	75	Loudest human scream ever recorded	123.2
Washing machine	78	50-hp siren at 100 ft.	125
Garbage disposal	80	Jet engine at 100 ft.	130
Alarm clock at 2 ft.	80	Gunshot blast	140
Heavy city traffic	80	Jet flyover at 50 ft.	140
Train at 100 ft.	83	Rocket launch pad	160
Diesel truck	84	Firecracker	160
Propeller aircraft at 1,000 ft.	88		

Noise Exposure: Safe Limits

The louder a noise is, the less time you can be exposed to it without harming your hearing. Relying on scientific evidence of noise damage, the Occupational Safety and Health Administration has set these standards for permissible daily exposure to noise. (If you choose to listen to rock music through 110-decibel headphones for 8 hours a day, it's not illegal, but it is foolhardy.)

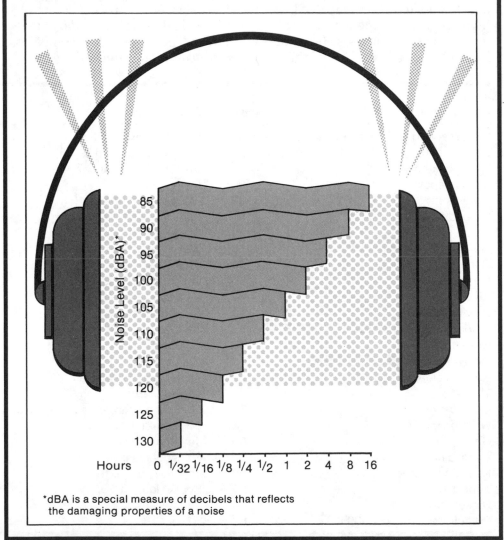

*dBA is a special measure of decibels that reflects the damaging properties of a noise

Comparing Ear Protectors

The two basic types of devices, earplugs and earmuffs, are compared in the chart. (Less sophisticated approaches such as stuffing cotton balls, tissue paper, or your fingers in your ears aren't as dependable. The cotton-or-tissue route will knock only 7 decibels off the decibel count; your fingers do a little better.)

Protector	How They Work	Best Used for	Noise Reduction	Comments
Earplugs	Fit into outer ear canal. Must totally block ear canal with an airtight seal to be effective. Available in a variety of shapes and sizes; some are pre-molded, some expand to fit ear canal.	Low-frequency noise	6–35 dB	May not seal if improperly fitted, dirty, or worn out; can irritate ear canal.
Earmuffs	Fit over entire outer ear to form seal; held in place with adjustable band; band must have sufficient tension to give a firm fit.	High-frequency noise	14–29 dB	Will not seal around eyeglasses or long hair; earplugs and earmuffs worn together recommended when noise level exceeds 105 dB—add 10–15 dB more protection.

University of Florida ceramics engineer Larry Hench, Ph.D., has developed a glass implant that can replace damaged bones of the middle ear. It can be shaped for a perfect fit within 12 minutes, contains calcium and phosphorus in the same proportions as bone, and bonds to the ear in ten days.

Ringing in the Years

The older you get, the more likely it is that you may hear ringing, buzzing, or other disturbing noises. Tinnitus affects nearly one in every ten Americans in the 65 to 74 age group.

Why It's Hard to Sleep in a Hospital

If you have to sleep in a hospital, be prepared for a restless night. The racket in intensive care units and wards can be more than double the Environmental Protection Agency's recommended hospital noise limit and can equal that of busy traffic or a noisy restaurant.

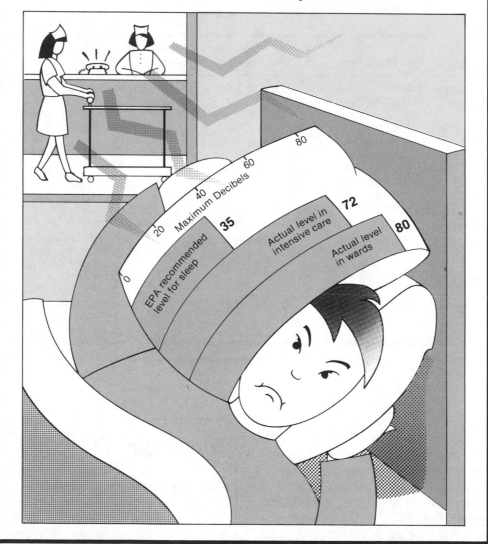

Maximum Decibels
0   20   40   60   80

EPA recommended level for sleep **35**

Actual level in intensive care **72**

Actual level in wards **80**

All about Otitis Media

Ot is ear; *itis* is inflammation; *media* is middle. This condition is a very common result of a very common infection of the middle ear. Children are especially susceptible, adults less so.

How you get it. Bacteria or viruses enter middle ear from nose or throat via eustachian tube, which is often inflamed from infection or allergy.

Symptoms. Earache, inflamed eardrum, and often fever. Pus and mucus can't drain from middle ear through swollen, inflamed eustachian tube. Fluid prevents the eardrum from vibrating, causing hearing loss.

Treatment. Antibiotics, antihistamines, decongestants, pain relievers; sometimes minor surgery to drain the fluid buildup. Promptness is necessary.

Complications. If not treated properly, otitis media can become chronic, lasting weeks, months, or even years. Hearing loss may become permanent.

Decibel Data

If a line representing 0 decibels were a tenth of an inch long, the length of a line representing 160 decibels would be: 15.7 billion miles.

Loudness of crowd in the Minnesota Metrodome during the second game of the 1987 World Series: 115 decibels.

Percentage of men over 50 living in rural areas, including farmers, who have some communication handicap: 50.

Percentage of farmers who consistently use ear protection around farm machinery: less than 20.

Cost in 1988 to train a hearing-ear dog: $3,000 to $4,000.

Length of time to train a hearing-ear dog: three to five months.

FILE ON THE FAMOUS

Silent Symphonies

The man many consider to be the greatest western composer, Ludwig van Beethoven, first noted a loss of hearing in 1798, when he was 28. Over the years his increasing deafness coincided with his increasing social isolation. During the same period, he composed his greatest works. By 1818 he had become virtually deaf and withdrawn from all but a small circle of friends, who wrote their remarks to him in "conversation books."

How Sign Language Works

Just because a person is hearing-impaired doesn't mean he or she can't talk with you. The different forms of sign language are expressive and versatile ways of communicating. The system illustrated here is Signed English, the easiest system to learn because most of its signs represent words instead of spellings or sounds, although some words are "fingerspelled." It is meant to be used in combination with body language and lipreading, as well as whatever sounds the hearing-impaired person can discern. The phrase depicted here is just an example of how Signed English works and the possibilities of expression it embodies.

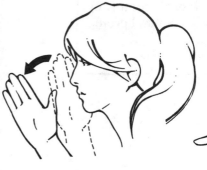

Would

Place palm of right hand near right cheek, then move out. Repeat.

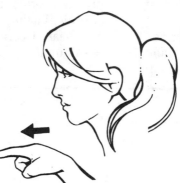

You

Point index finger at person being addressed.

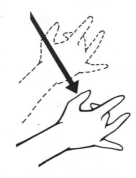

Like (verb)

Place right middle finger and thumb on upper chest, then draw out and close fingers.

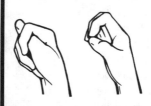

to T O

As part of an infinitive, to is often fingerspelled.

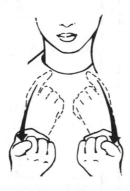

Go

Start with palms and index tips in. Flip index tips out, ending with palms up.

for

Place right index tip on forehead, twist wrist, and point tip forward.

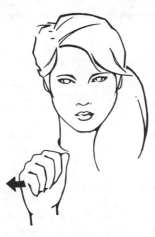

a
Cup right hand and move to right.

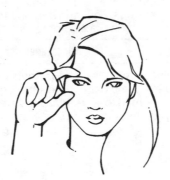

Moon
Form little C with right thumb and index finger. Place at side of right eye.

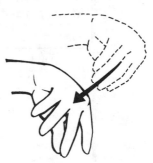

Light (noun)
Hold up hand at right side, then drop with fingers spread and palm down.

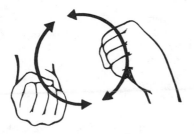

Drive
Move hands as if turning steering wheel of car.

question
Outline question mark in air with right index finger.

A study of mice suggests certain soft sounds may cause brain damage. Raised to the sound of soft but arrhythmic drumbeats, the mice were no good at mazes, developed vicious tempers, and had abnormal learning and memory centers in their brains. The theory is that the arrhythmic sound threw off the brain's natural rhythms, causing brain damage and malfunctions.

A Guide to Hearing Aids

Deciding to get a hearing aid is not an admission of defeat. It's a decision to preserve your remaining hearing by giving your ears the stimulation they need to keep from deteriorating further. These are some of the types available.

Type	Description	Advantages	Disadvantages
Canal aid	Battery powered; fits completely into ear canal; for mild to moderate hearing loss	Almost invisible; no interference with glasses or telephone use; can be worn during most physical activities	Cannot be adjusted to increasing hearing loss; small size makes it difficult to operate for those with limited manual dexterity; loaner models unavailable
In-the-ear aid	Battery powered; fits almost completely into ear canal; slightly larger than canal aid; for mild to moderate hearing loss	Useful for wider range of hearing loss than canal aid; easier to install and operate	Not recommended for people with moisture or skin problems in ear canal; loaners unavailable
Behind-the-ear aid	Battery powered; largest aid; worn behind the ear; for mild to severe hearing loss	Powerful and versatile aid; for those with rapidly deteriorating hearing, manual dexterity problems; loaners available during repairs	May interfere with glasses or telephone use
Eyeglass aid	Battery powered; similar to behind-the-ear aid; built into eyeglass frame; for mild to severe hearing loss	Same as behind-the-ear aids	No loaners available
Body aid	Battery powered; enclosed in cases carried in pockets or attached to clothing; receiver attaches to earmold inserted into ear canal, powered through cord connected to case	Powerful; controls easy to adjust	Bulky; may be inconvenient
Fully digital aid	For severe hearing loss (up to 85 dB); earpiece and pocket-size computer	High degree of control; reduces effect of background noise and high impact-noise (door slams, etc.)	Expensive (more than $1,500); size may be inconvenient

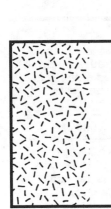

26

HERBS

Herbs have been used as healing agents for thousands of years. Literally defined as the leaves, roots, stems, or flowers of any nonwoody plant used for medicinal purposes, they are the forerunners and foundation of the modern pharmaceutical industry. Approximately 50 percent of all drugs prescribed by doctors today have their roots in medicinal plants that once grew down by a lake, over a hill, around the next bend, or outside the cottage of the local healer.

Several of the specific chemicals contained within these plants have been isolated and identified in laboratories around the world. In 1982, for example, German scientists discovered that hops —long used as an herbal remedy for insomnia—contain a volatile alcohol that becomes more potent when stored at room temperature for a couple of years. When the hops are then exposed to the air—stuffed in a pillow, perhaps —the alcohol acts like a sedative on anyone breathing its vapors. The result is a quick trip to the land of Nod.

It's this kind of scientifically confirmed effectiveness that has helped lead to something of an herbal renaissance in the United States. In 1988 health-food stores reportedly sold more than $265 million worth of herbs. Sales of herbal teas, which have jumped more than 19 percent each year since 1977, are expected to top $549 million by 1995. And common kitchen herbs—in all their variety—continue to enjoy tremendous popularity as healthful seasoning substitutes for salt.

Herbs That Heal

This table lists uses and effects of many traditional healing herbs for which there is now at least some scientific evidence. These effects were demonstrated primarily in the laboratory, not in clinical trials. The herbs should not be considered either safe or harmless. In most cases, they are actually potent drugs that should be treated with respect.

Common Name	Botanical Name	Part Used	Major Reported Effect
Aloe	*Aloe* spp.	Gel (used externally)	Encourages healing of wounds, burns, blisters, and scrapes; reduces frostbite damage
Arnica	*Arnica fulgens*	Flower heads (used externally)	Acts as an anti-inflammatory and analgesic for sore muscles and sprains
Barberry	*Berberis* spp.	Rhizome and roots	Kills bacteria; acts as an astringent
Bayberry	*Myrica cerifera*	Root bark	Controls diarrhea
Bearberry	*Arctostaphylos Uva-ursi*	Leaves	Acts as a diuretic, astringent, and urinary antiseptic
Black walnut	*Juglans nigra*	Juice	Kills bacteria, fungi
Boneset	*Eupatorium perfoliatum*	Leaves and tops	Relieves fever; promotes sweating, breaks up colds and flu
Butcher's broom	*Ruscus aculeatus*	Rhizome and roots	Improves circulation; reduces hemorrhoidal inflammation
Chamomile	*Matricaria Chamomilla* *Anthemis nobilis*	Flower heads	Reduces inflammation and infection
Camphor	*Cinnamomum Camphora*	Purified compound	Relieves itching when applied topically
Catnip	*Nepeta Cataria*	Leaves and tops	Induces sleep; aids digestion
Cayenne pepper	*Capsicum* spp.	Fruits	Aids digestion
Dandelion	*Taraxacum officinale*	Rhizome and roots; leaves	Aids digestion; acts as both laxative and diuretic
Dong Quai	*Angelica polymorpha*	Roots	Reduces muscle spasms
Evening primrose	*Oenothera biennis*	Seed oil	Soothes eczema; may relieve painful breasts
Fennel	*Foeniculum vulgare*	Fruits (seeds)	Aids digestion, relieves gas
Fenugreek	*Trigonella Foenum-graecum*	Seeds	Soothes stomach
Feverfew	*Chrysanthemum Parthenium*	Leaves	Prevents migraine headaches

Common Name	Botanical Name	Part Used	Major Reported Effect
Garlic	*Allium sativum*	Bulbs	Reduces cholesterol; reduces tendency of blood platelets to clot, thereby protects against atherosclerosis and stroke
Gentian	*Gentiana lutea*	Rhizome and roots	Aids digestion; stimulates appetite
Ginger	*Zingiber officinale*	Rhizome	Prevents motion sickness
Ginkgo	*Ginkgo biloba*	Leaves	Increases blood flow to the brain and other areas
Goldenseal	*Hydrastis canadensis*	Rhizome and roots	Aids digestion
Gotu kola	*Centella asiatica*	Leaves	Accelerates tissue healing
Hawthorn	*Crataegus Oxyacantha*	Fruits, leaves, flowers	Dilates blood vessels; lowers blood pressure
Hibiscus	*Hibiscus sabdariffa*	Flowers	Acts as a laxative and diuretic
Hops	*Humulus Lupulus*	Fruits	Induces sleep
Horehound	*Marrubium vulgare*	Leaves and tops	Acts as an expectorant
Horsetail	*Equisetum arvense*	Overground plant	Acts as a diuretic
Hyssop	*Hyssopus officinalis*	Leaves	Acts as an expectorant
Juniper	*Juniperus communis*	Fruit	Acts as a diuretic
Kelp	*Laminaria, Macrocystis, Nereocystis, and Fucus* spp.	Whole plant	Relieves constipation
Licorice	*Glycyrrhiza glabra*	Rhizome and roots	Acts as an expectorant and laxative; heals peptic ulcer
Linden	*Tilia* spp.	Flowers	Promotes sweating
Lovage	*Levisticum officinale*	Rhizome and roots	Relieves gas; acts as a diuretic
Marigold	*Calendula officinalis*	Flower parts	Encourages wound healing; reduces inflammation
Milk thistle	*Silybum Marianum*	Seeds	Protects the liver; accelerates regeneration of damaged liver
Milk vetch	*Astragalus membranaceaus*	Roots	Enhances immune system; acts as tonic
Mormon tea	*Ephedra nevadensis*	Stems	Acts as a diuretic; relieves diarrhea

(continued)

Herbs That Heal—*Continued*

Common Name	Botanical Name	Part Used	Major Reported Effect
Mullein	*Verbascum Thapsus*	Leaves and flowers	Acts as an expectorant and astringent
Myrrh	*Commiphora* spp.	Oleo-gum-resin	Acts as an antiseptic and astringent
Nettle	*Urtica dioica*	Overground plant	Acts as a diuretic
Oak, English	*Quercus robur*	Inner bark	Acts as an astringent
Onion	*Allium Cepa*	Bulb	Same as garlic
Parsley	*Petroselinum crispum*	Fruit (seeds)	Aids digestion; acts as a diuretic; stimulates menstrual flow
Passionflower	*Passiflora incarnata*	Top	Acts as a sedative
Pennyroyal	*Hedeoma pulegioides*	Leaves	Relieves gas; promotes sweating; stimulates menstrual flow
Peppermint	*Mentha × piperita*	Leaves	Aids digestion; relieves gas
Psyllium	*Plantago Psyllium*	Seeds	Acts as a laxative
Purple coneflower	*Echinacea angustifolia*	Rhizome and roots	Encourages wound healing; acts as a mild anti-infective agent; stimulates immune system
Raspberry	*Rubus idaeus*	Leaves	Alleviates diarrhea; acts as an astringent
Rose hips	*Rosa* spp.	Fruits	Acts as a diuretic; relieves constipation
Rosemary	*Rosmarinus officinalis*	Leaves and/or tops	Aids digestion; promotes sweating
Sarsaparilla	*Smilax* spp.	Roots	Acts as a diuretic
Savory	*Satureja hortensis*	Overground plant	Stimulates appetite; relieves gas and diarrhea
Senna	*Cassia acutifolia C. angustifola*	Leaflets	Acts as a laxative
Slippery elm	*Ulmus rubra*	Inner bark	Acts as an expectorant
St. John's wort	*Hypericum perforatum*	Leaves and tops	Reduces inflammation; acts as a tranquilizer
Valerian	*Valeriana officinalis*	Rhizome and roots	Acts as a tranquilizer
Witch hazel	*Hamamelis virginiana*	Leaves and bark	Acts as an astringent
Yarrow	*Achillea Millefolium*	Tops and leaves	Reduces inflammation, infections, spasms

Seven Ancient Immune Helpers

Many of the ancient herbs used in traditional Unani (Greek) and Ayurvedic (Indian) medicine were employed not so much as powerful drugs that destroyed disease-causing organisms but as more subtle modifiers of the body's own natural immune power.

The following table details seven ancient herbs that preliminary modern-day research suggests either stimulate the immune system, boost its ability to kill invaders or—in the case of diseases caused by an *over*active immune system—suppress its hyperactivity.

Botanical Name	Traditional Use
Aconitum heterophyllum	Treatment of debility, fever, inflammation, rheumatism
Hemidesmus indicus	Treatment of syphilis, rheumatism, skin problems
Holarrhena anti-dysenterica	Treatment of worms, chronic chest disease
Ocimum gratissimum	Treatment of bronchitis, rheumatism
Picrorhiza kurroa	Treatment of chronic dysentery, asthma, jaundice
Tinospora cordifolia	Treatment of rheumatism, skin diseases, protection of liver
Tylophora indica	Treatment of asthma, bronchitis

Some people who suffer from hay fever—actually an allergy to ragweed—have experienced severe reactions after drinking a cup of chamomile or chrysanthemum tea. Apparently individuals who are allergic to ragweed are frequently also allergic to chamomile and chrysanthemums.

Instead of Salt

Cutting down on excess salt is easy when you use herbs to flavor foods. Here's a list of some tried-and-true combinations that make good culinary—as well as nutritional—sense.

Try This Herb	On This Food
Basil	Beef
Caraway	Cabbage
Garlic	Eggplant
Nutmeg	Broccoli
Onion	Dried beans
Rosemary	Chicken
Savory	Fish
Tarragon	Eggs
Thyme	Green beans

70 Dangerous Herbs

The following plants are potentially dangerous, according to herb experts. Depending on amounts and duration of exposure, ingestion in one form or another has been known to cause negative effects, ranging from mild to severe or fatal.

	Moderate Danger	Greatest Danger		Moderate Danger	Greatest Danger
Akee		X	Mandrake, European		X
American hellebore		X	Marsh tea	X	
American mistletoe	X		Mayapple	X	
Annual mercury		X	Monkshood		X
Arrowpoison tree		X	Mountain laurel		X
Autumn crocus		X	Mountain tobacco	X	
Aztec tobacco		X	Mugwort	X	
Barberry	X		Nux-vomica		X
Belladonna		X	Oleander		X
Black cohosh	X		Opium poppy		X
Bloodroot	X		Pasque flower	X	
Blue cohosh	X		Pennyroyal	X	
California poppy	X		Periwinkle, common		X
Castor		X	Pinkroot		X
Chinaberry		X	Poison hemlock		X
Christmas rose		X	Pokeweed		X
Climbing onion		X	Rubber vine		X
Colocynth		X	Sabine	X	
Corkwood		X	Sandbox tree		X
Culebra		X	Sassybark		X
Daffodil		X	Scarlet poppy	X	
European mistletoe	X		Scotch broom	X	
Fools parsley		X	Southernwood	X	
Foxglove		X	Spurge		X
Glory lily		X	Squill		X
Golden chain		X	Sweet flag	X	
Goldenseal	X		Thornapple		X
Henbane		X	Traveler's joy	X	
Jamaican quassia		X	Tree tobacco		X
Jequerity		X	Water fennel		X
Jimsonweed		X	Water hemlock		X
Larkspur		X	White snakeroot		X
Licorice	X		Wormwood	X	
Lily-of-the-valley	X		Yellow jessamine		X
Luckynut		X	Yohimbe	X	

Seasoning with Super Nutrition

Although kitchen herbs and spices are generally used in small quantities to season foods, some have been found to contain enormous concentrations of trace minerals. Thyme, for example, contains 100 times as much chromium as does meat, and 400 times as much manganese—on a per weight basis. Black pepper, cloves, ginger, and bay leaves have also been tested and found to be extraordinarily rich in trace elements. In fact, scientists say their intensity of taste might be due to the concentration of such minerals.

Land of 1,000 Healing Herbs

The People's Republic of China has over 4,000 medicinal plants. Nearly 1,000 of these plants have been used as healing herbs for centuries, although Chinese scientists have just recently begun to isolate their active chemicals and document their utility.

The chart lists just a few of these ancient herbs and their scientifically validated uses.

Herb	Botanical Name	Use
Bitter melon	*Momordica charantia*	Suppresses the immune system
Chinese fumewart	*Corydalis yanhusuo*	Acts as a tranquilizer and painkiller
Indigo naturalis	Powdered mixture of *Baphicacanthus cusia, Indigofera suffruticosa, Polygonum tinctorium,* and *Isatis indigotica*	Treats psoriasis and granular leukemia
Mongolian snakegourd	*Trichosanthes kirilowii*	Kills some types of cancer cells
Yellow vine	*Tripterygium wilfordii*	Reduces arthritic inflammation, kills pain, may be a male contraceptive

~~~
**A** preliminary study of 21 non-insulin-dependent diabetics in Israel revealed that 15 grams of ground fenugreek seed—mixed with water then eaten with a meal—lowered the normally high after-meal blood sugar levels to which diabetics are prone.

# New Drugs, Old Ingredients

Herbs that have been around for centuries are popping up as the active constituent in many a modern-day drug. Here's a sampling.

| Herb | Botanical Name | Active Constituent/ Drug | Use |
|---|---|---|---|
| Belladonna | *Atropa belladonna* | Atropine/Donnatal | Relaxes spasms of the digestive tract |
| Bloodroot | *Sanguinaria canadensis* | Saguinarine/ Prunicodeine | Expectorant, emetic |
| Eucalyptus | *Eucalyptus globulus* | Eucalyptol/Vicks Vapo rub | Frees up breathing |
| Foxglove | *Digitalis purpurea* | Digitoxin/crystodi-gin/Digiglusin | Treats congestive heart failure |
| Madagascar periwinkle | *Catharanthus roseus* | Vincristine sulfate/ Vincasar | Fights cancer |
| | | Vinblastine sulfate/ Velban | Fights cancer |
| Snakeroot | *Rauwolfia serpentina* | Reserpine/Serpasil | Lowers blood pressure |
| Spurred rye | *Claviceps purpurea* | Ergonovine maleate/ Ergotrate maleate | Stimulates uterine contractions |
| Thea | *Camellia sinensis* | Theophylline/ Theospan | Relief of bronchial asthma |

~~~
S eventy percent of the 3,000 plants identified by the National Cancer Institute as offering potential cures for cancer are located in tropical rain forests. Rain forests are being destroyed at a rapid rate by encroaching civilization.

Toxic Tea

Most herbal teas provide a welcome alternative to caffeinated teas and coffees. The majority of these are believed to be safe. But Harvard Medical School researchers have identified the following 25 teas as having a potentially toxic effect.

Tea	Botanical Source	Clinical Toxicity
Buckthorn	*Hippophae rhamnoides*	Can cause severe watery diarrhea.
Burdock	*Arctium minus*	Blocks nerve impulses to organs— including the heart.
Comfrey	*Symphytum officinale*	Can cause liver disease (including cancer) or liver failure.
Foxglove	*Digitalis purpurea*	Can cause fatal heart rhythms or cardiac arrest.
Gordolobo	*Senecio longiflorus*	Can cause liver disease.
Groundsel	*S. vulgaris* *S. spartoides*	Can cause liver failure.
Hops	*Humulus lupulus*	May, under some conditions, destroy red blood cells.
Jimsonweed	*Datura Stramonium*	Can cause hallucinations, lack of muscle coordination, blurred vision, central nervous system intoxication.
Kava-kava	*Piper methysticum*	Can cause deafness, lack of muscle co-ordination, skin yellowing, central nervous system intoxication.
Lobelia	*Lobelia inflata*	May damage the liver.
Mandrake	*Mandragora officinarum*	Can block nerve impulses to organs.
Maté	*Ilex paraguariensis*	May cause liver disease or failure.
Melilot	*Melilotus officinalis*	Can cause increased clotting time and a tendency to hemorrhage.
Nutmeg	*Myristica fragrans*	Can cause hallucinations, visual disturbances, central nervous system intoxication, and perhaps liver damage.
Oleander	*Nerium Oleander*	Can cause cardiac arrest.
Pokeweed	*Phytolacca americana* *P. decandra*	Can cause intestinal infection, bloody diarrhea, and perhaps breathing difficulties.
Sassafras	*Sassafras albidum*	Can cause liver cancer.
Senna	*Cassia acutifolia* *C. angustifolia*	Can cause severe watery diarrhea.
Snakeroot	*Rauwolfia serpentina*	May affect the central nervous system.
Tansy ragwort	*Senecio jacobaea*	May cause liver disease or failure.
Thorn apple	*Datura* spp.	Can block nerve impulses to organs such as the heart.
Tonka bean	*Dipteryx odorata*	May create a tendency to hemorrhage.
T'u-san-chi	*Gynura segetum*	Can cause liver disease or failure.
Woodruff	*Galium odoratum*	May increase clotting time or cause a tendency to hemorrhage.
Yohimbe bark	*Corynanthe yohimbe*	Can block nerve transmission between cells.

27

HIGH

BLOOD PRESSURE

High blood pressure, or hypertension, is one of the most common chronic conditions in America, affecting more than 58 million people. But it is also one of the most mysterious. Doctors can find the cause only 10 percent of the time—then it's called secondary hypertension, linked to an underlying condition such as kidney disease, an adrenal gland tumor, or a congenital defect in the heart's main artery. But in essential hypertension—90 percent of the cases—the cause is unknown.

Everyone has blood pressure. The heart's pumping action makes the blood exert pressure against artery walls. These walls are elastic, and can expand or contract to maintain blood pressure at more or less consistent levels.

High blood pressure occurs when the pressure hits or exceeds 140 mm Hg (millimeters of mercury) systolic and/or 90 diastolic. It shows the heart is working harder than it should and the arteries are under greater strain than they should be. The results of high blood pressure are severe and often deadly: atherosclerosis, heart attacks, congestive heart failure, stroke, and kidney failure—hypertension contributes to about 250,000 deaths each year. Half of those having a first heart attack and two-thirds of those having a first stroke also have high blood pressure.

The American Heart Association estimates that high blood pressure costs the economy more than $12 billion annually. Hypertension is the number-one diagnosis in visits to doctors' offices, and the antihypertension drug dyazide is the number six prescription medicine.

Despite the mystery of high blood pressure, doctors do know what the risks are: Increasing age, being black, smoking cigarettes, abusing alcohol, and being overweight. And, again despite the mystery, many cases of high blood pressure can be controlled with lifestyle changes.

Defining the "High" in High Blood Pressure

There are degrees of high blood pressure, as this table of blood pressure ranges for adults and children shows. Less than 3% of American children have high blood pressure. As with adults, children should not be diagnosed as hypertensive on the basis of a single blood pressure reading. Repeated measurements are advisable.

Range	Category	Range	Category
Adults		124 or more systolic	Severe hypertension
Diastolic		84 or more diastolic	Severe hypertension
Less than 85	Normal	*6-9 years*	
85–89	High normal	Less than 122 systolic	Normal
90–104	Mild hypertension	Less than 78 diastolic	Normal
105–114	Moderate hypertension	122–129 systolic	Significant hypertension
115 or more	Severe hypertension		
Systolic, when diastolic is less than 90		78–85 diastolic	Significant hypertension
Less than 140	Normal		
140–159	Borderline isolated systolic hypertension	130 or more systolic	Severe hypertension
		86 or more diastolic	Severe hypertension
160 or more	Isolated systolic hypertension	*10-12 years*	
		Less than 126 systolic	Normal
Children		Less than 82 diastolic	Normal
Newborn — systolic (diastolic is not measured)		126–133 systolic	Significant hypertension
95 or less	Normal		
96–105	Significant hypertension	82–89 diastolic	Significant hypertension
106 or more	Severe hypertension	134 or more systolic	Severe hypertension
8-30 days — systolic (diastolic is not measured)		90 or more diastolic	Severe hypertension
Less than 104	Normal	*13-15 years*	
104–109	Significant hypertension	Less than 136 systolic	Normal
		Less than 86 diastolic	Normal
110 or more	Severe hypertension	136–143 systolic	Significant hypertension
30 days-2 years			
Less than 112 systolic	Normal	86–91 diastolic	Significant hypertension
Less than 74 diastolic	Normal		
112–117 systolic	Significant hypertension	144 or more systolic	Severe hypertension
		92 or more diastolic	Severe hypertension
74–81 diastolic	Significant hypertension	*16-18 years*	
		Less than 142 systolic	Normal
118 or more systolic	Severe hypertension	Less than 92 diastolic	Normal
82 or more diastolic	Severe hypertension	142–149 systolic	Significant hypertension
3-5 years			
Less than 116 systolic	Normal	92–97 diastolic	Significant hypertension
Less than 76 diastolic	Normal		
116–123 systolic	Significant hypertension	150 or more systolic	Severe hypertension
		98 or more diastolic	Severe hypertension
76–83 diastolic	Significant hypertension		

Who Has High Blood Pressure?

Hypertension is full of mysteries, beginning with why it even exists. Why should aging increase blood pressure? Why are black Americans 33 percent more likely to have high blood pressure than white Americans? Why do men start out with higher blood pressure, then get passed up by women? The answers are being sought, but for now the bottom lines are those on this chart. (For age groups 6 to 11 and 12 to 17, there is no sex or race breakdown.)

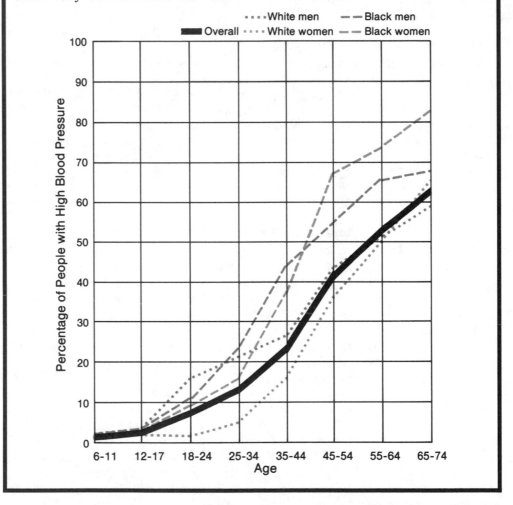

····White men   — — Black men
■■■ Overall ····White women — — Black women

Percentage of People with High Blood Pressure

Age: 6-11, 12-17, 18-24, 25-34, 35-44, 45-54, 55-64, 65-74

Studies show that the typical couch-type potato has a 35 to 52 percent greater risk of developing high blood pressure than someone who gets regular exercise. And if you're a fat potato, your risk is even higher.

What Do People Know about Hypertension?

Education about high blood pressure is apparently paying off, as this graph based on data from the National Heart, Lung, and Blood Institute illustrates.

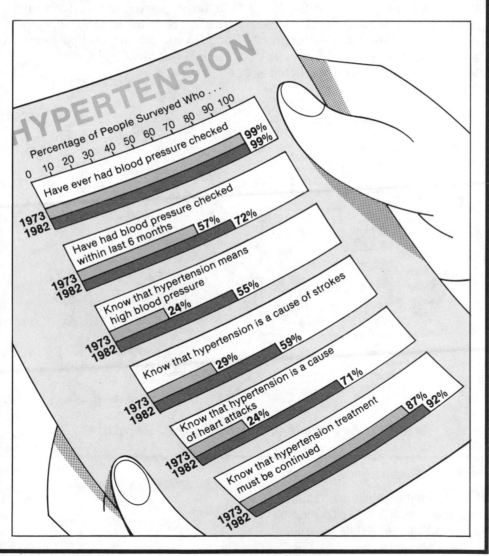

The Geography of High Blood Pressure

Take your typical westerner, and your typical American from anywhere else. The chance that the person from anywhere else has high blood pressure is about 25 percent greater. There seem to be good reasons for that: Number-crunchers at the National Center for Health Statistics note that the West has smaller proportions of the two main high-risk-for-hypertension groups, old people and blacks. Four other possible hypertension connections: Figures from the Centers for Disease Control indicate westerners are more physically active, don't smoke as much, and are less likely to be overweight; and a Roper survey shows westerners eat more heart-healthy vegetables and fresh fruits and less hypertension-linked red meat and salt.

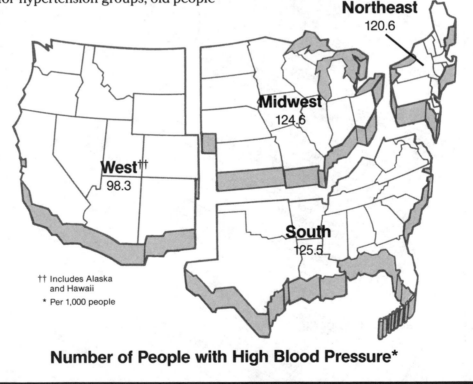

Northeast
120.6

Midwest
124.6

West††
98.3

South
125.5

†† Includes Alaska and Hawaii

* Per 1,000 people

Number of People with High Blood Pressure*

Hypertension in paradise: Melanesians and Micronesians are coming down with high blood pressure as they adopt a more western lifestyle that includes obesity, stress, and lack of exercise.

Is That a Fact?

People who drink alcohol are more susceptible to hypertension.

Yes. From 5 to 11 percent of all hypertension in men is attributed to alcohol. The most common cause of reversible hypertension in men is the consumption of more than 2 to 4 ounces of whiskey per day (or 8 to 16 ounces of wine, or 24 to 48 ounces of beer). One Harvard study found women who daily drank three or four beers or glasses of wine, or two mixed drinks, were 40 percent more likely to develop hypertension than abstainers. Drinking more than that upped their chances to 90 percent.

Elevated blood levels of creatinine—a by-product of muscle breakdown generally linked to impaired kidney function—raise a special warning flag for people with high blood pressure. For them, high creatinine is a stronger predictor of fatal heart attack or stroke than cholesterol is, some doctors say. Hypertensive people should have their creatinine levels checked yearly.

Some research points to sleep disorders as a cause of hypertension. Sleep apnea (a breathing interruption), snoring, violent tossing and turning, panic attacks, and daytime fatigue are found in a disproportionately high percentage of people with high blood pressure.

How Is Blood Pressure Measured?

With a sphyg-mo-ma-NOM-e-ter (Greek for "pulse-pressure measurer"). A rubber cuff wrapped around your upper arm is inflated to shut off the main artery; air is then slowly released. The nurse listens with a stethoscope to the artery for the first sound of blood flowing. That first sound is the thump of the heartbeat; at that sound, the nurse looks at the gauge to see what the *systolic* pressure is—the maximum pressure of blood flow. As the cuff loses more air, the thumping fades, and just before it disappears, another gauge reading is taken to get the *diastolic* pressure—the minimum pressure between beats. The pressure is measured in millimeters of mercury (mm Hg); systolic is always higher than diastolic. A systolic pressure higher than 140 and/or a diastolic pressure of 90 or more is high blood pressure.

The Risks Rise with Pressure

The association between high blood pressure and stroke, heart disease, and congestive heart failure is a close one, and the higher the pressure, the greater the danger.

Data indicate, for instance, that the risk of stroke is more than seven times greater in men with hypertension than in men with normal blood pressure.

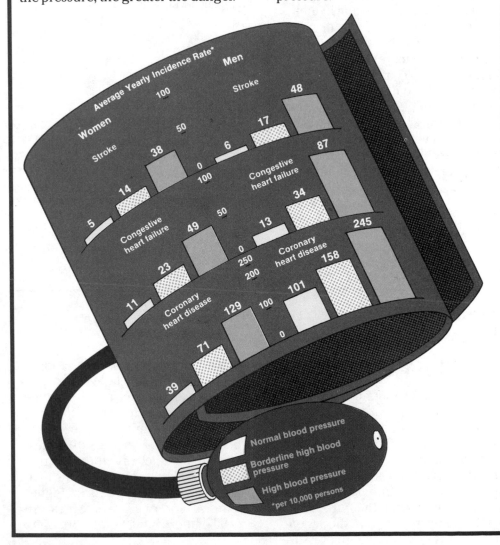

A Guide to Home Blood Pressure Monitors

It's been known for 50 years that home blood pressures are lower than doctor-office readings. A 1989 study found that people with "white-coat hypertension" actually had normal blood pressure when it was measured over a 24-hour period *away* from the doctor's office. Avoiding a false reading is just one good reason to do it yourself. Other reasons: If you do have hypertension, you can get immediate feedback on the effects of medication or other treatments—this can spur you to stick with your therapy and lets the doctor fine-tune it; and it's cheaper to take your own readings at home than to pay for office visits.

There are three types of sphygmomanometers. This chart describes their use, along with advantages and disadvantages. Test the device before buying; be sure the cuff is the right size, that you can get it on by yourself, that the gauge numbers are easy to read, that you can hear through the stethoscope, and that the unit has clear instructions. If you buy it in a drugstore, have your doctor or nurse show you how to use it. If you buy it in a medical supply store, there should be someone there to instruct you. Your local health department can also teach you.

Type	Features	Advantages	Disadvantages	Comments
Mercury	Inflatable cuff; mercury gauge; inflation bulb; control valve to adjust rate of deflation; separate stethoscope	Simple mechanism; consistent and accurate; easy to read; gauge doesn't need adjustment; parts easily replaceable; portable	Bulky, heavy; glass gauge is breakable; gauge must be upright on flat surface and near eye level; bulb difficult to squeeze rapidly; cuff hard to apply with one hand; may be unsuitable for hearing-impaired	Standard on which other types are readjusted; get D-ring cuff to put on single-handedly
Aneroid (without mercury)	Inflatable cuff; dial gauge; inflation bulb; control valve to adjust rate of deflation; separate stethoscope	Highly portable; lightweight; gauge functions in any position; inexpensive	Delicate, complicated mechanism; easily damaged; needs factory readjustment (at least yearly) and repair; cuff hard to apply with one hand; bulb difficult to squeeze rapidly; may not be suitable for hearing-impaired	Some models have large, easy-to-read gauge, built-in or attached stethoscope, self-deflating valve; get one with D-ring cuff; gauge should have no pin at "0" to stop needle from falling below zero, a sign that readjustment is needed
Digital	Inflatable cuff; digital readout; inflation bulb; control valve to adjust rate of deflation; built-in microphone instead of stethoscope	Easy to use; portable; good for hearing-impaired; minimizes human error	Accuracy affected by movement or noise; can be expensive; accuracy checks needed more than once a year; level surface needed for accuracy; mechanism is complex and sensitive	Get D-ring cuff; some models have automatic inflation/deflation, large, easy-to-read display, error indicator, printout of reading, built-in pulse measurement

The Salt Connection

Salt (sodium chloride) seems to have only a minor role in *causing* high blood pressure. But limiting salt can help with control of hypertension, although the exact mechanism is unknown. It's been known for some time that cutting back on salt can help many people lower their blood pressure. But restricting salt is hard for most people: In one study only 30 percent of those instructed in salt-restricted diets were able to match the diets' requirements. But success on the salt front can mean success on the drug front: Of those who managed to cut back, more than a third were also able to reduce their medication.

The salt/hypertension link exists only for those who are salt-sensitive—maybe 50 percent of all people with hypertension. As yet there is no test for salt-sensitivity, and it may develop without warning. Salt control may work best for the elderly, since people seem to become more salt-sensitive as they grow older. In one study, older people with hypertension had greater increases in blood pressure after "loading" themselves with salt than did younger hypertensives, and greater decreases after taking a diuretic to get rid of the salt in their systems.

Seven Successful Nondrug Therapies

There are several drugless ways to control high blood pressure. Their success varies from person to person, largely depending on how high the pressure is.

Weight loss. In one significant study, this was more effective over a longer period of time than the beta-blocker metoprolol; weight loss also decreased total cholesterol counts and increased HDL ("good") cholesterol, while the drug had just the opposite effect.

Sodium restriction. Virtually risk-free. Most studies show a modest drop in blood pressure—the higher the blood pressure, the bigger the fall—in salt-sensitive people when they cut back.

Potassium supplements. One study showed a five-point drop in blood pressure from potassium supplements.

Fiber. Thought to be a reason why vegetarians generally have a lower incidence of hypertension.

Alcohol moderation. Alcohol abuse is the most common cause of reversible hypertension.

Exercise. Studies repeatedly show a five- to ten-point fall in blood pressure due to exercise.

Relaxation techniques. Meditation, yoga, biofeedback, and psychotherapy have all been shown to reduce blood pressure in some hypertensives.

Where You'll Find the Sodium

The sodium found in salt plays a vital role in body chemistry, especially in the regulation of water balance. But too much sodium may contribute to blood pressure problems in sensitive individuals. American adults eat an average 3,000 to 7,000 milligrams of sodium a day—far above the daily allowance of about 1,100 to 3,300 milligrams. The foods listed here all contain substantial amounts of sodium. And table salt is about 39 percent sodium.

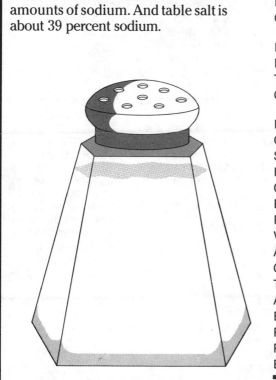

Food	Portion	Sodium (mg)
Salt	1 tsp.	2,300
Beef, dried, chipped	2 oz.	1,988
Sauerkraut, canned	1 cup	1,560
Crabmeat, Alaska king, cooked	1 cup	1,436
Potato salad	1 cup	1,322
Enchilada dinner, beef and cheese	8 oz.	1,260
Spaghetti and meatballs, canned	1 cup	1,220
Ham, canned	3 oz.	1,086
Cream of mushroom soup	1 cup	1,076
Refried beans	1 cup	1,071
Chop suey with beef and pork	1 cup	1,053
Bread stuffing from mix	1 cup	1,008
Dill pickle	1 med.	928
Tomato juice, canned	1 cup	881
Cashew nuts, dry roasted, salted	1 cup	877
Pizza, cheese	2 slices	811
Creamed corn, canned	1 cup	730
Smoked Chinook salmon	3 oz.	666
Hot dog, turkey	1	642
Green olives, canned	5 large	463
Bologna, beef	2 slices	460
Parmesan cheese, hard	1 oz.	451
Vanilla pudding, canned	½ cup	441
American cheese	1 oz.	406
Carrot cake	1 slice	373
Total cereal	1 oz.	352
All-Bran cereal	1 oz.	320
English muffin with butter	1	310
Pickled herring	1 oz.	262
Pita bread	1	215
Bagel	1	198

Blood pressure bottoms out around 3:00 A.M. It rises rapidly between 6:00 A.M. and noon, precisely the hours when heart attacks, strokes, and fatal heart failure occur most often.

Food Factors That May Take the Pressure Off

This table lists the food factors most often associated with lower blood pressure, and which foods contain them. Because these factors have complex interactions, and because supplements can have wide-ranging effects, it's best to get these nutrients from food. If you have high blood pressure—and especially if you're on medication—you should consult with your doctor before taking any supplements.

Nutrient	Possible Effects	Status of Evidence	Food Sources	Comments
Potassium	Potassium-sodium ratio regulates body's water balance; potassium acts a diuretic, increasing excretion of sodium and water; too little potassium means too much water is retained, leading to high blood pressure	Inconclusive, not as strong as sodium connection but becoming stronger; high dietary potassium linked with low blood pressure, low dietary potassium linked with high blood pressure; extra potassium in diets of people with mild hypertension lowers blood pressure	Unrefined foods rich in potassium and low sodium: baked potatoes, avocados, raisins, sardines, nuts, orange juice, winter squash, bananas, whole grains—in general, fresh fruits, vegetables, legumes	Black people with hypertension may benefit from increased potassium in diet; try to get three times more potassium than salt in diet; high potassium intake has adverse effects on kidney disease
Calcium	Counteracts high sodium levels in salt-sensitive people, those who excrete excess calcium in urine, or elderly whose kidneys allow retention of sodium; low blood calcium may increase parathyroid hormone levels, leading to high blood pressure	Major controversy; low dietary calcium linked to high blood pressure; high calcium blunts effects of high-salt diet in salt-sensitive people; most studies show adding 800–1,500 mg to diet lowers blood pressure about 5 points in one-third of patients; calcium/blood pressure link is weak because if calcium is insufficient, the body takes what it needs from bones	Low-fat dairy products, green leafy vegetables (except spinach), sardines and salmon (with bones), nuts	Most Americans do not get enough calcium in diet; calcium is used by the body to cause muscle contraction, including heart and artery muscles; excess calcium can cause kidney stones in some people; some people's pressure may actually worsen with increased calcium
Magnesium	Balances calcium's muscle-contraction function, preventing increased heartbeat strength	Inconclusive; high dietary magnesium linked to low blood pressure, low dietary mag-	Dried beans, nuts, whole grains, bananas, leafy greens, hard water	Most Americans do not get enough magnesium in diet; women should try to get 280 mg and

Nutrient	Possible Effects	Status of Evidence	Food Sources	Comments
	and thus higher blood pressure; may lower blood pressure in some people by helping regulate sodium; may help lower blood pressure further in people taking potassium-sparing diuretics	nesium linked to high blood pressure in women; deficiency may cause rise in blood pressure in people with family history of hypertension		men 350 mg of magnesium daily in diet
Unsaturated fat	Linoleic acid, an unsaturated fatty acid, may increase prostaglandin production—prostaglandins dilate blood vessels and may reduce blood pressure; eicosapentaenoic acid (EPA) from fish oil increases prostacyclins, which indirectly or directly may lower blood pressure	Inconclusive; linoleic acid and EPA have reduced blood pressure in some studies but not in others	Safflower and sunflower seed oils, olive oil, peanut oil, canola oil, nuts, fish (salmon, mackerel, tuna), fish oil	Increased consumption of unsaturated fat appears to offset blood pressure-raising effect of too much saturated fat; blood pressure-lowering effect seems to come from increased levels of unsaturated fat in diet; try to get more than half of fat from polyunsaturated and monounsaturated fats
Fiber	Prevents complete digestion of carbohydrates, keeping insulin levels lower and thereby keeping blood pressure down	Inconclusive; one study showed 10-point systolic and 5-point diastolic pressure drops	Raw fruits and vegetables, legumes, dried fruit, whole-grain cereals, oat bran, nuts, seeds	May also lower cholesterol and help weight loss, which can improve blood pressure
Vitamin C	Lowers blood level of sodium and ratio of sodium to potassium, which might help body excrete excess sodium and water, thereby lowering blood pressure	Inconclusive; 1,000 mg each day for 6 weeks did not affect blood pressure of subjects with normal blood pressure, only helped those with mild hypertension	Raw citrus fruits and juices, chili and sweet peppers, broccoli, greens, cauliflower	High doses of supplemental vitamin C may cause diarrhea

As Obesity Goes, So Goes Hypertension

The link between obesity and hypertension is shown no more clearly than in this chart: The mean blood pressure of obese people before, during, and after a weight-loss diet mirrors their initial loss, and then slight gain, of weight. All the people were at least 100 pounds overweight and had mild, unmedicated high blood pressure. Up to six months after the diet, they were no longer obese and their blood pressure was normal, even though they had gained some weight back.

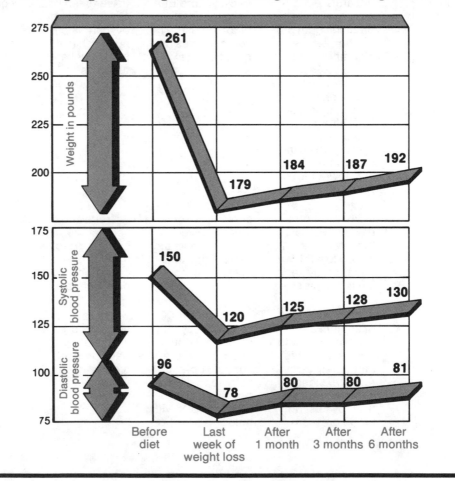

The Hypertension Pharmacy

The hypertension pharmacy is a huge one, full of tongue-twisting names, categories and subcategories of drugs, and combination prescriptions. If you and your doctor decide you need medication to control your high blood pressure, the next decision is which drug or drugs will help you most and produce the fewest side effects. For people with persistently high diastolic blood pressure, the benefits of drug therapy outweigh the risks, says the National High Blood Pressure Education Program. Your doctor can determine which categories of drugs are most likely to help you, and then it's a matter of trial and error to tailor the specific drug and dosage to your needs.

Category	Drugs	How They Work	Possible Side Effects	Comments
Diuretics	*Thiazide or thiazide-like:* Chlorthalidone, Indapamide, Metolazone, Quinethazone, and drugs ending in "thiazide"; *Loop diuretics:* Furosemide, Bumetanide, Ethacrynic acid; *Potassium-sparing:* Amiloride, Spironolactone, Triamterene	Increase kidney's excretion of sodium and water, reducing volume of blood in circulation; loop diuretics used when thiazides don't work or when kidney or heart problems are present; potassium-sparing helps retain potassium	Weakness, muscle cramps, joint pains (gout), sexual dysfunction, depression; can raise cholesterol and triglyceride levels; Spironolactone can cause development of breast tissue in males	Usually first drug given; often used in combination with other blood pressure drugs; more effective for people over 60; effective for blacks; good for people with heart failure; *success rate:* 40–50% when used alone, higher when used with other drugs
Beta-blockers	Acebutolol, Atenolol, Metoprolol, Nadolol, Penbutolol sulfate, Pindolol, Propranolol hydrochloride, Propranolol/long-acting, Timolol	Block nerve signals that increase heart rate, reducing amount of blood pumped with each beat	Insomnia, fatigue, nightmares, slow pulse, weakness, asthmatic attacks, cold hands and feet, dizziness, sexual dysfunction; may cause or exacerbate depression; decreases ability to exercise	Often first drug given; drug of choice for people who have had heart attack; more effective for people under 60; good for people with angina or episodes of rapid heartbeat; *success rate:* 40–50% when used alone, 80–85% when used with diuretic
ACE (angiotensin converting enzyme) inhibitors	Captopril, Enalapril maleate, Lisinopril	Prevent body's production of blood-vessel constrictor, causing dilation	Rash, loss of taste, weakness, cough, palpitations, headache	Often first drug given; new drugs, very effective; especially effective for people with heart failure or diabetes

(continued)

The Hypertension Pharmacy—*Continued*

Category	Drugs	How They Work	Possible Side Effects	Comments
Calcium-channel blockers	Diltazem hydro-chloride, Nicardipine, Nifedipine, Verapamil, Verapamil SR (all available in long-acting form)	Block entry of calcium into blood-vessel walls, relaxing and dilating vessels	Swelling of legs, dizziness, palpitations, headache, flushing, constipation	Often first drug given; more effective for people over 60; good for people with angina or episodes of rapid heartbeat; *success rate:* 30–40%
Vasodilators	Hydralazine, Minoxidil	Dilate arteries	Hirsutism (Minoxidil); Hydralazine can cause vitamin B_6 deficiency or drug-induced Lupus erythematosus	Usually combined with beta-blocker and diuretic; good for people with heart failure or kidney failure; not good for people with angina unless given with beta-blocker
Peripheral adrenergic antagonists	Guanadrel sulfate, Guanethidine monosulfate, Rauwolfia, Reserpine	Block release of adrenaline during stress	Diarrhea, problems with ejaculation; may exacerbate depression	Sedative effect; safe and effective for pregnant women; *success rate:* 40–50% when used alone, 70–80% when used with diuretic
Centrally acting alpha-stimulants	Clonidine, Clonidine TTS, Guanabenz, Guanfacine hydrochloride, Methyldopa	Dilate blood vessels; lower heart rate	Dry mouth, sedation; may cause or exacerbate depression; can cause dizziness or fainting	Good for people with heart failure; well-tolerated by diabetics; should be avoided by people who have had stroke; sudden cessation can cause pressure bound
Peripheral-acting alpha-blockers	Prazosin, Terazosin	Block nerve signals that constrict blood vessels, causing dilation	Fainting due to sudden drop in blood pressure when patients stand up quickly	Use caution when just starting use; used when other drugs don't control blood pressure, especially diastolic

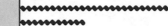

28

THE HUMAN BODY

With its miles of tubing, acres of living tissue, and dozens of specialized organs, the human body is a remarkable creation that we still only partially understand. Correct and perfect in design, it is simple yet baffling in form and function.

Eons of evolutionary development have shaped the human body to its present form. The upright posture and forward-facing eyes—coupled with the incredible thinking machine inside our skulls—give us the ability to manipulate our world like no other animal possibly can. Having used our brains and bodies to conquer the basics of survival, we now turn our strength and energy to higher pursuits and find once again that our unique human form is more than equal to the challenge.

We extract life-giving oxygen from the air that surrounds us, while gaining food energy to power ourselves from the other living things that share our environment. The body demands these things from its surroundings, as well as care and good treatment from its owner. In return, it allows us to experience a sunrise, climb a mountain, run a marathon, explore the limits of our world—in short, to enjoy all the benefits ownership has to offer.

From hair to heart, from bone to brain, each part of the human body has its own amazing story to tell, its own secrets to reveal. The charts and tables that follow show how each part compares to others, as well as how things fit together and why. Viewed separately, the parts help us understand the whole and, in so doing, better appreciate this assembly called the human body.

THE BIG PICTURE

A Full Range of Possible Sizes

The tallest human in the world was Robert Pershing Wadlow of Alton, Illinois. Born in 1918, he reached a height of 8 feet, 11.1 inches before his death in 1940. He reached a top weight of 491 pounds at age 21 and consumed 8,000 calories daily.

The shortest mature human was Pauline Musters, who measured only 23.2 inches tall before her death of pneumonia at age 19. Born in Holland in 1876, her heaviest mature weight was 9 pounds—a bit overweight for her size.

By contrast, the average man is about 5 feet, 10 inches tall and weighs 172 pounds. The average woman is a little over 5 feet, 3 inches tall and weighs 134 pounds.

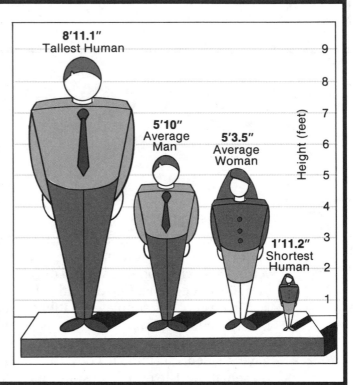

The Importance of Food and Water

The human body is made largely of water and needs a steady supply of it to survive. While humans can live for months without solid food, we perish after only a few days without water.

Longest survival time without food or water: 18 days

Longest survival time without solid food: 382 days

The Body You've Always Wanted

The body we have and the body we want are rarely the same.

~~~T~~~he distribution of American men by height shows a nation filled with more potential jockeys than basketball players. About 14 percent of American men measure less than 5 feet, 6 inches tall, while only a minuscule 2 percent are taller than 6 feet, 2 inches.

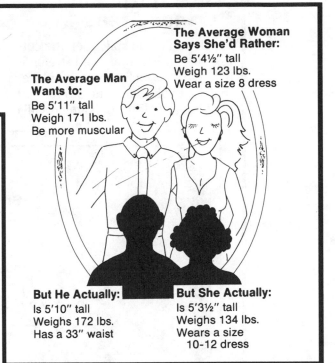

The Average Man Wants to:
Be 5'11" tall
Weigh 171 lbs.
Be more muscular

The Average Woman Says She'd Rather:
Be 5'4½" tall
Weigh 123 lbs.
Wear a size 8 dress

But He Actually:
Is 5'10" tall
Weighs 172 lbs.
Has a 33" waist

But She Actually:
Is 5'3½" tall
Weighs 134 lbs.
Wears a size 10-12 dress

The Major Organs Ranked by Weight

Though there's no such thing as an unimportant organ, the ones we tend to think of as being largest or most important are frequently smaller and lighter than we realize. Conversely, one organ that we rarely think of as such proves largest of all.

Organ	Weight
Skin	6 lb.
Liver	3 lb.
Brain	3 lb.
Lungs	1 lb. each
Heart	10 oz.
Kidneys	4.5 oz. each

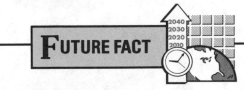

FUTURE FACT

How Tall?

Though man has grown remarkably since the days when our 3½-foot-tall ancestors roamed the Earth some 3 million years ago, it seems unlikely that we will see such continued growth during the next 3 million years. Experts say the optimal height man will reach in his current two-legged form is about 7 or 8 feet (anything taller, experts theorize, might place such stress on the thigh bones that we would have to start walking on all fours—again).

Some Surprising Surface Areas

If you could split open the cortex of a human brain and stretch it flat, you'd be lucky to cover a placemat. But split open and stretch out the billions of little folds (microvilli) that make up the insides of the small intestines, and you could cover the wings of a DC-10. Talk about food for thought!

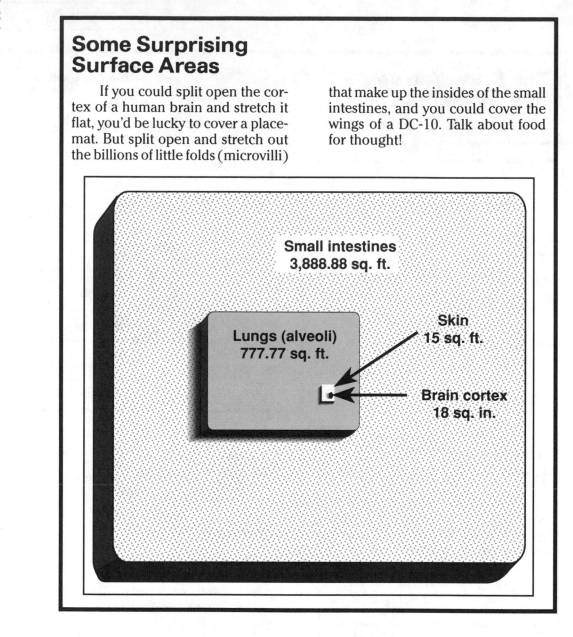

The human body has an active brain with a strong need for outside stimulation. According to the *Guinness Book of World Records,* the longest any volunteer has been able to withstand total deprivation of the senses is 92 hours.

Body Temperature: The Extremes

Human bodies function best inside a narrow range of internal temperatures that are neither too hot nor too cold for survival. Even so, some individuals have pushed these narrow limits far beyond the body's normal breaking point and still survived.

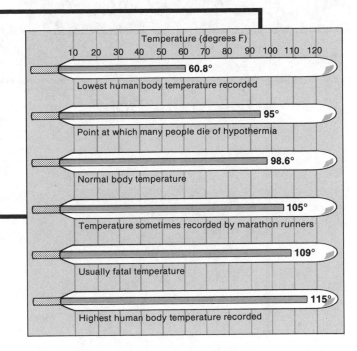

Temperature (degrees F)

10 20 30 40 50 60 70 80 90 100 110 120

60.8°
Lowest human body temperature recorded

95°
Point at which many people die of hypothermia

98.6°
Normal body temperature

105°
Temperature sometimes recorded by marathon runners

109°
Usually fatal temperature

115°
Highest human body temperature recorded

"If You Can't Stand the Heat . . ."

The human body can withstand some terrifying extremes of hot and cold. Here's what the U.S. Air Force found when it conducted a test to discover what the limit of human endurance is when it comes to hot air.

385° F
Temperature at which steak will fry

400° F
Hottest air temperature endured by unclothed human

500° F
Hottest air temperature endured by clothed human

During his lifetime, a typical male will eat about 50 tons of food in order to reach and then maintain a weight of 160 lbs.

MUSCLE AND BONE

The Major Bones

1. Skull
2. Mandible
3. Clavicle
4. Sternum
5. Ribs
6. Humerus
7. Radius
8. Hip bone
9. Sacrum
10. Carpus
11. Metacarpus
12. Phalanges
13. Femur
14. Tibia
15. Fibula
16. Scapula
17. Spinal vertebrae
18. Coccyx
19. Patella
20. Tarsus
21. Metatarsus
22. Phalanges

Your Two Skeletons

The human skeletal system has two major subdivisions. The axial skeleton, consisting of the skull, vertebrae, and ribs, supports and protects vital organs. The appendicular skeleton, consisting of the limb bones, is designed primarily for support and motion.

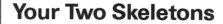The largest bone in the human body is the femur (thigh bone), with a length of 1.6 feet in a 6-foot-tall man, and a length of 1.3 feet in a 5-foot-tall woman. The smallest bone is the stapes of the middle ear, with an average length of 0.1 inches.

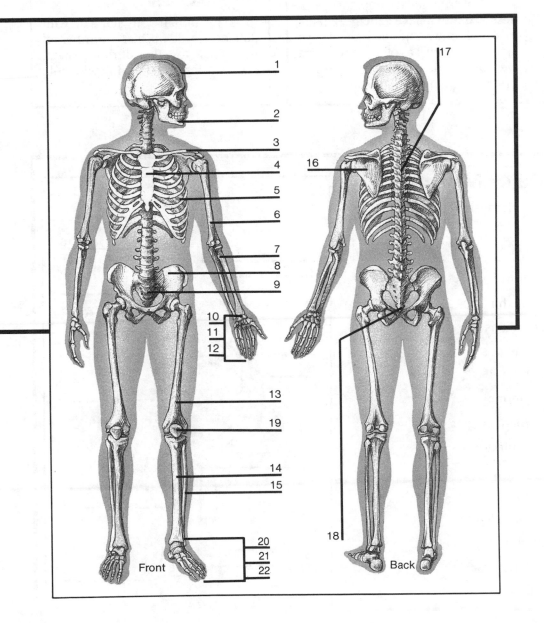

Front

Back

The Major Muscles

1. Sternocleidomastoid
2. Trapezius
3. Deltoid
4. Pectoralis major
5. Biceps brachii
6. Brachioradialis
7. Gluteus medius
8. Sartorius
9. Rectus femoris
10. Vastus medialis
11. Tibialis anterior
12. Soleus
13. Gastrocnemius
14. Vastus lateralis
15. Rectus abdominis
16. Orbicularis oris
17. Orbicularis oculi

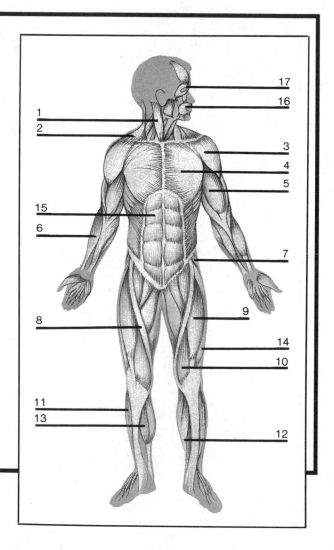

Muscles Outnumber Bones by Three to One

More than 650 muscles drape the 206 bones of our skeletons and power our movements. Muscle accounts for 40 percent of a man's total weight and 35 percent of a woman's. Muscles are made of muscle fibers, of which there are about 6 trillion in the entire body. Each fiber is thinner than a hair and can support up to 1,000 times its own weight.

The Three Types of Muscle

The human body contains three specialized muscle types. Skeletal muscle is under our voluntary control and helps us move about. Smooth muscle, which lines the blood vessels, stomach, and intestines, is not under our conscious control. It automatically constricts to keep blood pressure steady when we stand, and it also moves food along in the digestive tract. Cardiac muscle, found only in the heart, has a slow, rhythmic contraction that's controlled by the heart's natural pacemaker.

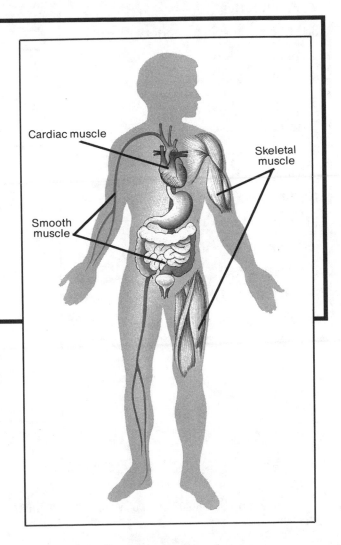

Cardiac muscle

Skeletal muscle

Smooth muscle

Music to the Ears

The smallest muscle in the human body is the stapedius. Associated with the stapes bone in the middle ear, it sends vibrations through the eardrum. The stapedius muscle, at 1/20 inch in length, is shorter than a dime is thick.

THE HEART
AND CIRCULATION

The Major Blood Vessels

1. Jugular vein
2. Carotid artery
3. Subclavian vein and artery
4. Brachial artery
5. Cephalic vein
6. Basilic vein
7. Inferior vena cava
8. Radial artery
9. Ulnar artery
10. Iliac artery and vein
11. Femoral artery
12. Saphenous vein
13. Aorta
14. Heart
15. Femoral vein

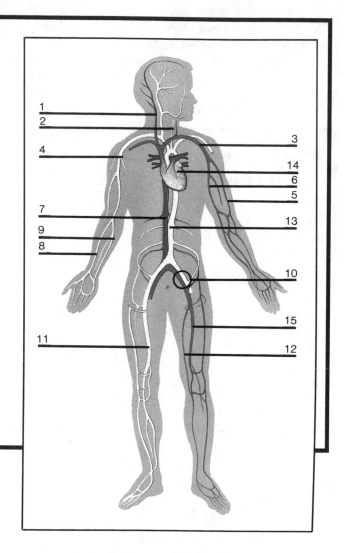

There are 80,000 miles of blood vessels inside the human body.

Baby's a Half-Pint, But Not for Long

Babies start life with but ½ pint of blood in their bodies. If the baby's a boy, however, he will produce another 8½ to 9½ pints by the time he reaches adulthood, depending on body size. If a girl, the baby will develop only another 5½ to 6½ pints of blood, except when pregnant. Women gain an extra pint at that time for baby.

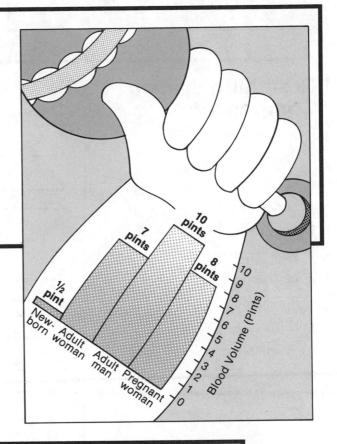

The aorta, with its 1-inch diameter, is the biggest blood vessel in the human body. Capillaries are the smallest, averaging only ½,₅₀₀ inch in diameter. But what capillaries lack in size they more than make up in number. While there's only one aorta, capillaries number 10 billion.

Where Your Blood Is (Mostly) Located

Veins hold most of the body's blood. In addition to returning blood to the heart, veins act as a blood reservoir in times of need. This can help ensure steady blood flow even when 25 percent of the blood is lost through injury. The diagram shows other major locations where blood is found.

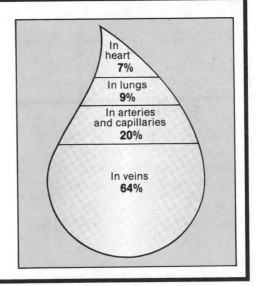

In heart
7%

In lungs
9%

In arteries and capillaries
20%

In veins
64%

THE LUNGS

Breathing System Components

1. Nasal cavity
2. Pharynx
3. Epiglottis
4. Larynx
5. Trachea
6. Right bronchus
7. Left bronchus
8. Right lung
9. Left lung
10. Diaphragm
11. Ribs

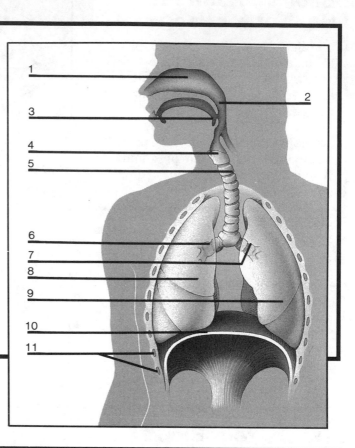

Take a Deep Breath Before Tackling These Terms

▼ The greatest amount of air that can be breathed in and out of the lungs—normally about 4.8 liters—is known as your *vital capacity.*

▼ The amount of air you take in with a normal breath (.5 liters) is called *tidal air.*

▼ You can force an additional 1.0 liter of air out of your lungs following normal exhalation; this is known as your *expiratory reserve.*

▼ *Residual volume* is the amount of air (1.2 liters) that always remains in your lungs after a forced exhalation.

▼ Because of residual volume, your vital capacity never equals your *total lung capacity* (generally about 6 liters).

Air Volume Increases with Activity

We breathe about 8 quarts of air a minute while lying quietly in bed. Simply sitting upright increases intake to 16 quarts. Walking raises breathing to 24 quarts a minute, while running causes that amount to more than double. Marathon runners can take in more than 60 quarts of air per minute.

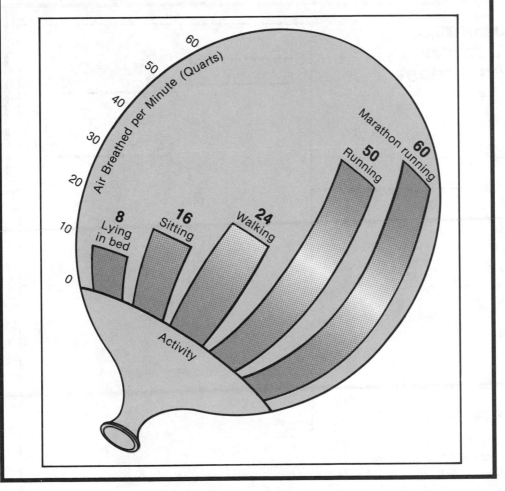

Every day we breathe in 5,000 gallons of air. Over a lifetime, the average person breathes in 13 million cubic feet of air.

THE BRAIN AND NERVOUS SYSTEM

Components of the Central Nervous System

1. Cerebrum
2. Cerebellum
3. Brain stem
4. Spinal cord

A Remarkable Cord

The spinal cord has about the same diameter as your index finger, is less than 2 feet long, and weighs less than an egg. Yet it contains about 10 billion nerve cells, many of which leave it through openings in the backbone and extend to the farthest reaches of your body.

The Brain's Major Parts

The brain is the largest and most complex part of the nervous system. It's composed of between 50 billion and 100 billion nerve cells and is made up of several distinct parts that work in harmony to produce what we know as thought.

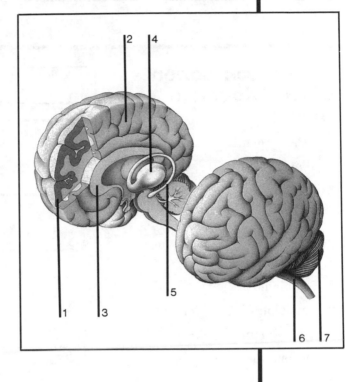

1. **The cortex.** A thin, wrinkled layer of about 8 billion nerve cells that has evolved over millions of years, the large cortex is what makes us uniquely human. Because of it, we are able to organize, remember, create, and understand.

2. **The corpus callosum.** A C-shaped band of millions of nerve cells, the corpus callosum forms a bridge connecting the left and right hemispheres. This bridge allows each half of your brain to stay in touch with the other half.

3. **The cerebrum.** The largest part of the human brain, the cerebrum is divided into two halves, called hemispheres, each of which controls the opposite side of the body.

4. **The thalamus.** Centrally located in the brain, the thalamus relays incoming information from the eyes, ears, mouth, and skin to the correct area of the brain for interpretation.

5. **The limbic system.** In addition to helping maintain several body functions, the limbic system is strongly involved in the emotional reactions that have to do with survival. It also plays a role in memory.

6. **The cerebellum.** Often called the "little brain," the cerebellum is responsible for balance and fine control of muscle movements. The cerebellum does not initiate movements, but makes sure they are carried out correctly.

7. **The brain stem.** In evolutionary terms the oldest part of the brain, it determines your general level of alertness and handles basic body functions such as breathing and heart rate.

THE DIGESTIVE SYSTEM

Major Components of the Digestive System

1. Salivary glands
2. Teeth
3. Esophagus
4. Stomach
5. Liver
6. Pancreas
7. Gallbladder
8. Small intestine
   - 8a. Duodenum
   - 8b. Jejunum
   - 8c. Ileum
9. Large intestine
   - 9a. Cecum
   - 9b. Colon
   - 9c. Appendix
10. Rectum

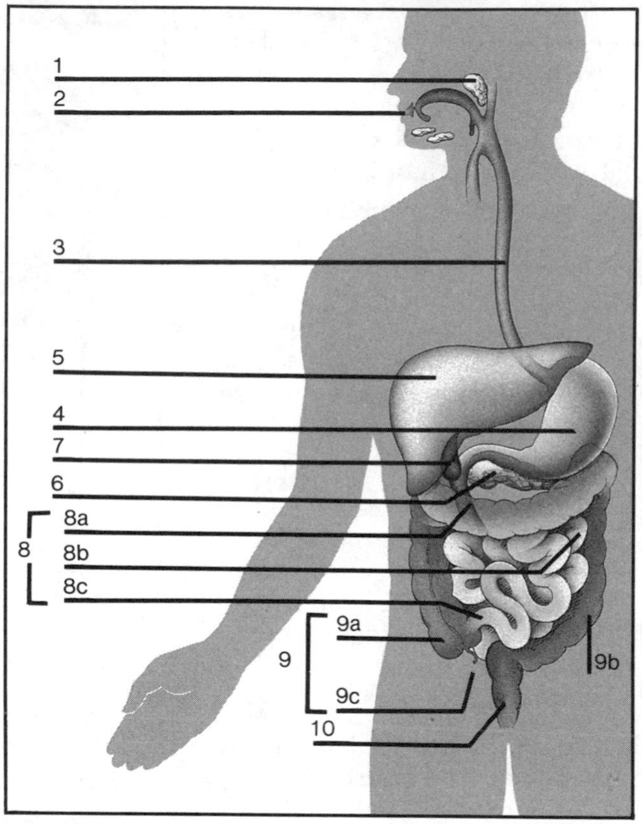

Between 7 and 11 quarts of gas enter or are formed in the large intestine daily. While it may sometimes seem like more, only about ½ quart of gas is actually expelled each day. The rest is reabsorbed into the body.

Digestion's Long and Winding Road

If it were not looped back and forth on itself, the small intestine would never fit inside the human abdomen. In the average adult, it measures from 18 to 23 feet long, making it roughly four times longer than the average person is tall.

The small intestine (so named because of its narrow, 1½-inch diameter) performs a number of functions along its incredible length. At the duodenum, partially digested food from the stomach is further broken down. Food then moves to the jejunum, where most nutrients are absorbed. The last stop inside the small intestine is the ileum, where remaining nutrients are absorbed before the residue is moved to the large intestine.

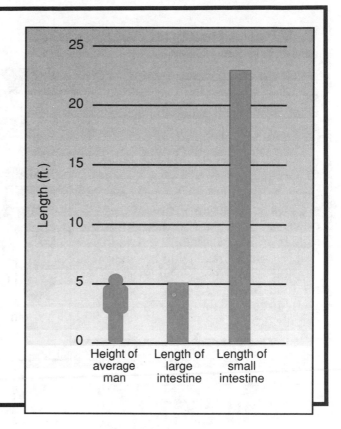

Two Blood Supplies for the Liver

It weighs 3 pounds, has at least 500 functions, and is served by two blood supplies—one that brings it fresh blood from the heart, another that brings it blood from the other digestive organs for processing. Over a pint of blood is in the liver at any one time—fully 13 percent of the body's total supply—and 2½ pints flow through it every minute. The liver's many activities produce enough heat to help keep our body temperature constant.

Food must come in contact with a large number of intestinal cells in order for us to absorb enough nutrients from the 2.5 gallons of food, liquid, and bodily secretions we process each day. To make sure that happens, the walls of our intestines are covered with small, fingerlike projections called villi. Each of these villi is studded with minute microvilli. In just one square inch of the small intestine, there are about 20,000 villi and 10 billion microvilli.

Where Digestion Sets the Juices Flowing

A starch-reducing enzyme in saliva begins the digestive process while food is still inside the mouth. After food moves to the stomach, secretions released there continue breaking it down before passing it to the small intestine. As food enters the small intestine, the pancreas secretes three enzymes to help break down starch, fats, and proteins. Bile salts from the gallbladder join in to help emulsify fats. Inside the small intestine several more enzymes attack the food, breaking it down into simpler forms that the large intestine can absorb.

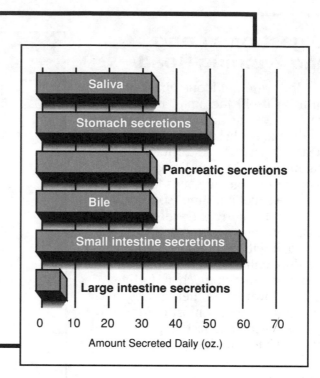

Amount Secreted Daily (oz.)

THE KIDNEYS AND BLADDER

Your Kidneys: Small but Powerful Filters

Though each one is only the size of a child's fist, up to 25 percent of the blood in your body is passing through the kidneys at any moment.

Although only a portion of that blood is actually cleansed by the kidneys at any one time, these organs filter every drop of blood inside you once every hour, separating harmful substances from useful ones.

Most of the fluid that passes through the filter portion of the kidneys (called "filtrate") is quickly reabsorbed by the body. In fact, of the 40 to 50 gallons of filtrate processed daily, only about 0.4 gallon is disposed of as urine. Worth noting: 48 gallons a day amounts to almost 1.3 million gallons in a lifetime of 73 years—enough filtrate to fill a small city's water tank.

Major Components of the Urinary System

1. Inferior vena cava (to heart)
2. Aorta (from heart)
3. Kidney
4. Ureter
5. Bladder

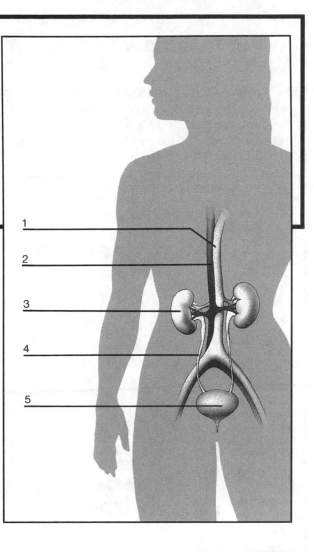

Your heart pumps about 1.5 gallons of blood through your body every minute, 87 gallons every hour, 2,100 gallons every day, 766,600 gallons every year.

Although the average adult bladder can hold 24 ounces of urine, the urge to void is felt when its capacity reaches about 10 to 16 ounces. Nerve impulses inside the bladder trigger the urge to urinate when their walls are stretched.

Water In Equals Water Out

If you take in eight glasses of water a day, then eight glasses must be eliminated to maintain the correct water balance inside your body. Actually, as the chart shows, we receive water from three sources and lose it in four ways. Even so, it's the kidneys' job to maintain the delicate balance between too little and too much internal water.

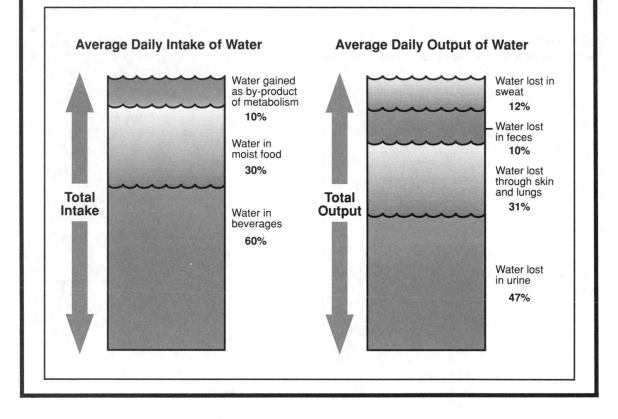

Average Daily Intake of Water

Water gained as by-product of metabolism
10%

Water in moist food
30%

Total Intake

Water in beverages
60%

Average Daily Output of Water

Water lost in sweat
12%

Water lost in feces
10%

Water lost through skin and lungs
31%

Total Output

Water lost in urine
47%

Awash in Water

About 95 pounds of a 150-pound man is water. Protein and stored fat together account for another 50 pounds. The rest is minerals, glycogen (blood sugar), and other substances, such as nucleic acids.

TO TASTE AND SMELL

The Components of Taste and Smell

1. Limbic cortex
2. Olfactory tract
3. Olfactory bulb
4. Olfactory nerves
5. Nasal cavity
6. Oral cavity
7. Tongue
8. Epiglottis
9. Trachea
10. Esophagus
11. Pharynx
12. Uvula
13. Palate

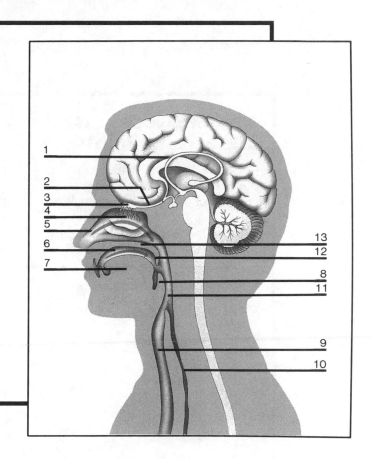

Four Tastes Make a Thousand Flavors

Four basic tastes—sweet, salty, sour, and bitter—combine to create the thousands of flavors we experience. Of the four, we are least sensitive to sweetness, which means we have to take in a lot of sugar before our tongue registers its flavor. The tongue is about five times as sensitive to saltiness, however. And it's even more sensitive to the acidic bite we associate with the taste of sourness. Bitterness is the most sensitive taste of all, for it acts as a warning system against possible poisons.

We are unable to taste anything until it's dissolved by saliva. An adult produces about 10,000 gallons of saliva during an average lifetime.

Why the Nose Is Not Our Strong Point

Small patches of tissue in the roof of the nasal cavities allow us to smell the odors in the air we breathe. But compared to most animals, humans live in a relatively odorless world. While our sensory patches are about the size of a postage stamp, those of a hunting dog measure 10 square inches. Sharks, which can smell blood in the water from great distances, have sensory patches measuring 24 square feet.

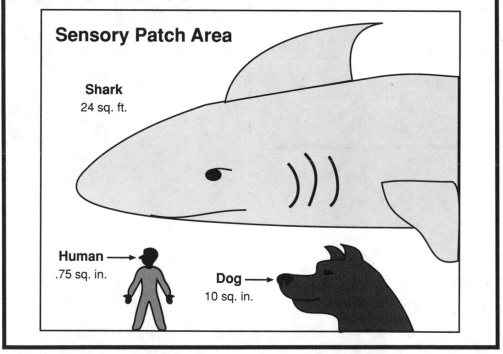

Sensory Patch Area

Shark
24 sq. ft.

Human →
.75 sq. in.

Dog →
10 sq. in.

Most of us can detect and recognize about 4,000 distinct scents. Some people can recognize up to 10,000.

TO SEE, HEAR, AND FEEL

The Organs of Sight, Sound, and Touch

1. Eyes. These are two jelly-filled balls in the front of the skull. Light entering the eye passes through the cornea, aqueous humor, pupil, and lens to the retina. From the retina impulses travel through the optic nerve to the brain for interpretation. Our eyes provide 80 percent of the data we receive from the outside world.

2. Ears. The organs of hearing have external, middle, and inner parts. In addition to making hearing possible, the ears provide a sense of equilibrium, or balance.

Hearing is functionally superior to sight. We can hear around corners and in complete darkness, for example, but we can't see in such situations.

3. Skin. When changes occur within or near the body, the sensory (or touch) receptors are stimulated. These receptors trigger nerve impulses that travel to the brain for interpretation. The skin, in which the sensory receptors are located, is the largest and first-to-develop sense organ of the body.

The Major Components of the Eye

1. Choroid
2. Retina
3. Optic nerve
4. Vitreous humor
5. Ciliary body
6. Sclera
7. Cornea
8. Iris
9. Lens

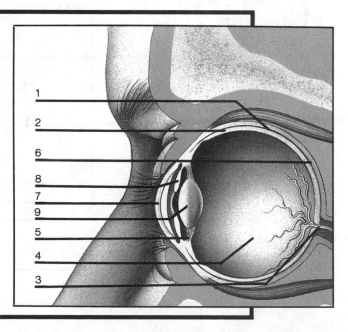

How Eyes Pierce the Darkness

The light-sensitive cells embedded in the retina of the eye are called rods and cones. Cones are responsible for color vision, while rods are responsible for night vision. Once immersed in darkness, the eye begins increasing its sensitivity to light, dilating the pupil to let in as much faint light as possible. After a lengthy period in darkness the human eye attains its greatest sensitivity to light, becoming 100,000 times more sensitive than before the lights went out.

The lens constantly changes shape to focus light as it enters your eye. The muscles that activate the lens move about 17,000 times a day.

If everyone in the world shouted at once and the resulting volume was concentrated at a single point, it would produce a level of sound equal to that of a jet engine at full throttle.

The Major Components of the Ear

1. Pinna
2. Ear canal
3. Hammer
4. Anvil
5. Stirrup
6. Semicircular canals
7. Vestibulocochlear nerve
8. Vestibule
9. Eardrum
10. Cochlea
11. Eustachian tube

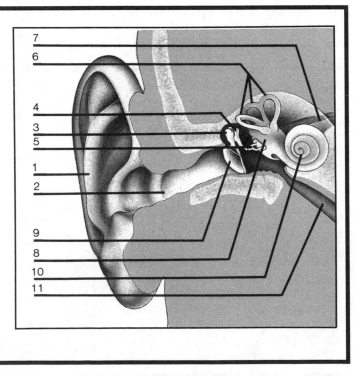

The Limits of Human Hearing

Babies have the most acute hearing. As we age, our sensitivity range starts to dwindle, primarily at the high-pitched end. As the chart shows, most human speech falls within a relatively narrow frequency range of 250 to 4,000 cycles per second.

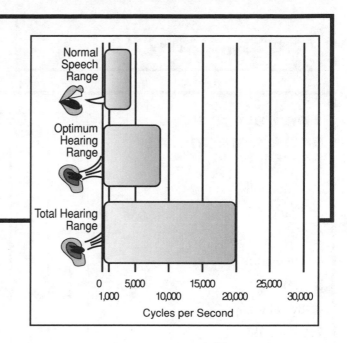

Normal Speech Range

Optimum Hearing Range

Total Hearing Range

0   5,000   15,000   25,000
1,000   10,000   20,000   30,000

Cycles per Second

Bad News Travels Fast

Two types of nerve fibers send signals of pain to the central nervous system for processing. Pricking pain zips along on one set of nerve fibers. Burning, aching, and tickling pains move at a relatively slow speed along another set of nerve fibers. Those slower messages "plod" along at 6½ feet per second or less.

The body of an adult has about 640,000 sensory receptors in the skin. Our fingertips are so sensitive that we can respond to a pressure of less than ¹/₁,₄₀₀ of an ounce, the weight of an average fly.

Maximum Speed in Feet per Second (fps)

115 fps

6 1/2 fps

3 fps

Tickle   Burning or aching pain   Pricking pain

THE SKIN AND HAIR

The Layers and Components of Skin

1. Hair shaft
2. Epidermis
3. Dermis
4. Oil gland
5. Hair muscle
6. Sweat gland
7. Hair bulb
8. Subcutaneous layer
9. Pacinian corpuscle (senses pressure)
10. Vein
11. Artery
12. Nerve fiber

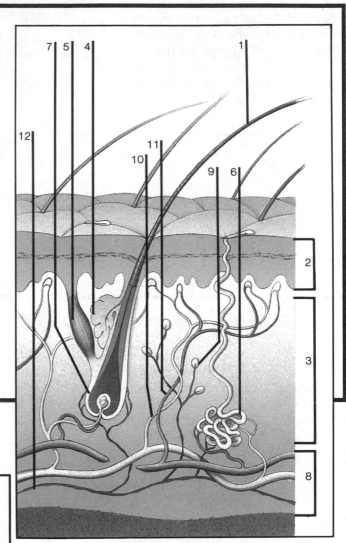

Don't Look Now, but You're Shedding

A fair-sized man or woman will shed about 1½ pounds of skin particles annually. At that rate, a person loses about 105 pounds of skin by age 70. Through shedding, all of us replace our outer skin about once a month, which gives us about 900 new coats of skin to wear in a lifetime.

Hair color depends on the amount of melanin, or pigment, present in an individual. As we age, less melanin is formed in the body, and small bubbles of air form in the hair shaft, making the hair appear gray or white.

A Nail's Pace

Ordinarily, your fingernails grow about 1½ inches a year. Your toenails only grow one-half to one-third that length in the same period of time. Compared to your nails, your hair gallops ahead at a blinding pace of 5 inches per year.

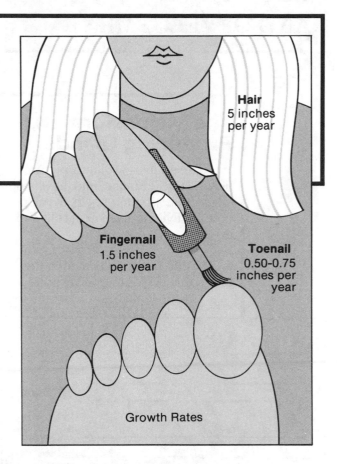

Hair
5 inches
per year

Fingernail
1.5 inches
per year

Toenail
0.50-0.75
inches per
year

Growth Rates

All about Sweat Glands

Some 2 to 3 million sweat glands cover the skin, excreting water, waste salts, and compounds such as urea. The evaporation of water helps keep us cool and regulates body temperature. There are two types of sweat glands. One kind, which is located throughout the body, responds to an increase in temperature. But the other kind responds to emotional stimulation. Those sweat glands are located on the palms of the hands, on the soles of the feet, and in the armpits.

If uncoiled, each sweat gland would measure about 50 inches long, giving you about 1,500 miles of sweat-gland ductwork in your body.

While blonds may have more fun, chances are *you'll* have to lighten your hair a bit to find out. Almost 70 percent of all Americans have brown hair, while only 15 percent are blond. Regardless of color, about 65 percent of us have straight hair, 25 percent boast wavy locks, and only 10 percent have curly hair.

The Major Hormone-Producing Glands

The endocrine glands pictured here secrete hormones into the blood which influence the growth, development, activity, and repair of cells and organs.

1. Hypothalamus. Located in the brain, this gland receives informa-tion from all parts of the body. It acts as the primary coordinating center between the nervous system and endocrine system, telling the pituitary gland when to release some of its numerous hormones.

2. Pituitary gland. Found at the base of the brain, the pituitary gland produces hormones that stimulate the thyroid, adrenal glands, ovaries, testes, smooth muscles, and the kidneys. Because of its ability to stimulate so many other glands, the pituitary is sometimes called the "master gland."

3. Pineal gland. The function of this small, oval structure located deep in the brain remains uncertain. It seems to be controlled by varying light conditions and may be involved in regulating circadian rhythms—patterns of behavior associated with day and night.

4. Thyroid gland. This gland, located at the front of the neck, produces hormones that maintain your metabolic rate and help determine your level of activity.

5. Parathyroid glands. These glands control the calcium level in the blood, increasing its absorption in the intestines and removing it from the bones.

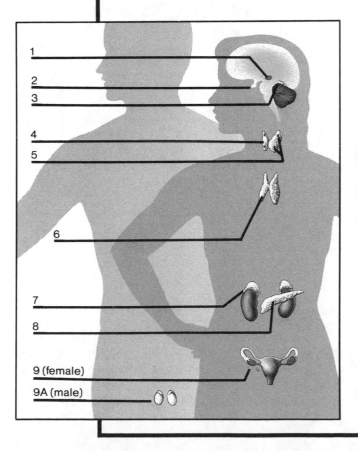

6. Thymus. The thymus lies behind the breastbone. While large in children, it shrinks with age. It may be important in the production of white blood cells.

7. Adrenal glands. The adrenals sit above the kidneys. They produce hormones that help maintain normal body chemistry, as well as the sex hormones androgen and estrogen. The adrenal glands also secrete epinephrine (adrenaline) and norepinephrine (noradrenaline), which prepare your body for "fight or flight."

8. Pancreas. The endocrine areas of the pancreas secrete the hormones insulin and glucagon. Insulin removes glucose from the blood, while glucagon releases glucose to the blood, keeping the body's fuel supply in balance.

9. Ovaries. In females from puberty onward, these produce the hormones estrogen and progesterone, which determine female secondary sexual characteristics and prepare the uterus for pregnancy.

9a. Testes. In males from puberty onward, these produce testosterone, responsible for secondary sexual characteristics such as facial hair.

Every minute 300 million cells in your body die and are replaced immediately by the division of living cells, so that the number of cells in your body remains constant throughout adult life.

Microscopic Facts

Cell sizes are measured in microns. A micron equals $1/1000$ of a millimeter. A human egg cell is about 140 microns in diameter, and is barely visible to the human eye. This may seem small, but the egg cell is a giant when compared to a red blood cell, which measures about 8 microns in diameter, or a white blood cell, which stretches the tape at 10 to 12 microns.

REPLACEMENT PARTS AND THE BODY OF TOMORROW

Man-made Parts Save Life and Limb

While unsurpassed in design and function, the human body is not indestructible. Whether through accident, illness, or birth defect, parts are sometimes lost, deformed, or rendered useless.

Fortunately, clever inventors have combined the wonders of modern technology and materials to bring hope where only despair once existed. Artificial legs, hands, fingers, and toes not only fill in for missing limbs, but function as well. Synthetic ligaments and blood vessels, plastic lenses, and implanted hearing aids all sustain life or help improve it when precious parts fail.

More than 3 million artificial body parts have been installed in American patients. If that trend continues, your chances of wearing an artificial body part in the next 15 years is about 1 in 12.

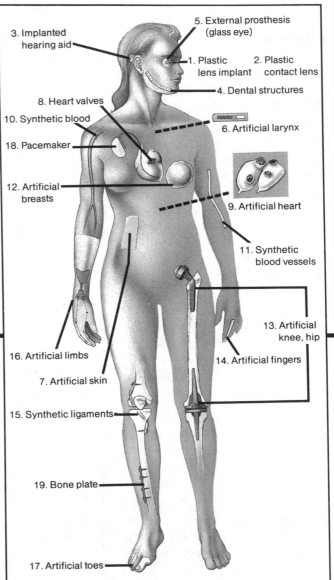

3. Implanted hearing aid
5. External prosthesis (glass eye)
1. Plastic lens implant
2. Plastic contact lens
4. Dental structures
8. Heart valves
10. Synthetic blood
6. Artificial larynx
18. Pacemaker
12. Artificial breasts
9. Artificial heart
11. Synthetic blood vessels
13. Artificial knee, hip
16. Artificial limbs
14. Artificial fingers
7. Artificial skin
15. Synthetic ligaments
19. Bone plate
17. Artificial toes

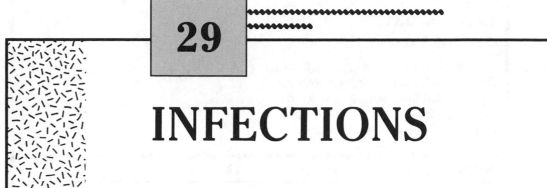

29

INFECTIONS

The human immune system could well be considered one of the world's wonders. Still, it is less than perfect. Everybody gets infections from time to time, and each year the average American adult sniffles through three to five colds.

But once you've had a particular cold virus your immune system protects you from that strain for a long time, maybe even forever. Unfortunately, there are more than 200 different cold viruses out there—the major reason a cure for the common cold may be a long time coming. In the meantime, Americans spend more than a billion dollars annually on over-the-counter cold medicines.

At least colds aren't killers—not literally, anyway. But influenza and pneumonia can be deadly. They combine to rank sixth among causes of death, with a mortality rate of 28.4 per 100,000 people. Yet we've come a long way in fighting infections. Vaccines have drastically reduced the incidence of everything from polio to measles. And in 1980 the World Health Organization finally declared small-pox eradicated.

While you can't seal off your body from invading infections, the amount of protection you can provide is largely up to you. Immunizations for many infectious diseases are widely available. And research indicates you may better resist infections by eating a nutritious diet, exercising regularly, and maintaining a positive attitude.

Is It a Cold or the Flu?

Both can make you miserable. But while the flu's worst symptoms typically last three to four days, colds hang on from seven to ten days. Here are some other differences.

Symptoms	Cold	Flu
Fever	Rare	Characteristic; high (102–104°F); sudden onset; lasts 3–4 days
Headache	Rare	Prominent
General aches and pain	Slight	Usual; often quite severe
Fatigue and weakness	Quite mild	Extreme; can last up to 2–3 weeks
Prostration	Never	Early and prominent
Runny, stuffy nose	Common	Sometimes
Sneezing	Usual	Sometimes
Sore throat	Common	Sometimes
Chest discomfort, cough	Mild to moderate; hacking cough	Common; can become severe
Complications	Sinus congestion or earache	Bronchitis, pneumonia; can be life-threatening

That Stuffed-Up Feeling

Once a cold virus makes itself at home in your nose it triggers release of inflammatory chemicals called kinins. This dramatically increases the blood flow to the nose, which in turn produces:

▼ Swelling

▼ Congestion

▼ Excessive amounts of mucus

Antihistamines and decongestants can help relieve those symptoms, but they can't cure the cold.

Older people are more susceptible to infections, and the infections they get tend to be more severe and more likely to cause death.

Colds tend to have an adverse effect on thinking, while the flu is more likely to disrupt visual perception.

How Colds Are Caught

Just how did you catch that cold anyway? Quite possibly, not the way you think you did.

▼ You can't catch a cold from sitting in a draft or from a sudden dip in temperature.

▼ You don't raise your chances of catching a cold by losing sleep or being fatigued.

▼ You probably won't catch a cold by kissing someone with a cold.

What probably happened instead was:

▼ You shook hands with a cold sufferer and then touched your eyes or nose.

▼ You touched an object such as a telephone or coffee cup used by a cold sufferer, and then you touched your eyes or nose.

▼ You got too close to a cold sufferer who sneezed or coughed the virus into the air and into your nasal passages.

Because there are so many different cold viruses—and because they can live outside the body for hours or even days—odds are that somebody else's cold will catch up you to every so often.

Ways to Ease the Misery

Time will eventually take care of your cold. But in the meantime . . .

Rest. Rushing full speed ahead, especially during the first few days of a cold, will probably just make matters worse. Bed rest, however, usually is not essential.

Drink hot liquids. This will help in three ways: by relieving congestion, soothing throat irritation, and replenishing body fluids.

Vaporize or humidify. Moistened air can make dry nasal passages more comfortable.

Rub down. Camphor/menthol rubs may make you feel better, and not just because of soothing memories of Mom. The Food and Drug Administration found that camphor and menthol can each be effective to calm a cough.

Consider over-the-counter drugs. The shelves are full of nonprescription cold remedies—antihistamines, decongestants, and even combinations of the two. They may help, but be careful: Many induce drowsiness.

Take vitamin C. Although test results are mixed, there appears to be some evidence extra vitamin C may reduce the length and severity of a cold in some people.

Consider zinc lozenges. Some studies indicate that sucking on a zinc tablet can speed a cold's journey through the body by several days. Zinc in large amounts can be toxic, though, so check with a doctor before trying this out.

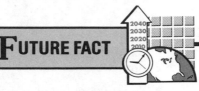

A Cold Shoulder for Cold Viruses

With more than 200 different viruses associated with the common cold, one vaccine for all seems unlikely. But scientists now see a different way to go after colds—by blocking the cellular receptor sites that the viruses need to enter the cell, replicate, and cause illness.

First, researchers discovered that there appear to be one or two major receptor sites to which rhinoviruses (the main type of cold virus) attach. They then reasoned that if they could block the major receptors with a special antibody, they could prevent infection by these viruses 80 to 90 percent of the time. When the special antibody was tested in humans, it tended to delay the onset of a cold and reduce its severity. But it did not actually prevent the cold. In the future, however, scientists believe it's possible that with further development, this approach may be able to totally block some cold viruses—and prevent the common cold.

Scientists are investigating the possibility that peptic ulcer disease is a bacterial infection.

The Negative Impact of Infections

The volume of infections in the United States each year—more than 700 million—is staggering in and of itself. But the effects are far-reaching —nearly 200,000 deaths, billions of lost workdays and schooldays, and a price tag in excess of $17 billion.

Cases: 742,248,261

Deaths: 194,700

Years of life lost before age 65: 2,192,370

Hospital days: 42,029,624

Days lost from work, school, preschool, housekeeping: 1,901,847,705

Cost (excluding costs of death, aftereffects of infections, home care, and reactions to treatment): $17,191,400,000

Flu Shots— Who Needs Them?

Each year scientists and researchers from the Food and Drug Administration, the Centers for Disease Control, and the National Institutes of Health determine which flu viruses to target with a vaccine. The different types of flu are generally identified as A, B, or C. Type A is the most common and often the most severe. Type C is the rarest and mildest. (Because flu germs change, there may be many different strains within one type at one time.)

The people who should get the influenza vaccine each year are those who are most at risk for complications. They are:

▼ Residents of nursing homes and other chronic-care facilities

▼ People 65 and older

▼ Adults and children (six months and older) with continuing medical problems such as anemia, asthma, diabetes, suppressed immunity, or heart, lung, or kidney disease

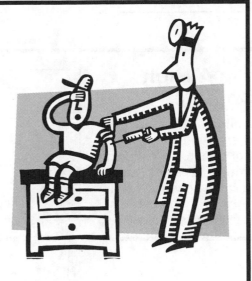

▼ Health workers who might pass the flu on to those at high risk for complications

Individuals *should not* get flu shots if they are allergic to eggs, because the flu vaccine contains egg protein. If you're pregnant, flu shots are generally safe after the first trimester, but it's a good idea to check with a doctor. People with colds or fever should wait until symptoms disappear before getting a flu shot.

Is That a Fact?

One flu epidemic killed millions of people.

It's hard to believe, but yes, in 1918 the flu accounted for at least 21 million deaths worldwide. Since the year 1510, 31 global epidemics of respiratory disease similar to modern influenza have been documented. And from 1968 to 1988 more than 500,000 deaths have occurred in the United States from epidemic influenza.

Day Care: A High Infection Rate

Young children in group care and day care situations tend to get more infections than do children cared for at home. The study results charted here show how many children in each category had at least six infections in their first year of life.

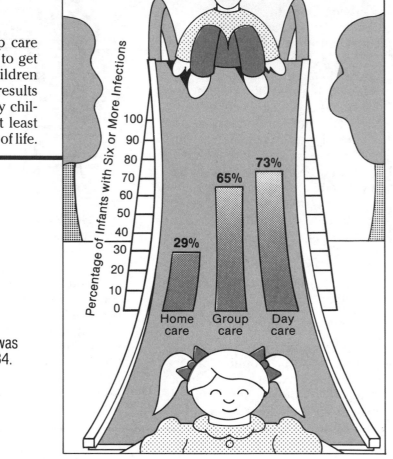

Only one case of diphtheria was reported in the United States in 1984.

IS THAT A FACT?

Cranberry juice can cure or prevent urinary tract infections.

By itself, cranberry juice is not a cure or safeguard against urinary tract infections. According to a study in the *Journal of Urology,* cranberry juice therapy may provide temporary relief by inhibiting the ability of some bacteria to stick to the lining of the bladder and urethra. But once the therapy is stopped, the infection generally reappears.

In a survey, about 60 percent of "high income" people considered immunizations in general to be very safe, but only 49 percent of "low income" people agreed.

A Guide to Childhood Immunizations

All states require proof of immunization before allowing a child to start school. The Centers for Disease Control recommend the following schedule.

Vaccine	Recommended Age	Comments
Diphtheria/pertussis/tetanus	2, 4, 6, and 15 months	Boosters of DPT should be given between the ages of 4 and 7; boosters for diphtheria and tetanus should be given again in 10 years.
Polio	2, 4, and 15 months	If the infant receives live polio vaccine, make sure that everyone in the family has been immunized against polio. In a few cases, the vaccine has caused polio in unprotected family members. A booster shot should be given between the ages of 4 and 7.
MMR (measles/mumps/rubella)	15 months	Can be given at the same time as DPT.
Hib (*Haemophilus influenzaea* type b; immunizes against the microbe that is the leading cause of meningitis in children)	25 months	Can be given at 18 months to children who may be at increased risk—those going to day care, for example.

Of the approximately 40 million people hospitalized each year in the United States, between 5 and 10 percent, or 2 to 4 million patients, develop an infection that was not present or incubating upon admission.

Putting the Chill on Food-Borne Infections

Food poisoning comes in many forms, the most common being salmonella infection. Approximately 50,000 cases of salmonella are reported annually by state health departments, but some experts estimate the actual count may be as much as 40 times higher. Staphylococcus infection is believed to be the second most common form of food poisoning. And unlike salmonella, this toxin is not destroyed by cooking, so proper handling and refrigeration are of even greater importance. Proper refrigeration is also critical in preventing other types of food poisoning—from bacteria such as bacillus and clostridium, for example. But even cold storage has its limits, as this table indicates. Times shown are the maximum periods that meat and poultry may be stored and subsequently eaten with safety.

Food	Refrigerator (Days at 40°F)	Freezer (Months at 0°F)	Food	Refrigerator (Days at 40°F)	Freezer (Months at 0°F)
Fresh meats			Gravy and meat broth	1–2	2–3
Beef roasts	3–5	6–12	*Fresh poultry*		
Beef steaks	3–5	6–12	Chicken and turkey, whole	1–2	12
Lamb chops	3–5	6–9	Chicken, pieces	1–2	9
Lamb roasts	3–5	6–9	Duck and goose, whole	1–2	6
Pork chops	3–5	3–4	Turkey, pieces	1–2	6
Pork or veal roasts	3–5	4–8	Giblets	1–2	3–4
Pork sausage	1–2	1–2	*Cooked poultry*		
Hamburger	1–2	3–4	Cooked poultry dishes	3–4	4–6
Variety meats (tongue, brain, kidneys, liver, and heart)	1–2	3–4	Fried chicken	3–4	4
Processed meats			Covered with broth or gravy	1–2	6
Sausage, dry, semidry	14–21	1–2	Pieces not in broth or gravy	3–4	1
Sausage, smoked	7	1–2	*Game*		
Bacon	7	1	Deer	3–5	6–12
Frankfurters	7	1–2	Rabbit	1–2	12
Ham, whole	7	1–2	Duck and goose, whole	1–2	6
Ham, half	3–5	1–2			
Ham, slices	3–4	1–2			
Luncheon meats	3–5	1–2			
Cooked meats					
Cooked meat and meat dishes	3–4	2–3			

Fish versus Chicken — An Infection Scorecard

Seafood—excluding shellfish—is less likely to transmit infection than chicken is, according to the Food and Drug Administration. The FDA reports:

▼ On a pound-for-pound basis, chicken is 7.8 to 11.5 times more likely than seafood to cause illness.

▼ About one illness occurs per 25,000 servings of chicken, compared with one illness per 250,000 servings of all seafood.

▼ Overall, the number of disease cases blamed on chicken ranges from 1.4 million to 2.1 million annually, with deaths ranging from 140 to 503.

▼ Shellfish and finfish account for about 64,230 cases of disease annually, and 22 deaths.

What You Can — and Can't — Catch

What is and isn't contagious may surprise you.

Acne. Look around a junior high and you would assume acne must be contagious, but it's not. Stress may trigger an outbreak in some people.

Athlete's foot. Yes, it's possible to "catch" athlete's foot. But some people resist the fungi and others don't, and dermatologists don't know why.

Canker sores. Painful, yes. Contagious, no. Some studies indicate canker sores may be associated with stress.

Eczema. The root cause of this skin disease is unknown. But you can't catch eczema from someone else.

Strep throat. This you can catch, by direct or indirect personal contact.

Warts. The good news: You can't catch warts from frogs. The bad news: You can catch warts from people. Warts are caused by a virus which enters the skin through a cut or scratch. As with other infections, a weakened immune system puts you at greater risk. Wart viruses can be picked up by direct contact or indirectly in moist environments such as showers or swimming pools.

Immunizations— Protection for Adults, Too

Widespread immunization has made the United States much safer from infectious diseases. Tetanus, for example, only strikes about 500 Americans each year. But illnesses such as tetanus and diphtheria still need to be taken seriously and immunized against. And other illnesses that people were not immunized against —or were inadequately immunized against—as children should be immunized against now in adulthood.

Immunization	Dosage Schedule	Comments
Routine use for all adults		
Tetanus	At least every 10 years	Management of wounds
Diphtheria	At least every 10 years	Management of contacts of cases of diphtheria
Use in selected populations		
Elderly persons; those with chronic disease		
Influenza	Annually	Annual immunization of high-risk individuals
Pneumococcal disease	Once	Immunization of high-risk persons over 2 years old
Postexposure treatment of animal bites		
Rabies	Five 1 ml doses	Preexposure treatment only in special situations
Adolescents and young adults		
Rubella	Once	Adolescent and adult females who are unimmunized or who have no serum antibodies; hospital workers
Measles	Once	Adolescents and young adults who have not had measles and have no serum antibodies to measles or have not received previous live virus vaccine; postexposure protection
Mumps	Once	Prepubetal and adolescent males who have not had mumps or mumps vaccine

Seven Nutrients for a Stronger Immune System

You already know that eating right—especially eating a lot of fruits and vegetables—is good for the immune system. Now it's time to take a closer look at individual nutrients and the role they play in intercepting and fighting infectious invaders:

Vitamin A. Think of vitamin A as a switch. It turns on the body's T-lymphocyte cells (or T-cells), which then signal antibodies to come and deactivate unwanted invaders. Beta-carotene, found in carrots and other yellow-orange foods, is a good way to get vitamin A.

Folate. This B vitamin is required to make special white blood cells such as the macrophages, the huge lymphocytes that eat infectious organisms. Leafy greens are a good source of folate. Alcohol may rob the body of folate to some degree.

Vitamin B6. White blood cells require B6 to produce antibodies, and the thymus gland needs it to make lymphocytes. Mice fed high doses of B6 showed higher immune responses. Foods rich in B6 include kidney beans, bananas, meat, and whole grain breads.

Vitamin C. Some studies indicate taking extra vitamin C can reduce severe cold symptoms. Other laboratory work has shown vitamin C stimulates the production of interferon, an aptly-named chemical that interferes with the reproduction of viruses. Citrus fruit and juices are good sources.

Vitamin E. Scientists believe this vitamin helps negate the effects of a hormone that suppresses the immune system as we age. Sunflower seeds and wheat germ are rich in vitamin E.

Iron. This mineral helps with the building of white blood cells. Low levels of iron have been associated with increased risk of virus infections. And an estimated 20 percent of women in the United States aren't getting enough iron. Good sources of iron are turkey dark meat, navy beans, and iron itself—use iron cookware when possible.

Zinc. According to some studies, zinc supplements increase resistance to antigens. On the flip side, zinc in very large quantities may actually depress the immune system. Best bet: Include zinc-rich foods, like beef, seafood, and pumpkin seeds in your diet.

Plastic prosthetic devices—including artificial joints and heart valves—are particularly inviting sites for staph infection.

30

MEDICAL CARE

In the world of medicine, time seems to tick away just a little bit faster. Consider all that until recently was merely fantasy, but is now fact: open heart surgery, kidney and liver transplants, lasers that burn through arterial blockages, and much more.

But time has also brought major changes outside the operating room. Consider that most doctors practicing today have never made an official house call, and they probably never will. The doctor-patient relationship has certainly changed. Consider, too, that more than half (54 percent) of all office visits to general and family practitioners now last 10 minutes or less. And while the average length of hospital stays is going down, health care costs for the consumer, as well as medical malpractice premiums for doctors, are going up.

Despite all the changes, the average American still seems reasonably satisfied with the quality of medical care. In a survey, 83 percent of people rated their doctors' competency as "excellent" or "very good." Sixteen percent rated their doctor only "fair," and just one percent ranked their doctor as "poor."

How Did You Select Your Current Doctor?

Most people rely on someone else's advice—be it a friend, a relative, or even another doctor. Another interesting finding: Most people don't shop around for a doctor. Once they get a recommendation, they tend to stick with that doctor, rather than trying several and then deciding. Americans aged 35 to 54 are the most likely to shop around for a physician (39 percent of them do it). And young adults aged 18 to 34 are the least likely to shop (18 percent do).

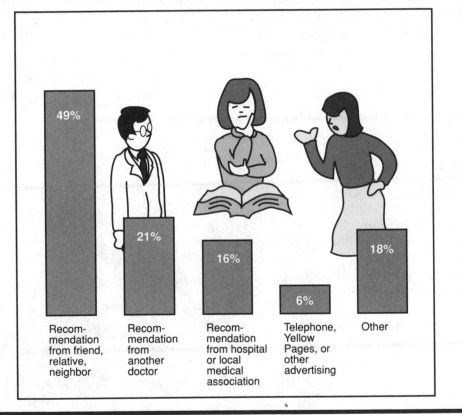

49% — Recommendation from friend, relative, neighbor

21% — Recommendation from another doctor

16% — Recommendation from hospital or local medical association

6% — Telephone, Yellow Pages, or other advertising

18% — Other

One study found that people who engage in self-care practices spend 26 percent less on hospital bills and 19 percent less on doctors' fees.

How Often, and Where, Do You Contact Your Doctor?

In 1987 in the United States there were 5.4 contacts with a doctor per person. And the majority of those contacts took place in doctors' offices. But telephone conversations and visits to hospital outpatient departments also contributed to the overall total.

In a survey of more than 200 hospitals, the Steiber Research Group found that in 1984, hospitals spent an average of $21,250 a year on advertising. By 1989, that figure had jumped to $142,975.

How Long Since Your Last Contact?

People aged 75 and older were the most likely to have had contact with a doctor within the previous year. People aged 15 to 44 were the most likely to have gone two or more years without doctor contact.

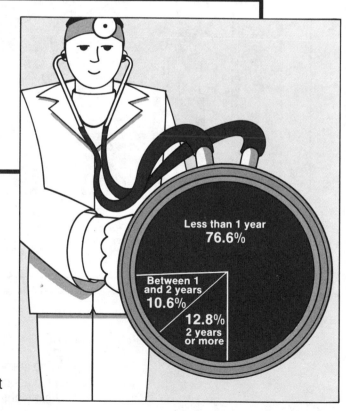

Less than 1 year
76.6%

Between 1 and 2 years
10.6%

12.8%
2 years or more

Between 1976 and 1987, enrollment in HMOs rose from 6 million to 29 million.

Hey, Doc, Tell Me More about . . .

A lot of things. Americans want more information from their doctors about everything from nutrition to psychology to new surgical procedures. But people most want their doctors to tell them how to better control stress.

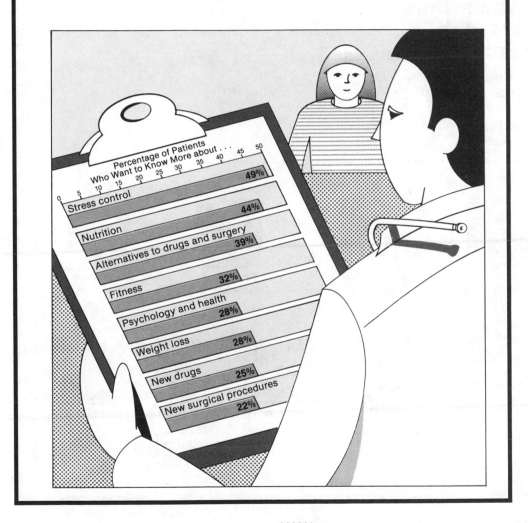

Percentage of Patients Who Want to Know More about . . .

Category	Percentage
Stress control	49%
Nutrition	44%
Alternatives to drugs and surgery	39%
Fitness	32%
Psychology and health	28%
Weight loss	28%
New drugs	25%
New surgical procedures	22%

On average, cancer doctors (oncologists) spend a half-day each week arguing with insurers for coverage of proven therapies.

In 1982 the average net income for physicians was about $98,000. By 1987, it had climbed to just over $132,000.

How Much Time Is Spent with Each Patient?

According to one survey, neurologists typically spend the most time with patients during office and hospital visits. General practitioners spend the least.

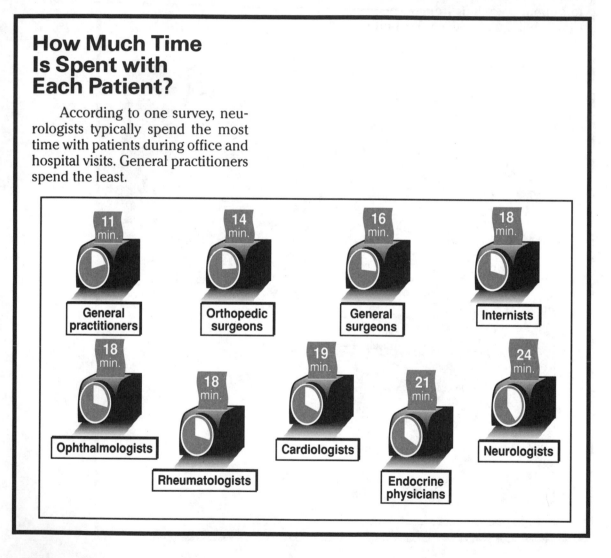

More high-risk surgery patients die on Wednesday — the doctors' traditional day off, than any other day, according to a study.

What Doctors Do That Their Patients Dislike

A lot of doctors make their patients do it, and a lot of people hate doing it . . . waiting. More than 40 percent of those surveyed said that bugged them most. Meanwhile, 32 percent of those surveyed said they had no complaints at all.

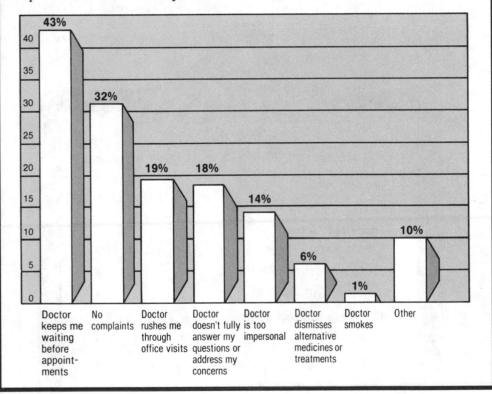

A year-long study of medical mishaps at teaching hospitals found more things go wrong in July than any other month. July is typically the month when new interns and residents replace more experienced hospital staff.

How Doctors Rate Each Other

Medical knowledge earns more respect from fellow doctors than any other single attribute, according to a national poll. Sixteen percent of doctors said that's the quality they admire most. The chart summarizes all their responses.

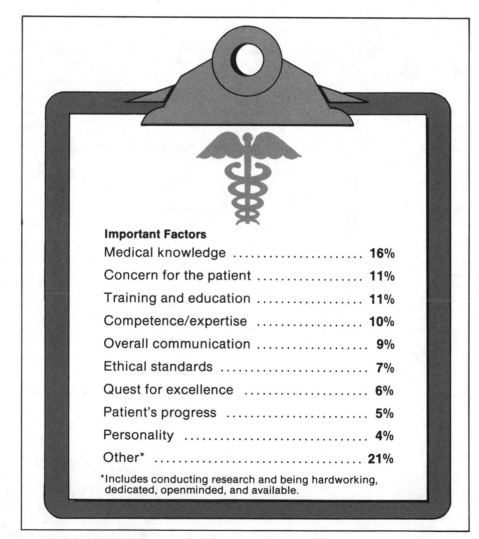

Important Factors

Medical knowledge	16%
Concern for the patient	11%
Training and education	11%
Competence/expertise	10%
Overall communication	9%
Ethical standards	7%
Quest for excellence	6%
Patient's progress	5%
Personality	4%
Other*	21%

*Includes conducting research and being hardworking, dedicated, openminded, and available.

The Number of Physicians Continues to Rise

In 1950, there were just under 220,000 medical doctors in the United States. By the year 2000, it's estimated there will be more than three times as many.

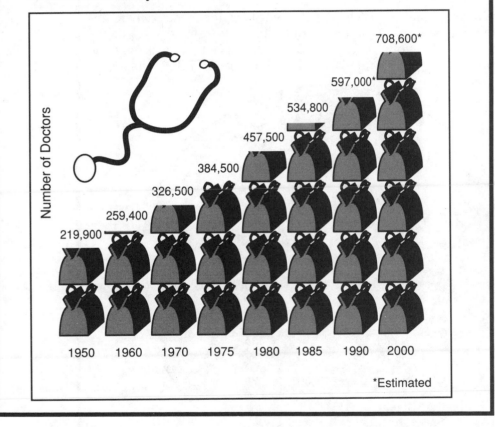

Number of Doctors

219,900 — 1950
259,400 — 1960
326,500 — 1970
384,500 — 1975
457,500 — 1980
534,800 — 1985
597,000* — 1990
708,600* — 2000

*Estimated

Did you know that both ECG and EKG are abbreviations used to describe electrocardiograms? No matter how it's abbreviated, the point of the test is to measure electrical impulses traveling through the heart.

Forty-one percent of hospitals offered outpatient rehabilitation services in 1987 — more than a three-fold increase from ten years earlier.

Where in the World Are the Doctors?

In high-income countries such as the United States, Canada, and Japan, there are usually enough doctors to go around. In 1984 in the United States, for example, there was one doctor for every 470 people. But in Ethiopia, there was only one doctor for every 77,360 persons.

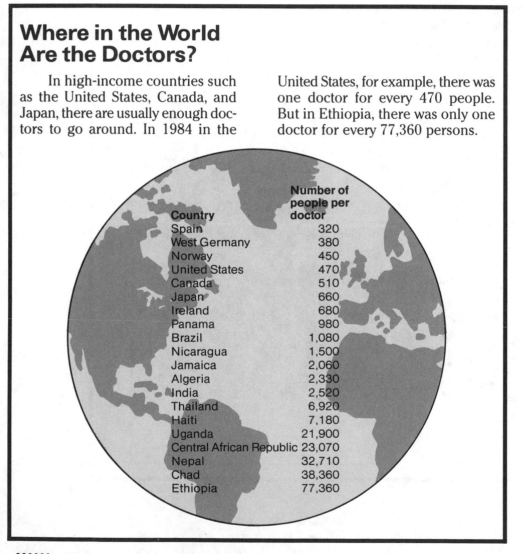

Country	Number of people per doctor
Spain	320
West Germany	380
Norway	450
United States	470
Canada	510
Japan	660
Ireland	680
Panama	980
Brazil	1,080
Nicaragua	1,500
Jamaica	2,060
Algeria	2,330
India	2,520
Thailand	6,920
Haiti	7,180
Uganda	21,900
Central African Republic	23,070
Nepal	32,710
Chad	38,360
Ethiopia	77,360

Percentage of adults surveyed who said they have a blood pressure reading taken at least once a year: 86.

A Guide to Modern Diagnostic Tests

Want to know if your unborn child is healthy? Amniocentesis can probably tell you. Suspect that awful pain is the result of gallstones? Cholecystography may give you the answer. Today, fortunately, modern medicine has a wide range of diagnostic tests at the ready. Listed here are some of the most common, along with a description of the procedures.

Test	Purpose	Procedure
Amniocentesis	Determination of health of the fetus; detection of many genetic defects and some hereditary disorders; generally used in pregnant women over 35 years of age.	A hollow needle is inserted through the abdominal wall into the uterus to remove a small amount of fluid from the amniotic sac. The placenta is located by ultrasound.
Biopsy	Examination of tissue samples and cells to determine abnormalities; indicated when cancer is suspected.	A small piece of tissue is removed for microscopic examination.
Bone marrow	Examination of specimen from bone interior to determine red and white blood cell balance and presence of iron.	A small amount of bone marrow is withdrawn with a syringe and special needle, usually from hip bone or sternum.
Bronchoscopy	Inspection of the interior of the tracheobronchial tree through a bronchoscope; helpful in diagnosing upper bronchial cancer, obtaining biopsy specimens, and removing obstructions; indicated in cases of severe, prolonged cough or coughing up of blood, and for an undiagnosed abnormality on chest x-ray.	A fiberoptic (a flexible material made of glass or plastic that transmits light along its course by reflecting it from the side or wall of the fiber) bronchoscope is passed from the mouth through the trachea and into the bronchi. Sedatives are administered before the test. A local or general anesthetic may also be administered.
Cholecystography	Examination of the gallbladder by x-ray study; useful in detecting gallstone or gallbladder dysfunction.	A radiopaque substance or contrast medium is given to make the gallbladder more visible. Then an x-ray is taken to determine the presence of gallstones. To test for gallbladder dysfunction, a fatty meal is eaten and another x-ray is taken.
Colonoscopy	Inspection of the colon above the rectum, obtaining tissue samples for biopsy, removal of polyps; used after repeated blood stool tests have been positive to look for suspected cancer or other disorders.	An endoscope is inserted into the anus and then threaded the entire length of the large intestine. Prior to test, the colon is cleansed by enemas, and a sedative is given.

(continued)

A Guide to Modern Diagnostic Tests—*Continued*

Test	Purpose	Procedure
Computerized Axial Tomography (CAT scan)	Imaging of internal structures, especially the brain; works only for parts of the body that can be completely immobilized; useful in diagnosing brain disorders and injuries, liver or pancreatic tumors.	Numerous parallel x-ray beams are projected through the body from various angles. These images are converted by a computer into cross-sectional views.
Culdoscopy	Endoscopic examination of the female internal organs and pelvic cavity; used in cases of suspected endometriosis (abnormal uterine tissue growth outside the uterus), infertility, and other disorders involving pelvic organs.	An endoscope (a flexible fiberoptic tube permitting visualization of a hollow organ) is inserted into the pelvic cavity through an incision in the vaginal wall.
Echocardiography	To record the size, motion, and composition of various cardiac structures; used in heart valve problems that are difficult to diagnose.	Use of ultrasound produces an image or photograph of an organ or tissue. Ultrasonic echoes are recorded as they strike tissues of different densities.
Fluoroscopy	Examination of inner parts of the body by means of the fluoroscope. Upper body: x-ray visualization of esophagus, stomach, and duodenum to detect ulcers. Indicated when such symptoms as indigestion, stomach pain, nausea, and loss of appetite become persistent. Lower body: x-ray visualization of large intestine. Useful in detecting diverticulosis (weakened outpouches in the colon wall) and colon tumors.	For an upper gastrointestinal (GI) series, a patient is given a barium drink. X-rays and fluoroscopic studies are then taken. For a lower GI series, barium mixture is fed into the empty colon via a tube inserted into the anus. While barium is being fed in, fluoroscopy (the projection of moving x-rays onto a special screen) is undertaken to look at the intestinal lining. Regular x-rays are taken after the large intestine is filled.
Gastroscopy	Examination of the stomach and abdominal cavity; collection of biopsy specimens and photographing of organs; used in cases where there is a suspicion of stomach ulcers and upper gastrointestinal tract bleeding of unknown origin or unexplained abnormalities.	This procedure calls for a flexible fiberoptic endoscope to be threaded from the mouth through the esophagus into the stomach and upper intestine. Air may be blown through the tube for better visualization. Either local anesthetic or mild sedative is administered.

Test	Purpose	Procedure
Nuclear Magnetic Resonance (NMR)	A new technique, NMR imaging is becoming available at large medical centers. It promises many of the advantages of the x-ray, CAT, and other scans without the hazard of ionizing radiation.	Various atoms in the body, acting like tiny magnets, can be caused to emit weak radiowaves as a result of a combined magnetic field and radio stimulation. These waves, computer detected and analyzed, project an image on a TV monitor.
Positron Emission Tomography (PET)	A scanner that makes images from radioactive isotopes introduced into the patient's body; these images are deciphered by the use of computers.	Specially prepared chemicals containing radioactive atoms that emit positrons, are injected or inhaled. A scanning device detects these radioactive isotopes within the body.
Radioisotope scanning	The study of the function and condition of internal organs, vessels, or body fluids. Used in patients with symptoms of various serious diseases. There are specific scans for virtually all the body organs.	A radioactive substance is injected into the blood and concentrates in the organ under study. The presence and location of this substance in the body is detected by special apparatus.
Sigmoidoscopy	Inspection, through a speculum, of the interior of the sigmoid colon; indicated for the detection of abnormalities in the lower 12 inches of bowel.	A tubular speculum is inserted through the anus to examine the sigmoid flexure (the lower part of the descending colon, shaped like the letter S).
Spinal tap	Lumbar puncture; used in cases of suspected meningitis, and in certain types of spinal cord or brain damage.	A needle is injected at the juncture between the third and fourth vertebrae to extract spinal fluid for lab analysis.
Thermography	A process for measuring temperature by means of a thermograph; the technique has been used to study blood flow in limbs and to detect cancer.	A regional temperature map of a body or organ is obtained with thermographic imaging. An infrared camera scans the body and the computer codes body temperature.
Ultrasonography	Use of ultrasound to produce an image or photograph of an organ or tissue. Used where there is a suspicion of thyroid or gallbladder dysfunction, and in hard-to-diagnose cases of heart and valve problems.	A transducer, placed over the area to be examined, sends ultrasonic waves into the body. The ultrasonic echoes are recorded by the transducer as they strike tissues of different densities, and are converted into visual images.

How to Avoid Unnecessary X-Rays

This year seven out of ten Americans will get a medical or dental x-ray. And in most cases, that will be just fine. The picture will help the doctor or dentist determine how they should be treated. But x-rays can do harm, too.

True, the amount of radiation in x-rays is low. But because x-rays may add slightly to the chances of getting cancer later on in life, it makes sense to avoid any unnecessary x-rays. The experts' advice is to:

▼ First ask your doctor how an x-ray will help with diagnosis and treatment.

▼ Tell the doctor if you are, or might be, pregnant before having an x-ray of the abdomen.

▼ Don't insist on an x-ray if the doctor says it's not needed.

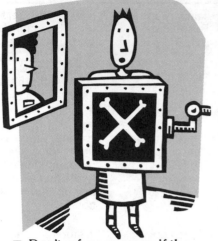

▼ Don't refuse an x-ray if the doctor says an x-ray is medically necessary—the risk is small.

▼ Keep an x-ray record card. When an x-ray is taken, fill in the type of exam, the date, and where the x-ray is kept. If another doctor suggests an x-ray of the same part of your body, tell him about the previous x-ray.

Hospital Infection Rates Compared

Unfortunately, infections seem to like hospitals. As a result, many patients wind up with an illness they didn't have when they checked in. Overall, hospitals have an infection rate of about 33.5 cases per 1,000 patient discharges. The rate of infection in large teaching hospitals is even higher—41.4 cases per 1,000—because they take care of more seriously ill patients requiring more complicated medical procedures.

A Timetable of Medical Checkups

The best way to avoid medical problems is to follow a healthy lifestyle and to get regular checkups. That way, if a problem is developing it can be diagnosed and treated early. The following guide comes from the American Medical Association.

Test and Purpose	When Recommended	When to Begin if Healthy	Frequency of Follow-Ups
Complete physical examination			
To check on the general health of your heart, lungs, brain, and major internal organs	If you have a family history of disorders of any of these organs and as a preventive measure	From the age of 20 onward	Every 3–5 years
Blood pressure			
To check the condition of your heart and arteries; if there is any rise in blood pressure, this may cause serious medical problems	If you have a family history of high blood pressure, heart or kidney disease, stroke or diabetes, or if you are overweight or taking the contraceptive pill	From the age of 20 onward	At least 3–5 years or annually if in a high-risk group or taking the contraceptive pill
Rectal examination			
To detect rectal or prostate cancer	If you have a family history of colon or rectal cancer	Annual digital exam after age 20	General exam every 3–5 years; annual stool test after age 50
Vaginal examination			
To examine the pelvic floor, perineum, and pelvic organs	Before you start any new contraceptive, if you are pregnant, or if you have a vaginal or pelvic infection	Regular checkups are not needed unless stated otherwise	Annually
Cervical (Pap) smear			
To detect any premalignant or malignant changes in the cervix	If you bleed between periods or have irregular periods	From the age of 25 onward, or as soon as you are sexually active	Annually
Mammography (breast x-ray)			
To detect signs of breast cancer before it becomes noticeable through physical exam	If you have a family history of breast cancer	Once between the ages of 35 and 40	Every 1–2 years between the ages of 40 and 50; annually thereafter

(continued)

A Timetable of Medical Checkups—*Continued*

Test and Purpose	When Recommended	When to Begin if Healthy	Frequency of Follow-Ups
Eye tests			
Even if you can see well you should have regular vision tests to detect problems at an early stage	If you have difficulty with vision or a family history of glaucoma	From the age of 40 onward	Annually
Dental checkups			
Regular inspections are vital to detect any early signs of decay, or for signs of infection of the mouth and gums	If you have not had regular checkups, start now rather than waiting until you have a tooth-ache or painful gums	From childhood	Every 6 months before the age of 21, then every 1–2 years
Serum cholesterol, triglyceride, and HDL level			
To detect people at high risk for development of coronary artery disease	If you have a family history of coronary artery disease, diabetes, high blood pressure, or large weight gain	In your 20s	No follow-up if first test is normal, unless at physician's recommendation

From *The American Medical Association Home Medical Adviser*. Copyright © 1988 by The American Medical Association. Reprinted by permission of Random House, Inc.

A Shortage of Nurses

In 1970 there were 750,000 registered nurses in the United States. By 1986, that figure had more than doubled—to 1,593,000. But, hospitals and other facilities are still short of nurses.

The shortage is partly due to the increasing number of older people in the country. When they become ill, they tend to need more skilled nursing care than younger patients. But a national survey also found that many hospitals are having difficulty recruiting registered nurses for evening, night, and rotating shifts.

Further, the American Hospital Association reports that since 1984, enrollment in nursing schools has dropped by 26 percent. The nursing shortage was so bad in 1987 that more than 60 percent of hospitals had to work nurses overtime to meet patients' needs.

Hospital Stays Are Getting Shorter

Overall, the average length of hospital stays decreased in the 1980s. By age, it declined for all groups except children 15 and younger. The most dramatic change was in the 65-and-older category, where the average length of stay was nearly 11 days in 1980, but down to about 8½ days in 1987.

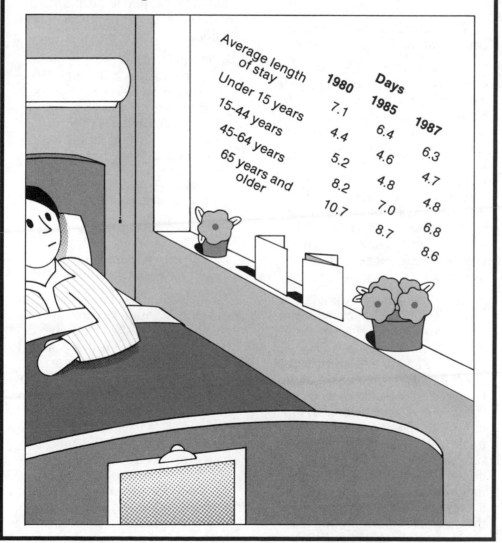

Average length of stay	1980	Days 1985	1987
Under 15 years	7.1	6.4	6.3
15–44 years	4.4	4.6	4.7
45–64 years	5.2	4.8	4.8
65 years and older	8.2	7.0	6.8
	10.7	8.7	8.6

A Hospital Patient's Bill of Rights

When you check into a hospital for care, you may temporarily surrender some of your freedom—and even some of your dignity. But you still retain certain rights, as listed here by the American Hospital Association.

1. The patient has the right to considerate and respectful care.

2. The patient has the right to obtain from his physician complete, current information concerning his diagnosis, treatment, and prognosis in terms the patient can reasonably be expected to understand. When it is not medically advisable to give such information to the patient, the information should be made available to an appropriate person in his behalf. He has the right to know, by name, the physician responsible for coordinating his care.

3. The patient has the right to receive from his physician information necessary to give informed consent prior to the start of any procedure and/or treatment. Except in emergencies, such information for informed consent should include but not necessarily be limited to the specific procedure and/or treatment, the medically significant risks involved, and the probable duration of incapacitation. Where medically significant alternatives for care or treatment exist, or when the patient requests information concerning medical alternatives, the patient has the right to such information. The patient also has the right to know the name of the person responsible for the procedures and/or treatment.

4. The patient has the right to refuse treatment to the extent permitted by law and to be informed of the medical consequences of his action.

5. The patient has the right to every consideration of his privacy concerning his own medical care program. Case discussion, consultation, examination, and treatment are confidential and should be conducted discreetly. Those not directly involved in his care must have the permission of the patient to be present.

6. The patient has the right to expect that all communications and records pertaining to his care should be treated as confidential.

7. The patient has the right to expect that within its capacity a hospital must make reasonable response to the request of a patient for services. The hospital must provide evaluation, service, and/or referral as indicated by the urgency of the case. When medically permissible, a patient may be transferred to another facility only after he has received complete information and explanation concerning the needs for and alternatives to such a transfer. The institution to which the patient is to be transferred must first have accepted the patient for transfer.

8. The patient has the right to obtain information as to any relationship of his hospital to other health care and educational institutions insofar as his care is concerned. The patient has the right to obtain information as to the existence of any professional relationships among individuals, by name, who are treating him.

9. The patient has the right to be advised if the hospital proposed to engage in or perform human experimentation affecting his care or treatment. The patient has the right to refuse to participate in such research projects.

10. The patient has the right to expect reasonable continuity of care. He has the right to know in advance what appointment times and physicians are available and where. The patient has the right to expect that the hospital will provide a mechanism whereby he is informed by his physician or a delegate of the physician of the patient's continuing health care requirements following discharge.

11. The patient has the right to examine and receive an explanation of his bill, regardless of source of payment.

12. The patient has the right to know what hospital rules and regulations apply to his conduct as a patient.

Reprinted with permission of the American Hospital Association, copyright 1972.

The Most Common Hospital Infections

For those unlucky enough to contract an infection during a hospital stay, odds are that they will develop a urinary tract infection. Regardless of the type of hospital surveyed, urinary tract infection rates were more than double those of the next most common infection—lower respiratory infection.

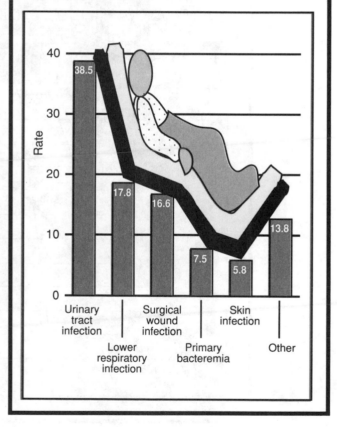

In a survey of adult women, more than three-fourths (78 percent) said they received a Pap smear test every one or two years.

Nursing Home Population Soars

The number of nursing home residents almost tripled from 1963 to 1985. The increase was especially dramatic in the age 85-and-older category—from 148,700 residents in 1963 to nearly 600,000 in 1985.

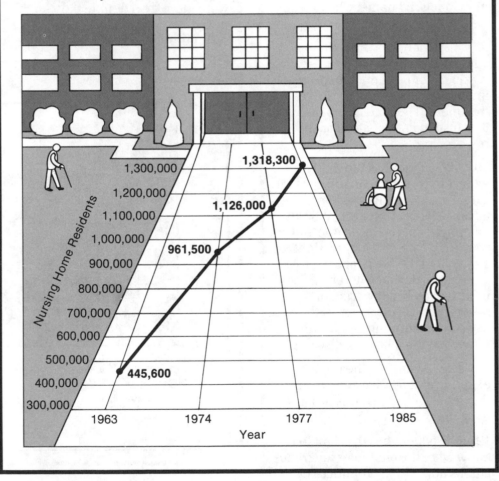

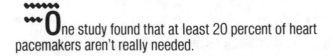
One study found that at least 20 percent of heart pacemakers aren't really needed.

The Most Frequently Performed Operations

Biopsy—the removal and examination of body tissue for diagnostic purposes—was the most frequently performed surgery in the United States in 1987. The top ten procedures, as reported by the American College of Surgeons, are listed here.

Surgery (1987)	Number*	Rate†
1. Biopsy	1,378	5.7
2. Cesarean section	953	3.9
3. Repair of current obstetric laceration	660	2.7
4. Hysterectomy	655	2.7
5. Operations on spinal cord and spinal canal structures	588	2.4
6. Removal of lesion of skin or tissue	568	2.4
7. Plastic surgery of the joints	556	2.3
8. Removal of gallbladder	536	2.2
9. Removal of one or both ovaries, or of a uterine tube and ovary	490	2.0
10. Surgical setting of a bone	481	2.0

*in thousands
†per 1,000 persons

More Women Are Becoming Surgeons

Not that long ago the only women in the OR were nurses and patients. But that's changing. As of 1987, there were more than five times as many female surgeons in the United States as there were in 1970.

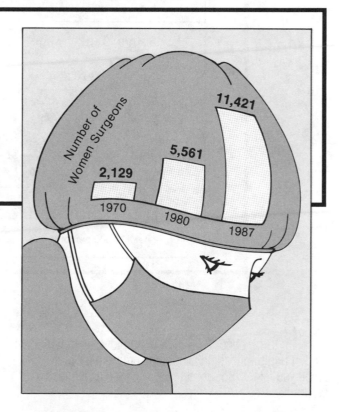

Number of Women Surgeons

2,129 — 1970
5,561 — 1980
11,421 — 1987

As of 1987, 19 percent of all hospitals had outpatient alcoholism and chemical dependency programs.

Who Undergoes Surgery?

Women have a higher rate of surgery than men, largely due to procedures associated with childbirth. And people 65 and older are more than three times as likely to have an operation as people aged 15 to 44.

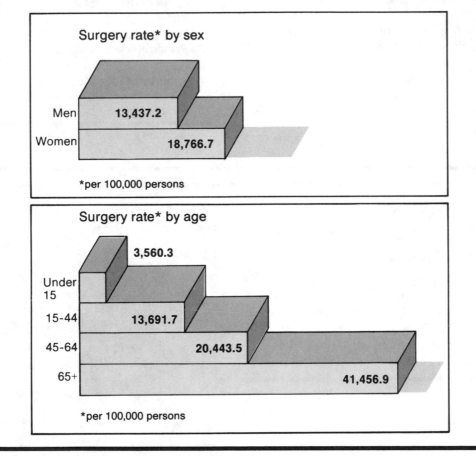

Surgery rate* by sex

Men 13,437.2
Women 18,766.7

*per 100,000 persons

Surgery rate* by age

Under 15 3,560.3
15-44 13,691.7
45-64 20,443.5
65+ 41,456.9

*per 100,000 persons

In 1982, about 5 percent of employers offered some kind of health-enhancing wellness program for their employees. In 1986, 36 percent provided a wellness program.

Transplant Trends

What once was impossible now seems almost commonplace. Organ transplants, though still medical miracles, are no longer rare. From 1983 to 1987, the number of organ transplants in the United States increased sigificantly.

Organ	1983	1984	1985	1986	1987
Heart	172	346	719	1,368	1,512
Kidney	6,112	6,968	7,695	8,976	8,967
Liver	164	308	602	924	1,182
Pancreas/islet cells	61	87	130	140	180
Heart/lung	20	22	30	45	41
Cornea	21,250	24,000	26,300	28,000	35,000

The Ten Most Frequent Malpractice Suits

The following are the most common liability allegations, based on a survey of the claims experience of 40,000 U.S. physicians.

1. Surgery: postoperative complications

2. Improper treatment: birth related

3. Failure to diagnose: cancer

4. Surgery: inadvertent act

5. Failure to diagnose: fracture-dislocation

6. Improper treatment: fracture-dislocation

7. Improper treatment: drug side effect

8. Failure to diagnose: infection

9. Surgery: inappropriate procedure

10. Improper treatment: infection

How Surgical Risk Can Vary

All surgery carries some risk, but that risk can vary considerably depending on where the surgery is performed and who does it. A study of coronary artery bypass surgeries, for example, found that the risk increases when relatively less experienced doctors are operating in hospitals which have not previously hosted large numbers of this type of surgery.

Hospital Volume (No. of Procedures)	Less Experienced Doctors: Mortality Rate (%)	More Experienced Doctors: Mortality Rate (%)
Less than 223	5.7	5.5
224–309	5.1	3.9
310–650	5.1	4.4
651–1,081	3.8	3.2
Total	4.9	4.0

What It Takes to Win a Malpractice Case

A plaintiff's lawyer must show four things to win a malpractice case:

▼ That there was an applicable standard of care

▼ That the standard was breached

▼ That the patient was harmed

▼ That the doctor's violation of the standard of care directly caused harm to the patient

The Most Important Health Care Issues

Depending on who you ask—the general public or doctors—you'll get a different set of priorities, as this survey shows.

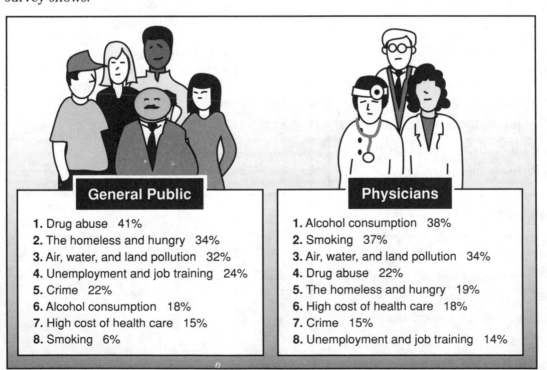

General Public

1. Drug abuse 41%
2. The homeless and hungry 34%
3. Air, water, and land pollution 32%
4. Unemployment and job training 24%
5. Crime 22%
6. Alcohol consumption 18%
7. High cost of health care 15%
8. Smoking 6%

Physicians

1. Alcohol consumption 38%
2. Smoking 37%
3. Air, water, and land pollution 34%
4. Drug abuse 22%
5. The homeless and hungry 19%
6. High cost of health care 18%
7. Crime 15%
8. Unemployment and job training 14%

Health Care Coverage—Where the Gaps Are

More than 15 percent of people under age 65 in the United States do not have health care coverage. Not surprisingly, those with an annual family income of $10,000 or less are most likely to be affected. Of those with coverage, 75.9 percent have private insurance and 5.9 percent rely on Medicaid.

A new device, called a flash pump dye laser, can destroy the hemoglobin in the skin that causes purplish birthmarks. The treatment is available at major medical centers.

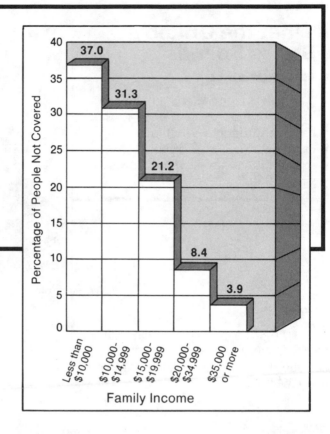

HMOs Are on the Rise

Health Maintenance Organizations—now simply known as HMOs—have become a staple of the health care industry in a very short time. Though individual HMOs vary somewhat, their basic premise is the same. People enrolling in an HMO enter into a contract in which they agree to pay, or have paid on their behalf, a fixed sum in return for access to health personnel facilities and services. If they choose to see a doctor outside the HMO, they will have to pay for it out of their own pocket.

Medical Costs on a Fast Track

Be it food, housing, or medical care, the prices continue to rise. But the consumer price index for medical care easily outdistanced cost increases in all other major categories over the last 30 years.

In 1986, Medicare funds reimbursed an average of $2,870 per person served.

What the United States Spends for Health

The United States spent $500.3 billion, or 11.1 percent of its gross national product (GNP), on health care in 1987. Here's a look at how expenditures have surged upward since 1950.

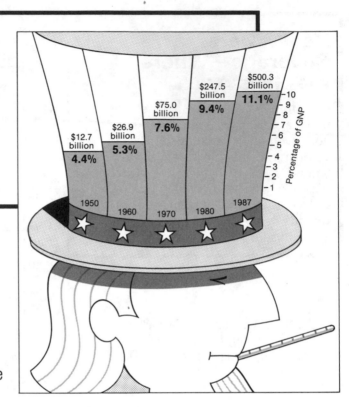

In 1988 Congress passed the Medicare Catastrophic Coverage Act, providing catastrophic health care insurance coverage under Medicare.

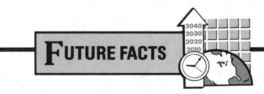

FUTURE FACTS

Computerized Patients Predicted

By the year 2000, or perhaps sooner, "computer patients" may be an integral part of medical training. According to the National Library of Medicine, a computer-generated hypothetical patient with a variety of symptoms and a full life history already has been developed. By using voice commands, a medical student can check the patient's medical history, order tests, and get results of those tests. Afterward, the computer evaluates the student's performance, and reports on how the patient fared.

31

MEDICAL ODDITIES

In medicine, as in life, truth is often stranger than fiction. Just consider the case of a patient who complained of hearing crunching sounds in the ear when chewing or swallowing. At first, the specialists at the Cleveland Clinic Hospital in Ohio were mystified. They tested, they probed, and they touched. They had heard that hair growing in the ear canal might cause problems. But they hadn't counted on hair *clippings*. It seems the patient had just gotten a haircut, and after the doctors removed a ¼-inch-long piece of hair from the ear—using snare forceps and an operating microscope—the noise was gone.

Then there's the case of the 34-year-old munitions worker in Israel who spent ten years in an explosives factory working with nitroglycerin—the same material heart patients depend on to dilate their arteries and banish

angina pain. He began complaining of weekend chest pains when he was away from his job. Eventually he suffered a heart attack on a Sunday morning and had to be hospitalized. Doctors ruled the case "a classic example of nitroglycerin withdrawal syndrome."

For every puzzle that scientists solve, a thousand astonishing occurrences and intriguing mysteries remain. Why, for example, do left-handers suffer from more allergies than right-handers? Why do some people decide to perform do-it-yourself surgery on themselves—successfully? What makes a person get a case of hiccups that never goes away?

The facts that follow may be unusual, even bizarre. But as Ripley himself never tired of telling us, the world really is a strange place—believe it or not.

The Story of Siamese Twins

On May 11, 1811, twin boys Chang and Eng Bunker were born on a houseboat in Meklong in Siam (now Thailand). They slid from their mother Nok's birth canal in one compact package—the head of one between the legs of the other.

The midwife laid the babies on a small bamboo mat for all to see—it was a prize to have two sons at once in a land where a woman's worth was determined by the number of children she bore. But the midwife's joy turned to horror as she prepared to separate the two to give them their first baths.

These weren't normal twin boys. They were joined at the chest by a band of cartilage. And even though the Bunkers weren't the first joined twins ever born, the term "Siamese twins" was coined.

This kind of medical oddity, conjoined twins, has actually occurred throughout history. The year A.D. 945 saw the birth of Armenian twins who were connected at the abdomen. An effort to separate them killed one immediately; the other died three days later. In 1100, Mary and Eliza Chuckhurst were born in Biddenden, Kent, England, joined at the hips and possibly at the shoulders. They lived to age 34. In 1475, Scottish brothers were born joined at the back —two people from the waist up and one from the waist down. King James III took them in, educated and raised them, and they lived to age 28. In 1701, Hungarian sisters were born who shared a pair of legs and whose bodies were back to back. They were exhibited at county fairs until age 9, then lived in a convent until they died at age 22.

The Bunkers, who might have spent their lives on display in a circus sideshow, didn't spend their lives as medical oddities. As young men, they moved to North Carolina, where they married sisters and fathered 22 children. The men died within 3 hours of each other at age 62. They were buried as they lived their whole lives, joined at the chest.

If you are prone to heartburn from esophageal reflux, you'd better think twice about giving in to the allure of a water bed. A study showed that people with an inflamed esophagus are more likely to be sleeping in water beds than are people with a healthy esophagus. Reflux occurs when acid that exists naturally in the stomach flows back up into the esophagus, resulting in a burning sensation. The position you lie in when sleeping in a water bed can inhibit acid clearing and allow the reflux action.

When Baron Rothschild was told his red blood corpuscles showed a tendency to form "money rouleaux" (a medical condition in which red blood corpuscles were rolled together like a pile of coins), he is said to have replied, "What is bred in the bone will out in the blood."

Six Offbeat but On-Target Treatments

Not too long ago, if you had told people that oil from certain kinds of fish might lower the risk of heart attack, they would probably have laughed. But yesterday's you've-got-to-be-kidding experiments have a way of turning into today's we-knew-it-all-along treatments. Here are eight offbeat but promising treatment ideas that are still in the eyebrow-raising stage. Some have already been tried clinically with humans, others only in test-tube or animal tests.

1. Kiss a frog and get a small dose of magainin, an infection-fighting substance that could be the penicillin of the 1990s. Magainin is the magic ingredient discovered in frog skin by Michael A. Zasloff, M.D., Ph.D. It speeds frog healing after surgery.

2. Cure cancer with a tobacco leaf? Perhaps, if you could turn the tobacco plant into a genetic factory for cancer-fighting substances. Using a plant virus that attacks only tobacco but that can also carry genes to make specific, useful proteins, scientists hope to force the tobacco leaf to make cancer-fighting agents such as interleukin-2.

3. Plug in your electric bandage to fight pain. The new device is an adhesive-backed fabric bandage impregnated with metal particles. As the bandage touches skin and perspiration, the metal particles react to each other, resulting in an extremely low-level electrical charge that works directly on the muscle. The charge relieves pain while relaxing the muscle.

4. A virus that makes cows sick may help keep skin cancer patients well. Cowpox virus, the same virus that was used to provide immunity against smallpox, can be turned into a vaccine intended to halt cancer recurrence in people who have had surgery for malignant melanoma, the deadliest form of skin cancer. Researchers have combined four different strains of melanoma cells with the relatively harmless cowpox virus. The resultant vaccine induces the immune system to form antibodies against melanoma cells, reinforcing the body's defensive response to the initial cancer.

5. A medication derived from the Western yew tree may be an ally for women with ovarian cancer. Taxol, a new drug made from the bark of the Western yew tree, inhibits production of cells.

6. The "catch of the day" could soon refer to heat-toughened sea coral, which may be used in bone replacement. Some types of sea coral are very similar to bone in pore structure. The coral must be combined with phosphates and water to convert it to hydroxyapatite, a calcium phosphate that is the major component of bone. Coral implants don't shrink, and their porous structure allows adjacent bone to grow into them, strengthening them over time.

The Case of the Refriger-Raider

A 37-year-old man visited his doctor complaining that he climbed out of bed three to five times a night to go to the kitchen to eat and drink —about once every 1½ hours. He wanted to quit his nocturnal nipping, but since he was *sleeping* through the snacking, he couldn't control himself.

A few times he woke up during his forays for food; one time he caught himself drinking sunflower oil. Most mornings he couldn't remember having gotten up during the night.

The eager eater was placed in a sleep laboratory for six nights. Researchers stocked his bedside table with two bottles of soft drink, a pork pie, and packages of potato chips and cookies.

Records show he slept an average of 439 minutes a night with normal stages of sleeping, including dreams. But on 31 occasions he ate, with 28 of these episodes occurring just before, in the middle of, or just after having a dream.

Scientists say babies on demand-feeding schedules eat according to this same pattern. And the man who was raiding his refrigerator ultimately decided it didn't bother him after all.

People Who *Really* Get the Blues

When people around Trouble-some Creek, Kentucky, say they're feeling a little bit blue, they aren't talking about feeling emotionally down and out. For more than 160 years, some of the inhabitants have had blue skin, caused by a recessive gene. These people, believed to be related to Martin Fugate, a French-born orphan who arrived in the United States six generations ago, are lacking the enzyme diaphorase. Normally, this enzyme turns the blue protein methemoglobin into the red protein hemoglobin in the blood. Community inbreeding in Trouble-some Creek has produced healthy but odd-looking blue people. There is a treatment for the condition, however. Pills containing the dye methylene blue allow the body of these true blue bloods to convert the methemoglobin back to hemoglobin, turning the skin pink. The one drawback is that the dye turns the urine blue.

A Directory of Out-of-the-Ordinary Ailments

Tennis players refer to the pain in their elbows as "tennis elbow." (It's caused by swinging a racket.) And anyone who has scrubbed a floor on their hands and knees knows about the pain called "housemaid's knee." Here are some even odder ailments that you may not have heard of but may have experienced.

Assembly headache. A headache due to exhaustion and poor ventilation in crowded areas such as theaters and exhibitions.

Backpacker's diarrhea. Gastroenteritis caused by the parasite *Giardia lamblia,* found in streams and ponds where a backpacker stops to drink.

Back-to-school syndrome. Tiredness and weight loss among mothers who rush to and from school with their young.

Bongo drum disease. An anthrax infection contracted from playing goat-hide bongo drums.

Bulb fingers. A tingling tenderness of the fingertips of people who handle large quantities of tulip, hyacinth, onion, and garlic bulbs.

Cinematic neurosis. A traumatic feeling brought on by movies with strong emotional effects, such as *Jaws* and *The Exorcist.*

Credit-card-itis. A sciatic nerve irritation causing pain over the buttock and down the thigh due to the pressure of a wallet stuffed with credit cards.

Driver's thigh. An irritation of the sciatic nerve caused by pressure from the car seat. Most often seen in people who drive for long periods of time.

Expressway blues. Headaches, caused by exhaust fumes and nervous tension, suffered by drivers on congested expressways.

Flip-flop dermatitis. Skin rash over the tops of the feet caused by wearing rubber flip-flops.

Fourth of July tetanus. A tetanus infection following wounds from fireworks or blank pistol cartridges.

Jet tummy. Abdominal swelling among airline hostesses due to the expansion of internal gases at high altitudes.

Listening-in dermatitis. An irritation of the ear from listening too long on the telephone.

Me-too syndrome. When one worker receives compensation for a work-related illness, other workers complain of the same problem.

Museum fatigue. What children and bored spouses feel after a long museum tour.

Quick-draw leg. A bullet wound in the leg, often sustained while practicing a fast draw.

Railway brain. Nervousness after a railroad accident.

Road rash. Scrapes, sores, and burns from skateboard, bicycle, and motorcycle accidents.

Sideswipe fracture. What auto drivers get from hanging their left elbow out the car window just before their car is sideswiped.

Stamp-licker's tongue. Ulcers found on the tongue and in the mouth of people who lick lots of gummed stamps.

Video voodoo. The "disease" people get from watching TV doctor shows, then imagining themselves sick.

Records in Childbearing

According to the *Guinness Book of World Records,* the record for the greatest number of children goes to a Russian peasant woman from Shuya, about 150 miles from Moscow. She lived in the mid-1700s and reportedly gave birth 27 times. Her efforts produced 16 pairs of twins, 7 sets of triplets and 4 sets of quadruplets. At least 67 of these children, who were born between 1725 and 1765, survived infancy.

The oldest mother on record is Ruth Alice Kistler, who lived from 1899 to 1982. In 1956, at the age of 57 years and 129 days, she gave birth to a daughter, Suzan, in Glendale, California.

The two heaviest babies born weighed in at 22 pounds, 8 ounces. One was a boy born in Aversa, Italy, in September 1955. The other boy was delivered May 24, 1982 in Transkei, South Africa. (The second child weighed 77 pounds at 16 months and 112 pounds at age 5.)

The first baby conceived in a test tube was Louise Brown, in Oldham General Hospital, Lancashire, England. She was conceived on November 10, 1977 and born July 25, 1978.

IS THAT A FACT?

The purpose of yawning is to funnel more oxygen into the body.

Scientists aren't so sure about that anymore. Dr. Robert Provine of the University of Maryland and Ronald Baenninger of Temple University theorize yawning might actually be your body's way of keeping you alert. After studying yawners and yawn-producing situations, they suggest this contagious, open-mouthed sigh is "the body's way of promoting arousal in situations where you have to stay awake."

Students in a calculus class had the highest yawning rates recorded. But the researchers found that emotionally excited people, as well as

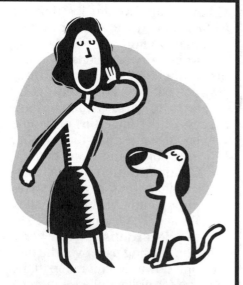

those who are highly aroused or stressed, also yawn frequently. One concert violinist yawns repeatedly before performances, claiming it helps him relax.

Medication by Proxy

A young woman doctor complained of excessive facial hair growth that was taking on a distinctly male pattern. She was taking an oral contraceptive but no other drugs, and doctors couldn't find any endocrine abnormalities that might explain her hirsute face. Her husband, however, was using a testosterone cream. When her husband quit using the cream, her hair growth stopped.

A man who was in good health complained that he was growing breasts. A checkup showed nothing that could cause the problems. His wife was using a cream containing estrogen for menopausal symptoms. When she used the cream in the morning rather than the evening, the man's breast enlargement subsided.

Death Under Odd Circumstances

Not everyone dies the way they might expect. Here are some people who met death under very unusual circumstances.

▼ Zeuxis (fifth century B.C.), a Greek painter, died from laughing so hard he broke a blood vessel.

▼ Alexander the Great (356–323 B.C.), Macedonian king and conqueror, died of a fever after two days of partying.

▼ Marcus Licinius Crassus (115–53 B.C.), Roman politician, died when molten gold was poured down his throat.

▼ Claudius I (10 B.C.–A.D. 54), emperor of Rome, choked to death on a feather meant to cause vomiting.

▼ Allan Pinkerton (1819–1884), founder of the detective agency, stumbled, bit his tongue, and died of gangrene.

▼ Arnold Bennett (1867–1931), a British novelist, died in Paris of typhoid from the local water, which he drank to demonstrate that the water in Paris was safe.

▼ Lionel Johnson (1867–1902), British critic and poet, died of injuries from falling off a barstool.

▼ Isadora Duncan (1878–1927), an American dancer, was strangled to death when her long scarf became entangled in a rear wheel of her car, breaking her neck.

▼ Jerome Napoleon Bonaparte (1878–1945), tripped over the leash of his wife's dog in Central Park, New York City, and died of injuries.

▼ Langley Collyer (1886–1947), recluse, was crushed to death by a booby trap he set in his home.

Giraffe-Necked Women of Burma

The women of the Padaung branch of the Kareni people in upland Burma wear brass rings around their neck from an early age. Five rings are fixed around the neck first, then more are added yearly until 22 or 24 encircle their necks.

Each ring stretches the neck of these women; at least one woman has been recorded as having a 15¾-inch-long neck. Because the cervical muscles are stretched and the neck vertebrae are pulled apart abnormally, medical experts speculate that if the brass rings were removed, the women probably couldn't hold their heads up and it might kill them.

Handicapped, but Gifted

One hundred years ago, Dr. J. Langdon Down of London discovered that some people with IQs of less than 25—called idiots at the time —also had amazing capabilities in learning. He coined the term *idiot savant* to describe these people who have a major mental illness or intellectual handicap, yet also have a spectacular talent or ability.

Here are some present-day examples cited by Darold A. Treffert, M.D., in his book *Extraordinary People.*

▼ George and his identical twin brother Charles are calendar calculators who can tell you all the years in which your birthday fell on a Thursday over a span of 80,000 years. Yet neither can add simple numbers.

▼ Leslie Lemke has never had formal musical training. But after he heard Tchaikovsky's Piano Concerto No. 1 on the piano the first time, he could play it flawlessly. He can do the same with any musical piece. He is blind, severely mentally handicapped, and has cerebral palsy.

▼ Kenneth can give the population of every city in the United States with a population over 5,000; the names, number of rooms, and locations of 2,000 hotels in America; the distance from each city and town to the largest city in each state; statistics about 3,000 mountains and rivers; and the dates and facts about more than 2,000 inventions and discoveries. Yet his mental age is 11 (his actual age is 38), and his vocabulary consists of just 58 words.

▼ Alonzo Clemons has earned national and international acclaim for his sculptures, which typically sell for $350 to $3,000 each. Some pieces cost as much as $45,000. One glimpse of any animal is all he needs to mold a lump of clay into a perfect three-dimensional replica. He has an IQ of 50 and a vocabulary of about that many words.

When Knots in the Stomach Are Real

Do you feel as if you sometimes have a knot in your stomach? Well, for some people that knot—the medical term is *bezoar*—is real. Many times it is formed by densely entangled residue of raw fruit, such as raisins, cherries, apples, coconuts, or peaches, or bulky balls of matted, stringy vegetables, such as cabbage, pumpkin, sauerkraut, or collard greens.

Scientists say bezoars can be caused by inadequate chewing and swallowing chunks of food that are too large. Or sometimes stomach juices can cause the tannin and cellulose in the fruits and vegetables to decompose into a sticky mass that hardens against the walls of the stomach.

Bezoars can also be made of inedibles. About 55 percent of all bezoars consist of hair, wool strands, carpet fibers, and similar material. Doctors say girls with a history of chewing or eating hair are most at risk.

But perhaps the most unusual bezoar found was composed of 290 shoestrings. It was discovered in the gullet of a psychiatric patient. Weighing in at 1 pound, 12 ounces, it formed a stringy, cordlike trail from the esophagus to the colon.

A Vitamin for Hard-to-Comb Hair

One old German fairy tale tells the story of a boy named "Stuwel Peter" or messy Peter, whose hair looked as if it had never been combed and perhaps had been stirred by static.

In 1973, scientists discovered the fairy tale was real for three children with short, sparse, straw-colored hair. They named it "uncombable hair syndrome," and since then have discovered more than 46 cases.

Hair from people with this syndrome appears normal under a light microscope. But under a high-powered electron microscope, scientists found canal-shaped indentations in the sides of the hair shaft, and cross sections of hair were triangular instead of round.

One cure for this kind of hair problem, researchers have found, is supplementation with the B vitamin biotin.

Did They or Didn't They? A Burning Question

Sometimes people seem to catch fire without any obvious cause. In the eighteenth century, for instance, Countess Cornelia Di Bandi of Cesena, Italy, was found burned to death, but her legs and stockings were untouched by the fire. The furniture and the floor in her room were unharmed.

Experts call it spontaneous combustion. In 1957 a 27-year-old welder in Pontiac, Michigan, was discovered in his car burned to death. His left arm, face, and genitals were badly burned. But the hairs on his body, his eyebrows, and the top of his head were unharmed. His clothes weren't even singed.

Here's a more recent report from *Fate* magazine. In the late fall of 1974, traveling salesman Jack B. Angel arrived at the Ramada Inn in Savannah, Georgia, to meet a clothing buyer. Angel was an hour late, and there was no room for him at the hotel. He decided to spend the night in his mobile showroom, a converted motor home.

The next day, Angel stepped into the bathroom for a shower. He doesn't remember what happened between then and when he awoke in bed at noon the following day covered with burns. He had third-degree burns on his right hand and on the inside of his arm, which later had to be amputated, a second-degree burn on his scrotum, and a 3- by 4-centimeter hole in his chest.

Doctors who examined Angel said he wasn't burned externally, only *internally*. Also, at least one doctor said the salesman's burns looked like the result of contact with an electrical source.

"The description of the burn and the findings in surgery are very typical of an electric-type injury," said one doctor. "This generates a high-powered heat source because of the resistance of the skin and the underlying tissue."

What could that heat source have been?

One Savannah physician said Angel was the victim of a bizarre molecular reaction that causes people to burn up inside.

Not everyone agreed. Other theories for the burns were suggested, then disproved. An engineering laboratory inspected the motor home but found no electrical problems. And, while some thought Angel might have been scalded, there was no evidence that hot water could have caused the burns.

One doctor at the burn unit at Washington Hospital Center in Washington, D.C., thought Angel might have had an adverse reaction to an antibiotic containing sulfur, which can shrink skin and blood vessels and create the appearance of a burn.

What experts do know is that something did burn Angel, creating explosion-like wounds in his chest but failing to singe his pajamas, the sheets on his bed, or the garments hanging all around him.

Fingerprints Never Forget

Fingerprints come in three basic patterns, the arch, the loop, and the whorl. Loops are most common and arches least common. Some studies show people with primarily looped patterns have the greatest tactile (touch) sensitivity.

Fingerprint experts pay attention to the tiniest details. They count ridges and look for "lakes," "islands," "spurs," "crossovers," and "bifurcations" to identify individual prints.

No two fingerprints have ever been found to be alike; experts say even identical twins do not have identical fingerprints.

Surprisingly, criminals who try to alter their fingerprints will never succeed. Fingerprints never forget. And they don't change with age. Even after being worn away, they grow back with their original loops, whorls, and arches.

Could Ties That Bind Make You Blind?

If you wear a tie to work every day and don't like it, check your neck size, say Cornell University researchers. Even if you *don't* mind it, check your neck size. Why? Because when they tested 94 white-collar workers, the researchers found that more than half (67 percent) of these men had wedged themselves into tightened collars that were smaller than their necks. And that didn't just make their necks hurt. It also affected their vision by restricting the blood flow through the neck arteries to their eyes.

This visual impairment didn't improve immediately after the men loosened their ties; it took a while for the blood flow to be reestablished. A discrepancy of even half an inch between your neck and collar sizes could cause measurable impairment, the researchers say.

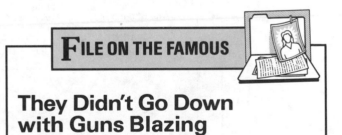

FILE ON THE FAMOUS

They Didn't Go Down with Guns Blazing

Despite six-shooting folklore, the real causes of death of famous gunfighters, according to the Hope Heart Institute, were:

- ▼ Wyatt Earp: cancer
- ▼ Doc Holliday: tuberculosis
- ▼ Bat Masterson: heart attack
- ▼ Calamity Jane: pneumonia
- ▼ Luke Short: damaged kidneys
- ▼ Clay Alison: broken neck

Making the Most of Multiple Births

Are there more triplets, quadruplets, and even quintuplets in America's future? Since 1980, the number of multiple births has been rising. The rate of plural births, 21 per 1,000 for all live births, reached a 30-year-high in the mid-1980s. Reasons cited include the increasing number of women who have used oral contraceptives, an increased use of fertility drugs, and the fact that more women are delaying childbirth until their thirties or later.

This chart shows the frequency of multiple births in the United States, according to the age of the mother.

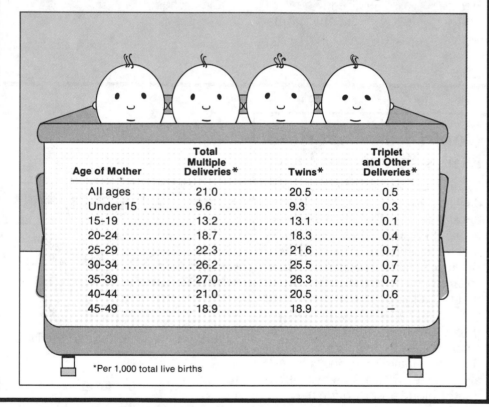

Age of Mother	Total Multiple Deliveries*	Twins*	Triplet and Other Deliveries*
All ages	21.0	20.5	0.5
Under 15	9.6	9.3	0.3
15-19	13.2	13.1	0.1
20-24	18.7	18.3	0.4
25-29	22.3	21.6	0.7
30-34	26.2	25.5	0.7
35-39	27.0	26.3	0.7
40-44	21.0	20.5	0.6
45-49	18.9	18.9	—

*Per 1,000 total live births

Stand on a ladder long enough—as a house painter, electrician, or window washer might—and you'll develop ladder leg, or painter's bosses, or stepladder bumps. They are all the same thing—bumps, like calluses, on the front of the leg just above the ankle, where legs and ladder rung meet.

The Yam Diet: It Has Twin Benefits

If you want to encourage twins in your family tree, eat a lot of yams. The 18-million-member Yoruba tribe of western Nigeria has the highest twin-producing rate in the world—about 3 percent of total births. They also consume large quantities of yams, a staple in their diet. Coincidence? Maybe not. It seems the vegetable contains high amounts of a substance similar to the female hormone estrogen, which scientists believe may stimulate other hormones to trigger the release of more than one egg from the ovaries. Note, however, that their yams are a different type than those grown in the United States.

The rarest blood group in the ABO system, one of 14 systems, is AB. The rarest blood type of all is Bombay blood (subtype h-h) found only in a Czechoslovakian nurse in 1961 and in a brother and sister living in Massachusetts in 1968.

Do-It-Yourself Surgery

Doctors have reported strange phenomena over the years, but perhaps nothing stranger than people who operate on themselves. At home.

One man, according to medical reports, fancied himself quite good at self-surgery and, indeed, removed his testicles successfully. Two months later he tried to remove his adrenal glands but became tired and found the pain to be a bit too much. So he admitted himself to the hospital for wound closure and postoperative care.

Sinister Findings for Lefties

Left-handed people are likely to die sooner than right-handed people, say Diane Halpern, Ph.D., of the University of California, San Diego, and Stanley Coren, Ph.D., of the University of British Columbia.

Southpaws, the researchers say, are more likely to be born prematurely and with a low birth weight. They are also more likely to have immune system and sleeping disorders, asthma, and allergies. After the age of 33, these conditions, as well as the fact that lefties are more accident-prone, make them 1 to 2 percent more likely than righties to die prematurely.

Hiccups That Just Won't Give Up

Charles Osborne of Anthon, Iowa, had the hiccups for more than 65 years. According to the *Guinness Book of World Records,* his first hiccup caught him during a 1923 hog slaughtering, and he estimates he's hiccuped 430 million times since. That's about 19,000 times a day or 12 times per minute. During those years he had two wives and fathered eight children. But he could not keep his false teeth in place.

More than 100 cases of persistent hiccups have been recorded. Hiccup epidemics were recorded during the 1919, 1922, and 1924 influenza/encephalitis outbreaks in Winnipeg, Canada, and other parts of the world. During those epidemics, bouts of hiccups lasted between 45 minutes and an hour and occurred every 2 or 3 hours.

"Normal" bouts of hiccups contain either just under 7 or more than 63 hiccups, according to one study. Unusually persistent hiccups occur more often in men (82 percent) than women (18 percent).

Here are some suggested remedies for everyday hiccups.

1. Yank forcefully on the tongue.

2. Lift the uvula (the little "boxing bag" at the back of the mouth) with a spoon.

3. Using a cotton-tipped swab, tickle the roof of your mouth where the hard and soft palate meet.

4. Swallow a teaspoon of sugar.

5. Swallow dry bread or crushed ice.

6. Drink from the far side of a glass.

7. Suck a lemon wedge soaked in Angostura bitters or vinegar.

8. Gasp, due to sudden fright or exposure to smelling salts.

9. Compress the chest by pulling the knees up or leaning forward.

10. Gargle with water.

11. Sneeze.

12. Hold your breath.

13. Rebreathe into a paper bag.

Take a long look at your ears in the mirror. Studies show a diagonal crease across the earlobe occurs nearly twice as often in men and women at risk for cardiovascular disease and hypertensive heart disease as in those who are not at risk.

Wasp-Waisted Women

Tight corsets did more than lend sex appeal to Victorian women. They bound and gagged vital organs. When a woman swooned, one remedy was to "cut her laces," allowing her organs to be unbound and enabling her to breathe normally. The illustration shows what happens to the internal organs of a tightly corseted woman.

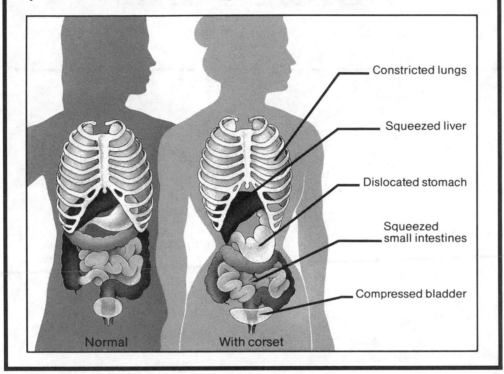

Constricted lungs

Squeezed liver

Dislocated stomach

Squeezed small intestines

Compressed bladder

Normal   With corset

Pricer's Palsy

A right-handed grocery clerk entered the Medical College of Wisconsin in Milwaukee complaining that she had had numbness in her left hand for two months. It seemed especially bad, she said, when she was at work, pushing and rubbing food items with UPC pricing codes over the code-sensing machine at the checkout counter. After examination, doctors named her condition "pricer's palsy" because they said the fast, repetitive movements of the pricer's left hand over the machine irritated the ulnar nerve, just above the wrist.

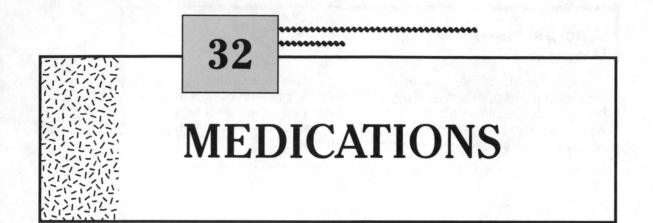

32

MEDICATIONS

Seventy-five million adult Americans take one or more drugs every week. They spend an average $16.62 per prescription order. Each year approximately 1.5 billion prescriptions are filled by 161,765 pharmacists across the United States.

Additionally, Americans spend $8.8 billion yearly on over-the-counter medicines, including $1.7 billion on painkillers and $1.6 billion on cough and cold remedies.

Who takes all these drugs? While older Americans—people aged 60 and over—account for just 16.6 percent of the total population of the United States, they use almost 40 percent of all prescription drugs.

Older adults swallow more than a third of the minor tranquilizers, a third of the antipsychotics, half of the sleeping pills, and a third of the antidepressants sold in the United States. About 65 percent of all high blood pressure drugs are taken by older adults, and 84 percent of all blood vessel dilating drugs are used by older adults.

The Ten Most Prescribed Drugs

Prescription in hand, you walk into the pharmacy. But what do you walk out with? Quite possibly one of these ten medicines—the most-often prescribed drugs in the United States.

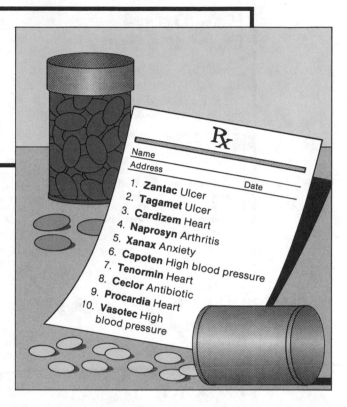

℞

Name

Address

Date

1. **Zantac** Ulcer
2. **Tagamet** Ulcer
3. **Cardizem** Heart
4. **Naprosyn** Arthritis
5. **Xanax** Anxiety
6. **Capoten** High blood pressure
7. **Tenormin** Heart
8. **Ceclor** Antibiotic
9. **Procardia** Heart
10. **Vasotec** High blood pressure

When to Discard Drugs

Old medicines and medicines that you no longer take should be flushed down the toilet or returned to the pharmacist for disposal. Do not place them in the garbage where children or animals may find them and eat them. Here are some likely candidates.

▼ Aspirin and acetaminophen tablets that smell like vinegar.

▼ Chipped, cracked, or discolored tablets.

▼ Soft, cracked, or sticky capsules.

▼ Liquids that have thickened or discolored. Also, those that taste or smell different than they did originally.

▼ Cracked, leaky, or hard tubes.

▼ Ointments and creams that have changed in color, odor, or softness and those that have separated.

▼ Tablets or capsules more than two years old.

Is THAT A FACT?

Prescription drugs are more potent and effective than over-the-counter drugs.

Technically, at least, that's not the case. According to the policy of the U.S. Food and Drug Administration, all drugs are offered for over-the-counter sale *unless* it is considered impossible to write a label that will be understood by the consumer and ensure that the drug will be used safely without medical supervision. Drugs in the latter category become prescription items.

How Drugs Enter the Body

Drugs can be administered in many different ways, as illustrated here. The speed with which a medication is absorbed depends on the means of delivery. Most drugs are taken by mouth and then absorbed into the bloodstream through the walls of the intestine.

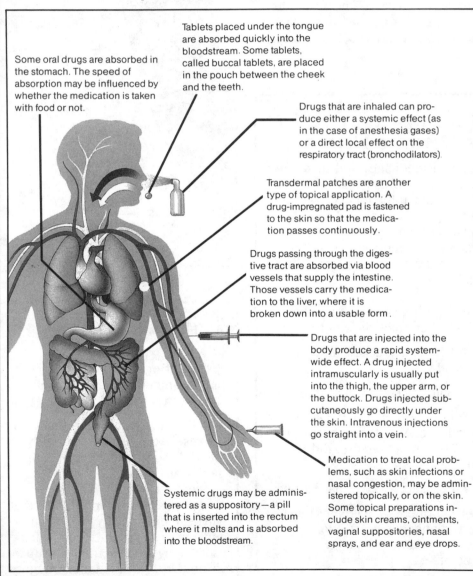

Some oral drugs are absorbed in the stomach. The speed of absorption may be influenced by whether the medication is taken with food or not.

Tablets placed under the tongue are absorbed quickly into the bloodstream. Some tablets, called buccal tablets, are placed in the pouch between the cheek and the teeth.

Drugs that are inhaled can produce either a systemic effect (as in the case of anesthesia gases) or a direct local effect on the respiratory tract (bronchodilators).

Transdermal patches are another type of topical application. A drug-impregnated pad is fastened to the skin so that the medication passes continuously.

Drugs passing through the digestive tract are absorbed via blood vessels that supply the intestine. Those vessels carry the medication to the liver, where it is broken down into a usable form.

Drugs that are injected into the body produce a rapid system-wide effect. A drug injected intramuscularly is usually put into the thigh, the upper arm, or the buttock. Drugs injected subcutaneously go directly under the skin. Intravenous injections go straight into a vein.

Medication to treat local problems, such as skin infections or nasal congestion, may be administered topically, or on the skin. Some topical preparations include skin creams, ointments, vaginal suppositories, nasal sprays, and ear and eye drops.

Systemic drugs may be administered as a suppository—a pill that is inserted into the rectum where it melts and is absorbed into the bloodstream.

Decoding Your Prescription

What does that doctor's prescription that you hand to your pharmacist really say?

Your prescription tells the pharmacist which medication and how much of that drug to supply. It tells the pharmacist the information that should appear on the container label, such as how often the drug should be taken and whether it should be taken before or after meals. It also tells the pharmacist if a generic sub-stitution for the prescribed drug is allowed.

Often, however, this information is transmitted in coded form. Along with the sample prescription reproduced here, you'll find an explanation of the most common Rx codes. You may want to use this information to check your prescription, comparing the instructions from your doctor to those that end up on the drug container.

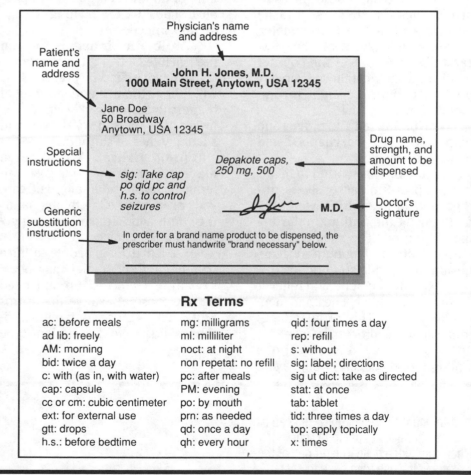

Physician's name and address

Patient's name and address

John H. Jones, M.D.
1000 Main Street, Anytown, USA 12345

Jane Doe
50 Broadway
Anytown, USA 12345

Special instructions

sig: Take cap po qid pc and h.s. to control seizures

Depakote caps, 250 mg, 500

Drug name, strength, and amount to be dispensed

_____ **M.D.**

Doctor's signature

Generic substitution instructions

In order for a brand name product to be dispensed, the prescriber must handwrite "brand necessary" below.

Rx Terms

ac: before meals	mg: milligrams	qid: four times a day
ad lib: freely	ml: milliliter	rep: refill
AM: morning	noct: at night	s: without
bid: twice a day	non repetat: no refill	sig: label; directions
c: with (as in, with water)	pc: after meals	sig ut dict: take as directed
cap: capsule	PM: evening	stat: at once
cc or cm: cubic centimeter	po: by mouth	tab: tablet
ext: for external use	prn: as needed	tid: three times a day
gtt: drops	qd: once a day	top: apply topically
h.s.: before bedtime	qh: every hour	x: times

Studies show that people who use tranquilizers are up to five times more likely than the average to be involved in a serious auto accident.

Eight Items That Belong in Every Medicine Cabinet

You don't need to keep something on hand for *every* ache and pain. If you do, you'll have a cabinet of out-of-date and seldom-used medications. Experts say stick to the essentials, such as a thermometer, tweezers, and first-aid kit, plus a few carefully chosen over-the-counter medications to treat those everyday problems. Here are eight recommended items.

Petroleum jelly. To protect and help heal dry, chafed, chapped, and wind-burned skin.

Antacid. This soother of heartburn, upset stomach, ulcers, indigestion, and gastritis works by neutralizing the acid and relieving the discomfort. The most common antacids contain aluminum and magnesium hydroxide compounds.

Aspirin. A potent pain reliever for headaches, toothaches, and menstrual cramps. This drug reduces inflammation, providing relief for arthritis, strains, and sprains. (Note: Children or teenagers should avoid aspirin because of a possible link with Reye's syndrome.)

Athlete's foot powder. At one time or another, 50 percent of people test positive for the fungus causing this infection.

Antibiotic ointment. This can prevent infection in cuts and scrapes.

Hydrocortisone cream. This will relieve the itch and swelling of hemorrhoids, minor skin irritations, insect bites, poison ivy or oak, and small patches of sunburn.

Antidiarrheal. A medication like this can soothe your gastrointestinal tract, stop cramping, and ease your discomfort. One that contains the combination of kaolin and pectin is a good choice.

Laxative. Even people eating a healthy, high-fiber diet may occasionally get blocked up and need help. Choose a laxative that forms bulk, such as those containing psyllium seeds. Avoid stimulant-type laxatives.

Forgetful about taking your medication? You can buy a rub-off dot label at the pharmacy to paste to your medicine bottle. When you take a dose, rub off one of the dots to keep track of medicine use from dose to dose.

The Most Easily Overdosed Drugs

This is a list of drugs that have been given a high overdose rating in drug profiles, meaning they are the drugs most easily overdosed. If you think someone has taken an overdose of one of these drugs, you must immediately call for medical help.

Acebutolol

Acetaminophen

Acetohexamide

Aminophylline

Amitriptyline

Aspirin

Belladonna

Chloral hydrate

Chloroquine

Chlorpropamide

Codeine

Colchicine

Cyclobenzaprine

Desipramine

Dicumarol

Digitoxin

Digoxin

Epinephrine

Ergonovine

Glipizide

Glyburide

Guanethidine

Heparin

Hydralazine

Imipramine

Insulin

Interferon

Isocarbonxazid

Isoniazid

Isoproterenol

Lithium

Maprotiline

Meperidine

Methotrexate

Minoxidil

Morphine

Nadolol

Orphendrine

Oxtriphylline

Phenobarbital

Phenylbutazone

Phenylpropanolamine

Primidone

Procyclidine

Propranolol

Pseudoephedrine

Quinine

Secobarbital

Theophylline

Tolazamide

Tolbutamide

Vasopressin

Warfarin

Drugs That Contain Alcohol

Many over-the-counter drugs and some prescription medications —including tonics, bronchodilators, cough and cold medicines, diarrhea medicines, and analgesics—may contain alcohol. Some people may have adverse reactions to these medicines, especially children, the frail elderly, or alcoholics who are also taking an alcohol-aversion drug. This chart lists some common products and the percentage of alcohol in each dose.

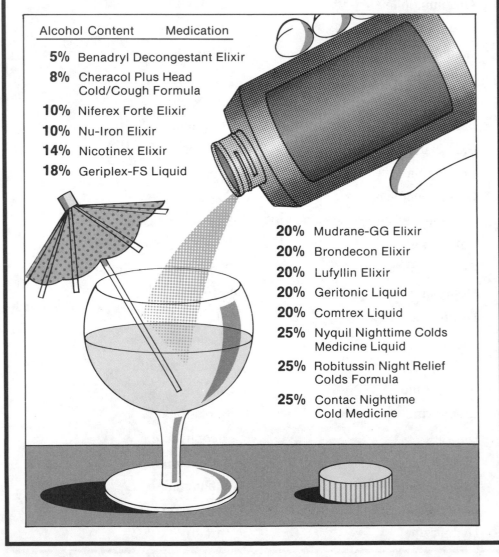

Alcohol Content	Medication
5%	Benadryl Decongestant Elixir
8%	Cheracol Plus Head Cold/Cough Formula
10%	Niferex Forte Elixir
10%	Nu-Iron Elixir
14%	Nicotinex Elixir
18%	Geriplex-FS Liquid
20%	Mudrane-GG Elixir
20%	Brondecon Elixir
20%	Lufyllin Elixir
20%	Geritonic Liquid
20%	Comtrex Liquid
25%	Nyquil Nighttime Colds Medicine Liquid
25%	Robitussin Night Relief Colds Formula
25%	Contac Nighttime Cold Medicine

Side Effects of Common Prescription Drugs

The right drug can work miracles—relieving the pain, infection, or whatever's ailing you. But in some instances, the right medication can also cause new or different symptoms, called side effects. The following table lists some of the popular prescription drugs (brand name first) and their possible side effects.

Drug	Use	Possible Side Effects
Aldomet (methyldopa)	Antihypertensive	Drowsiness, headache, nasal congestion, dry mouth, dizziness, diarrhea, nausea, constipation, muscle aches, skin rash, breast enlargement, impotence, jaundice, anemia
Aldoril (hydrochlorothiazide/ methyldopa)	Diuretic/ antihypertensive	Frequent urination, muscle weakness or cramps, headache, dizziness, skin rash, nausea, vomiting, reduced appetite, diarrhea, blurred vision, dry mouth, nightmares, depression, jaundice, breast enlargement, impotence, elevated blood sugar, elevated uric acid
Amoxil (amoxicillin)	Antibiotic	Nausea, vomiting, diarrhea, irritation of mouth and tongue, rash, itching, fever, sore throat, anemia, swollen glands
Ativan (lorazepam)	Tranquilizer	Dizziness, weakness, headache, disorientation, depression, nausea, sleep disturbances, agitation, eye function disturbance
Benadryl (diphenhydramine hydrochloride)	Antihistamine	Drowsiness, dizziness, blurred vision, upset stomach, difficult urination, dry mouth and throat, headache, loss of appetite, skin rash, fast heartbeat
Ceclor (cephalosporin)	Antibiotic	Nausea, vomiting, diarrhea, stomach cramps, rash, itching, joint pain, fever, swollen glands
Dalmane (flurazepam hydrochloride)	Hypnotic	Dizziness, lightheadedness, unsteadiness, drowsiness, headache, constipation, diarrhea, heartburn, nausea, vomiting, chest pains, irritability, nervousness
Darvocet-N (propoxyphene napsylate/ acetaminophen)	Analgesic	Nausea, vomiting, constipation, drowsiness, dizziness, lightheadedness, euphoria, skin rash, headache
Diabinese (chlorpropamide)	Antidiabetic agent	Loss of appetite, diarrhea, nausea, vomiting, weakness, headache, heartburn, skin rash, jaundice, low blood sugar, anemia, low-grade fever, sore throat

(continued)

Side Effects of Common Prescription Drugs—*Continued*

Drug	Use	Possible Side Effects
Dilantin (phenytoin)	Anticonvulsant	Swollen gums, nausea, vomiting, drowsiness, skin rash, slurred speech, mental confusion, dizziness, insomnia, headache
Dyazide (triamterene hydrochlorothiazide)	Diuretic/anti-hypertensive	Frequent urination, nausea, vomiting, diarrhea, skin rash, headache, weakness, dizziness, muscle cramps, dry mouth, constipation
Inderal (propranolol hydrochloride)	Beta-adrenergic blocking agent	Lightheadedness, insomnia, weakness, fatigue, mood swings, depression, hallucinations, vomiting, diarrhea, constipation, slow heart rate, tingling of fingers, hair loss
Indocin (indomethacin)	Anti-inflammatory	Headache, indigestion, heartburn, nausea, diarrhea, bloating, constipation, blurred vision, depression, drowsiness
Isordil (isosorbide dinitrate)	Antianginal agent	Dizziness, weakness, flushing, severe headache, restlessness, perspiration, collapse, low blood pressure, rash
Keflex (cephalexin)	Antibiotic	Diarrhea, indigestion, abdominal pain, skin rash, itching, dizziness, fatigue, headache, vaginitis, vaginal discharge
Lanoxin (digoxin)	Cardiotonic	Loss of appetite, nausea, vomiting, diarrhea, blurred vision, headache, weakness, apathy, palpitations, slow heart rate
Lo/Ovral (norgestrel ethinyl estradiol)	Contraceptive	Abdominal cramps, nausea, bloating, breakthrough bleeding, change in menstrual flow, fluid retention, breast tenderness or enlargement, weight loss or gain, rash, depression, migraine, jaundice
Lopressor (metoprolol tartrate)	Antihypertensive/beta-blocker	Fatigue, dizziness, depression, headache, insomnia, nightmares, wheezing, cold extremities, palpitations, heart failure, diarrhea, nausea, constipation, dry mouth
Mellaril (thioridazine)	Tranquilizer	Dry mouth, blurred vision, constipation, drowsiness, nasal congestion, nausea, diarrhea, difficult urination, impotence, swollen breasts
Norinyl (norethindrone, ethinyl estradiol)	Contraceptive	Breast tenderness or enlargement, weight gain or loss, nausea, vomiting, spotting, fluid retention, rash, depression, migraine

Drug	Use	Possible Side Effects
Omnipen (ampicillin)	Antibiotic	Diarrhea, nausea, vomiting, swollen tongue, abdominal discomfort, mouth and throat irritation, rash, anemia
Ortho-Novum (norethindrone mestranol, norethindrone ethinyl)	Contraceptive	Abdominal cramps, bloating, breakthrough bleeding, spotting, amenorrhea, breast tenderness or enlargement, weight loss or gain, migraine, rash, depression
Persantine (dipyridamole)	Vasodilator	Headache, dizziness, flushing, nausea, vomiting, diarrhea, stomach irritation
Premarin (conjugated estrogens)	Estrogen replacement therapy	Nausea, vomiting, abdominal cramps, bloating, breast tenderness or enlargement, breakthrough bleeding, migraine, headache, dizziness, depression, skin rash, blood clots in legs
Slow-K (potassium chloride)	Potassium supplement	Nausea, vomiting, abdominal discomfort, diarrhea, obstruction, bleeding, ulceration, perforation
Tagamet (cimetidine)	Anti-ulcer agent	Diarrhea, dizziness, rash, muscular pain, drowsiness, headache, may prolong effects of other medication
Theo-Dur (theophylline, anhydrous)	Bronchodilator	Nausea, vomiting, stomach pain, diarrhea, headache, irritability, restlessness, insomnia, convulsions, palpitations, flushing, rapid heartbeat
Timoptic (timolol maleate)	Antiglaucoma agent	Ocular irritation, conjunctivitis, inflammation of the eyelids and/or cornea, localized and generalized rash, irregular heartbeat, difficulty breathing
Tranxene (clorazepate dipotassium)	Tranquilizer	Drowsiness, dizziness, nervousness, headache, fatigue, irritability, insomnia, dry mouth, blurred vision, mental confusion, skin rash, depression
Valium (diazepam)	Tranquilizer	Drowsiness, fatigue, weakness, dry mouth, headache, mental confusion, depression, skin rash, itching, insomnia, nervousness, double vision, jaundice, difficult urination

How Beta-Blockers Work

Beta-blockers are medications that treat angina, high blood pressure, and irregular heart rhythms. They can also prevent migraine headaches, reduce anxiety, or control an overactive thyroid. Sometimes they are even added to eyedrops to treat glaucoma.

Beta-blockers work by blocking the flow of norepinephrine (a neurotransmitter produced in the adrenal glands and at the ends of sympathetic nerve fibers) thereby reducing the force and speed of the heartbeat. There are two types of beta-blockers. One works mostly in the heart muscle. The other works in the airways and blood vessels.

Here's how beta-blockers work in various parts of the body.

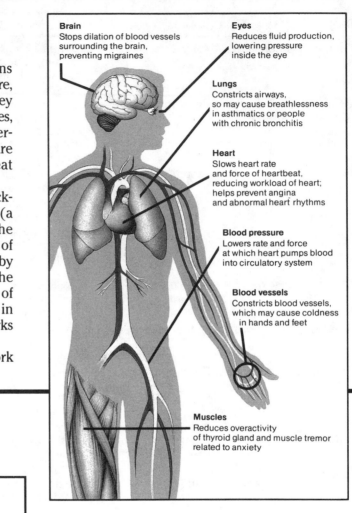

Brain
Stops dilation of blood vessels surrounding the brain, preventing migraines

Eyes
Reduces fluid production, lowering pressure inside the eye

Lungs
Constricts airways, so may cause breathlessness in asthmatics or people with chronic bronchitis

Heart
Slows heart rate and force of heartbeat, reducing workload of heart; helps prevent angina and abnormal heart rhythms

Blood pressure
Lowers rate and force at which heart pumps blood into circulatory system

Blood vessels
Constricts blood vessels, which may cause coldness in hands and feet

Muscles
Reduces overactivity of thyroid gland and muscle tremor related to anxiety

The Logic behind Antihistamines

Antihistamines are commonly used to treat allergic reactions. If you are allergic, your body releases histamine, which attaches to special receptor cells. Those dilate the blood vessels, inflame tissues, and narrow air passages, bringing on sniffling, sneezing, and worse. An antihistamine prevents the histamine from attaching to the receptor, so the body doesn't respond to the allergen.

Tell your doctor about any medications you're taking before you get a lab test done. Some medications will alter the results of certain lab tests, rendering them inaccurate.

Choosing an Antihistamine

Antihistamines are among the most widely used drugs. But there are important differences between them. This table lists some common antihistamines, what they are used for, and the possible side effects you might expect from the medication.

Drug	Used for	Duration of Action	Drowsiness Level
Azatadine	Allergic rhinitis, skin allergy	More than 12 hours	High
Brompheniramine	Allergic rhinitis, skin allergy	4–6 hours	Medium
Chlorpheniramine	Allergic rhinitis, skin allergy	6–12 hours	Medium
Dimenhydrinate	Nausea, vomiting	4–6 hours	Medium
Diphenhydramine	Sedation, Parkinson's disease, nausea, vomiting	4–6 hours	High
Hydroxyzine	Skin allergy, sedation	4–6 hours	Medium
Meclizine	Nausea, vomiting	More than 12 hours	Medium
Promethazine	Allergic rhinitis, skin allergy, sedation	4–6 hours	High
Terfenadine	Allergic rhinitis, skin allergy	More than 12 hours	Low
Trimeprazine	Skin allergy, sedation	6–12 hours	High
Triprolidine	Allergic rhinitis, skin allergy	6–12 hours	Medium

Taken as Prescribed?

Whether patients underdose, overdose, or take their medications erratically, it all adds up to a serious and common problem. And doctors have a name for it: patient noncompliance. A Connecticut study of epileptic patients receiving medication found that an average of 24 percent of all their pills never get taken. Researchers noted that the more doses of a medication needed daily, the less likely it is that all doses will be taken as directed.

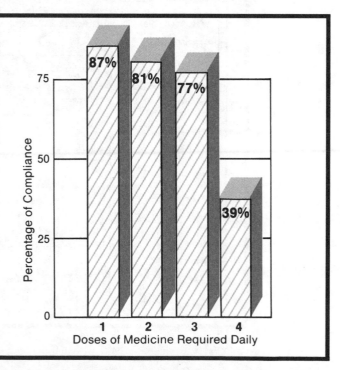

First-Aid Products Compared

The pharmacy shelves are loaded with first-aid creams, antiseptic sprays, and antibiotic ointments. Which ones work best? A study at the University of Pennsylvania showed which products produced the fastest results.

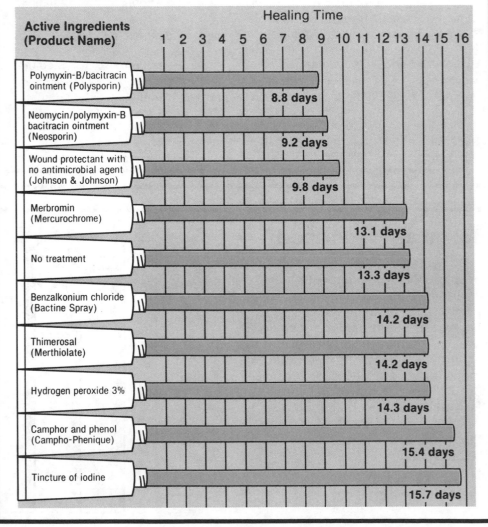

Active Ingredients (Product Name) — Healing Time

Active Ingredients (Product Name)	Healing Time
Polymyxin-B/bacitracin ointment (Polysporin)	8.8 days
Neomycin/polymyxin-B bacitracin ointment (Neosporin)	9.2 days
Wound protectant with no antimicrobial agent (Johnson & Johnson)	9.8 days
Merbromin (Mercurochrome)	13.1 days
No treatment	13.3 days
Benzalkonium chloride (Bactine Spray)	14.2 days
Thimerosal (Merthiolate)	14.2 days
Hydrogen peroxide 3%	14.3 days
Camphor and phenol (Campho-Phenique)	15.4 days
Tincture of iodine	15.7 days

Finding the Right Antibiotic for the Job

In 1928, something special was discovered growing in mold in a petri dish. It was penicillin, the first modern antibiotic. Now, there are hundreds of antibiotics, accounting for about 15 percent of the billion prescriptions written in the United States each year. Because not every antibiotic is effective against every strain of bacteria, these drugs have found special treatment niches, depending on their individual properties. Some of the common drug/disease match-ups are summarized here.

Antibiotic	Site of Infection									
	Ear, nose, throat, and mouth	Respira-tory tract	Skin and soft tissue	Gastro-intestinal tract	Eye	Kidney and urinary tract	Brain and nervous system	Heart	Bones and joints	Genital tract
Penicillins										
Amoxicillin	X	X		X		X		X	X	X
Ampicillin	X	X		X		X	X	X	X	X
Cloxacillin		X	X						X	
Penicillin G	X	X	X				X	X	X	X
Penicillin V	X	X	X							
Cephalosporins										
Cefaclor	X	X				X				
Cefazolin		X	X			X		X	X	
Cefoperazone		X	X	X		X	X		X	X
Cefoxitin		X	X	X		X				X
Cephalexin		X	X			X				
Cephalothin		X	X			X		X	X	
Aminoglycosides										
Gentamicin		X	X	X	X	X	X	X	X	
Neomycin		X	X							
Netilmicin		X	X	X		X	X		X	
Streptomycin		X						X		
Tobramycin		X	X	X		X	X		X	
Tetracyclines										
Doxycycline	X	X		X		X				X
Oxytetracycline	X	X								

(continued)

Finding the Right Antibiotic for the Job—*Continued*

Antibiotic	Site of Infection									
	Ear, nose, throat, and mouth	Respiratory tract	Skin and soft tissue	Gastrointestinal tract	Eye	Kidney and urinary tract	Brain and nervous system	Heart	Bones and joints	Genital tract
Tetracycline	X	X			X	X				X
Sulfonamides										
Sulfacetamide					X					
Sulfamethoxasole						X				
Sulfisoxasole	X	X				X				
Lincosamides										
Clindamycin		X	X	X					X	
Lincomycin		X	X						X	
Other drugs										
Bacitracin			X							
Chloramphenicol	X			X	X		X			
Colistin		X				X				
Dapsone			X							
Erythromycin	X	X	X			X			X	X
Gramicidin					X					
Metronidazole	X		X	X			X	X	X	X
Nalidixic acid						X				
Nitrofurantoin						X				
Trimethoprim						X				
Trimethoprim/ sulfamethoxasole	X	X		X		X				

From *The American Medical Association Guide to Prescription and Over-the-Counter Drugs,* edited by Charles B. Clayman, M.D. Copyright © 1988 by Random House, Inc. Reprinted by permission of the publisher.

When your prescription calls for bedtime medication, be sure to take it with plenty of fluids. In a study at Walter Reed Army Medical Center in Washington, D.C., doctors found some pills with little or no fluid could settle in the throat, melt, and cause esophageal injury.

Generics versus Brand Names

Would you rather pay $27.80 or $4.50 for your diazepam prescription? If you choose the lower amount, you get the same amount of active ingredients as the higher-priced medication. What you don't get is the brand name, but a *generic* equivalent to the drug Valium, made by drug manufacturer Hoffmann-LaRoche.

Since 1970, the Food and Drug Administration has approved more than 8,000 generic drugs, drugs that are chemically equal to brand-name versions of medications. Generics often cost 30 to 80 percent less than name brands.

Not all medications have generic equivalents. Generic drugs are usually offered after the patent on the original brand-name drug expires. About half the drugs available today are also offered generically. And about 25 percent of all prescriptions are for generic drugs. You can get a generic medication by asking your doctor to sign your prescription allowing substitution.

The table compares 1990 retail prices of generic and brand-name drugs. Each prescription is for 100 tablets or capsules except for Doxycycline Hyclate, which is for 14 tablets. Though prices do vary, and will of course change over time, the percentage of savings—which averaged 68 percent overall—can be expected to remain similar.

Generic/(Brand name)	Brand Name Price	Generic Price	Percentage of Savings
Allopurinol (Zyloprim) 300 mg	$47.00	$18.55	60
Amitriptyline HCL (Elavil) 25 mg	$33.55	$ 5.55	83
Chlorpropamide (Diabinese) 250 mg	$59.20	$ 6.35	89
Clonidine HCL (Catapres) 0.1 mg	$40.15	$12.20	70
Doxycycline hyclate (Vibramycin) 100 mg	$46.05	$14.65	68
Imipramine HCL (Tofranil) 25 mg	$43.90	$10.15	77
Indomethacin (Indocin) 25 mg	$49.80	$16.20	67
Hydroxyzine HCL (Atarax) 25 mg	$65.20	$14.30	78
Methyldopa (Aldomet) 250 mg	$27.30	$17.05	38
Propranolol HCL (Inderal) 20 mg	$27.60	$10.55	62

33

MENTAL ILLNESS

You can't "catch" mental illness like you can the flu—most of us know that —but neither is anyone immune to the problem. In any given six-month period, one in five Americans—30 to 45 million people—suffer some form of mental illness. Depression is especially common, with 9 to 20 percent of the U.S. population experiencing depressive symptoms at any one time.

Researchers believe an imbalance of chemical messages in the brain is to blame for some mental illnesses. Traumatic events that a person has trouble coping with may also play a role in some cases. Still other mental illnesses may be linked to the abuse of drugs and alcohol or other conditions that damage the brain.

Whatever the cause, mental illness is more likely to strike women than men, and people under 45 are more likely targets than people over 45. In a National Institute of Mental Health study, women had a 16.6 percent rate of mental disorder in the preceding month compared with a rate of 14 percent for men. In comparing ages, those 25 to 44 had the highest rate (17.3 percent), followed by 18- to 24-year-olds (16.9 percent), 45- to 64-year-olds (13.3 percent), and then those 65 years and older (12.3 percent).

Fortunately, professional treatment of mental illness is effective in most cases. In fact, eight of ten people who seek treatment for mental illness go on to lead productive lives. However, only one in five people with a mental illness ever seeks treatment.

The Risks: In the Course of a Lifetime

Each of us faces a one-in-three chance of suffering some form of mental illness during the course of our lives. As these National Institute of Mental Health study results indicate, anxiety disorders are the most common.

Illness	Rate*
Any disorder	32.2
Anxiety disorders (total)	14.6
Phobia	12.5
Obsessive-compulsive	2.5
Panic	1.6
Affective disorders (total)	8.3
Major depression	5.8
Manic episode	0.8
Schizophrenia	1.3

*Prevalence rate per 100 persons aged 18 or older

The Risks: In the Course of a Month

In the month preceding this National Institute of Mental Health study, 15.4 percent of the more than 18,000 persons interviewed had suffered a mental illness. Rates for specific disorders are listed here.

Illness	Rate*
Any disorder	15.4
Anxiety disorders (total)	7.3
Phobia	6.2
Obsessive-compulsive	1.3
Panic	0.5
Affective disorders (total)	5.1
Major depression	2.2
Manic episode	0.4
Schizophrenia	0.6

*Prevalence rate per 100 persons aged 18 or older

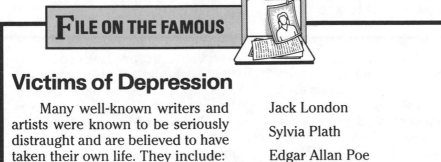

FILE ON THE FAMOUS

Victims of Depression

Many well-known writers and artists were known to be seriously distraught and are believed to have taken their own life. They include:

Hart Crane

Ernest Hemingway

Jack London

Sylvia Plath

Edgar Allan Poe

Vincent van Gogh

Virginia Woolf

The Major Mental Illnesses

Affective Disorder

Description: Mood disturbances characterized by manic or depressive symptoms or both.

Risk: In any six-month period, 9.4 million Americans suffer from depression. One in 4 women and 1 in 10 men can expect to develop "major depression" during their lifetime. Nearly 1 in 100 people will suffer from manic-depressive disorder, which is also known as bipolar illness.

Symptoms: Depression brings overwhelming feelings of sadness, helplessness, hopelessness, and irritibility. Other symptoms to look for include changes in appetite and sleep patterns, fatigue, feelings of guilt or worthlessness, and recurring thoughts of death or suicide. With manic-depressive disorder, depressive symptoms alternate with cycles of euphoria. Victims may express unwarranted optimism and even exhibit grandiose delusions—perhaps believing they have a special connection with God, movie stars, or political leaders. Their thoughts may become very scattered, and they may need little or no sleep for days.

Cause: Researchers have not pinpointed the trigger for affective disorders, but numerous studies report a family link in depression. If one identical twin suffers from depression or manic-depressive disorder, for instance, the other twin has a 70 percent chance of also having the illness. Further, scientists have discovered a marker for genes that make people susceptible to manic-depressive illness. Imbalances of brain chemicals, certain medications, and even environmental factors may also contribute to the incidence of affective disorders.

Treatment: A combination of medication and psychotherapy is the usual course of treatment. Psychotherapy involves verbal interaction between a trained professional and a patient with emotional or behavioral problems. Lithium carbonate is usually the drug of choice for treating manic-depressive disorder. It successfully reduces the frequency and intensity of manic episodes for 70 percent of its users.

Anxiety Disorders

Description: Characterized by overwhelming fears that interfere with daily living. Common types of anxiety disorders are phobias (fear of a particular object, situation, or activity), panic disorder (feeling terrified for no apparent reason), and obsessive-compulsive disorder (repeated, unwanted thoughts or compulsive behaviors).

Risk: Over their lifetime, 12.5 percent of Americans will be afflicted with a phobia of one kind or another. Panic disorder affects 1.2 million Americans, while 2.4 million suffer from obsessive-compulsive disorder.

Symptoms: In general, anxiety disorders bring trembling, sweating, muscle aches, dizziness, tension, fatigue, dry mouth, upset stomach, and a high pulse and/or breathing rate. Two of the most common phobias are social phobia (fear of being watched by others) and agoraphobia (fear of being alone or in a public place without an escape hatch). Victims of obsessive-compulsive disorder act out rituals, such as excessive cleaning or bathing.

Cause: Scientists believe no one situation or condition causes anxiety disorders, but rather a mix of physical and environmental factors is responsible. Studies indicate biochemical imbalances could also be partly to blame, as well as stressful childhood events.

Treatment: Phobias and obsessive-compulsive disorders are frequently treated by behavior therapy: The person is exposed to the feared object or situation under controlled conditions until the fear is removed or drastically reduced. About 90 percent of people with phobias or obsessive-compulsive disorder who cooperate with a therapist will recover. Medication is effective for about half of those suffering from obsessive-compulsive disorder.

Schizophrenia

Description: A disease that disrupts thought patterns, often affecting the five senses and causing an overall deterioration of mental processes.

Risk: About 150 in every 100,000 persons have schizophrenia.

Symptoms: Typically, symptoms begin gradually in adolescence or young adulthood and initially may not appear all that unusual. Victims experience trouble concentrating and sleeping, and feel increased tension. But over time they will start to exhibit strange behavior—saying things that don't make sense and seeing things that aren't there. In many cases, sufferers hear voices that issue commands. There are different kinds of schizophrenia—paranoid and disorganized, for example—and symptoms may vary. Some schizophrenics are able to behave normally much of the time.

Cause: As with other mental disorders, researchers have found a family link. In families where both parents have schizophrenia, a child's risk rises to between 15 and 50 percent. Some scientists think genetics, autoimmune illness, and viral infections combine to cause schizophrenia. According to this theory, a schizophrenic's genes tell the immune system to attack the brain after a viral infection. Since many schizophrenics were born in late winter or early spring, it's been suggested that their mothers may have suffered from a slow virus during the winter months of their pregnancy.

Treatment: A number of antipsychotic medications can bring biochemical imbalances closer to normal and reduce delusions and hallucinations. Side effects of the medication, such as dry mouth, blurred vision, and drowsiness, may persist for several weeks. Once medication is working well, psychotherapy can provide further help.

Christmas Isn't Necessarily Blue

Every year we hear about the "holiday blues syndrome," so it must exist, right? Well, not necessarily. Several studies have examined the issue, and their findings are summarized here.

▼ A study of more than 3,000 admissions to a Veterans' Administration Hospital Psychiatry Service found no significant increase in admissions during the holidays.

▼ Another study found holiday suicide rates in the United States to be lower than on other days.

▼ Still another study found that suicides are most likely to occur in spring, but not during the Easter holiday season.

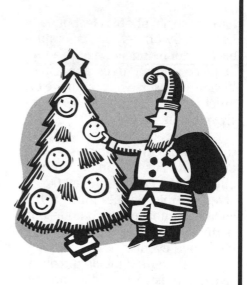

▼ In contrast, homicide rates do tend to be higher on holidays, when people spend more time than usual with their families.

The Top Eight Reasons Why People Turn to Counseling

A *USA Today* poll of mental health professionals asked the reasons why Americans seek counseling. The results, in order of frequency, were:

1. Marriage or intimate relationships
2. Depression
3. Relationships with parents, children, co-workers
4. Lack of self-esteem, excessive insecurity
5. Anxiety
6. Alcohol or drug dependence
7. Personality or character disorders
8. Sexual matters

On the Couch, by the Hour

Visiting a psychiatrist, like most everything else, has gotten a lot more expensive. In 1973, 1 minute of psychotherapy cost just over 58 cents. By 1986, 1 minute cost about $1.43. Here are the hourly amounts.

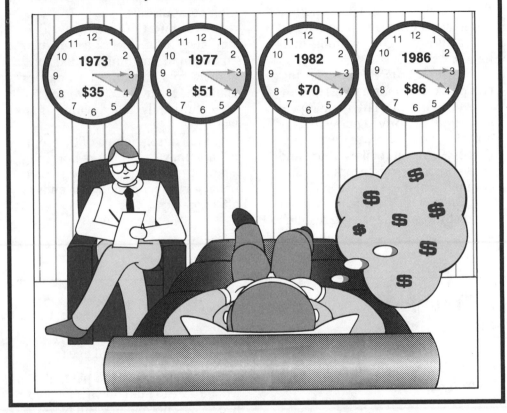

Is That a Fact?

People who are mentally ill act "crazy" all the time.

Even people suffering from severe psychiatric disorders seldom act "crazy" if they receive adequate medical care. Further, many mentally ill people can exercise some control. A person who falsely believes a movie star is in love with him, for instance, isn't likely to act on that belief in his normal work setting.

The Many Varieties of Compulsive Behavior

People suffering obsessive-compulsive disorders can find themselves trapped by their compulsive rituals, which may take many forms:

Cleaning: Afraid they may be contaminated by germs or dirt, some obsessive-compulsive people spend hours showering or washing their hands.

Completing: People with this compulsion perform a series of complex tasks in exact order and repeat them until performed perfectly. Any mistake, and they will repeat the process—even if it takes hours and causes them to miss work or other commitments.

Checking: They fear harming others by forgetting safeguards such as turning off an iron. Men are more likely to be checkers than women.

Hoarding: Collecting everything from chewing gum wrappers to bottle caps. This is one of the less common compulsions.

Avoiding: Compulsive avoiders stay away from the cause of their anxiety and anything related to it. One woman became so anxious about chocolate that she avoided not only the candy but anything that was brown.

Slowness: Victims of this compulsion may spend hours polishing a table or shaving themselves. Such behavior is uncommon and tends to affect men.

A Fresh Look at Autism

If you saw the movie *Rainman,* starring Dustin Hoffman, you already know that people with autism may be capable of some amazing things, such as multiplying and dividing huge numbers in their heads. Now here are a few more insights.

▼ Autism is rare. This developmental disorder occurs in only 1 out of 3,000 children.

▼ Children with autism look normal but do not act normal. They don't respond to their environment. They fail to make eye contact, refuse affection, and repeat the same behavior over and over.

▼ As adults, about 15 percent will be able to hold down a job and live a fairly normal life. But two-thirds will require lifelong care and supervision.

▼ One study of more than 5,000 autistic children from 40 countries found that 10 percent of them possessed abilities far beyond their general intelligence level. These extraordinary abilities centered around mathematics, memory, music, art, and physical coordination.

Where Are the Seriously Mentally Ill?

Maybe not where you thought. Five times as many live at home with their families, for example, than are confined to hospitals.

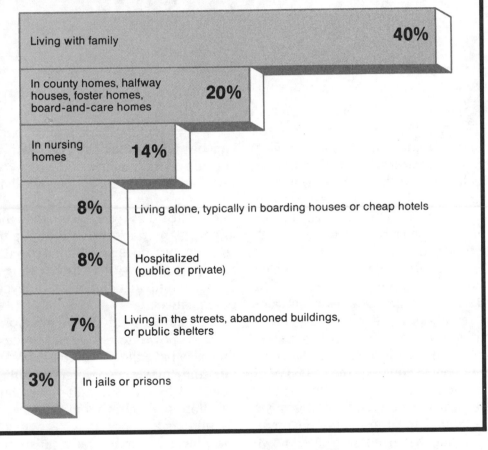

Living with family — **40%**

In county homes, halfway houses, foster homes, board-and-care homes — **20%**

In nursing homes — **14%**

8% Living alone, typically in boarding houses or cheap hotels

8% Hospitalized (public or private)

7% Living in the streets, abandoned buildings, or public shelters

3% In jails or prisons

Since 1963 when President Kennedy proposed the Community Mental Health Center Network, the federal government has spent more than $3 billion to fund nearly 800 community mental health centers.

34

MIND/BODY INTERACTIONS

At the University of Rochester, among women undergoing cervical biopsies after abnormal Pap smears, doctors found they could predict accurately, *before* biopsy results were known, the women most likely to have cancer—based solely on measurements of hopelessness.

Though the Rochester physicians may not have been aware of it, the Greek physician Galen made that same observation about his breast-cancer patients in the second century. Before Galen, Chinese doctors made the mind-body connection more than 4,000 years ago, noting that physical illness could follow frustration. Hippocrates made the connection, too, cautioning physicians that they needed to have knowledge of the mind as well as the body. But Western medicine succeeded in separating mind from matter, and the role of emotions and mood in health and disease was very nearly forgotten —until recently.

Now we know that rage and anger can be deadly, making those with a "hostile heart" 5.5 times more likely to die than those without. Science has also uncovered a "Type C (or Type 1) personality." Less well known than the angry, heart-attack-prone Type A personality, but no less lethal, Type C's tend to suppress their true feelings. They wind up at a high risk for developing cancer.

While the mind and our emotions have the power to ravage our bodies, they also have the power to heal. Witness the "newly discovered" positive power of hypnosis, meditation, visualization, and other mental focusing techniques. Science now recognizes the power of emotionally satisfying ties with family and friends to stave off illness and protect us from disease and injury. Even the emotional support of a pet can extend human life in some cases.

Where the Body Is Targeted by Stress

Research has shown that as stresses accumulate, a person becomes increasingly susceptible to physical illness, mental and emotional problems, and accidental injuries. Shown here are the parts of the body that are susceptible to stress-related diseases.

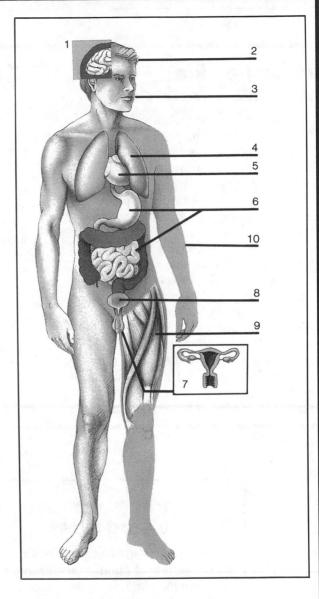

1. Brain: Many mental and emotional problems, among them anxiety and depression, may be triggered by stress.

2. Hair: Some forms of baldness, among them alopecia areata, have been linked to high levels of stress.

3. Mouth: Certain mouth problems, such as mouth ulcers and oral lichen planus, often seem to crop up under stess.

4. Lungs: Asthmatics often find that their condition worsens when they are subjected to high levels of mental or emotional stress.

5. Heart: Attacks of angina and disturbances of heart rate and rhythm often occur at the same time or shortly after a period of stress.

6. Digestive tract: Diseases of the digestive tract that may be either caused or aggravated by stress include gastritis, stomach and duodenal ulcers, ulcerative colitis, and irritable colon.

7. Reproductive organs: Stress-related problems in this part of the body include menstrual disorders, such as absence of periods in women, and impotence in men.

8. Bladder: The bladders of many people react to stress by becoming "irritable."

9. Muscles: Various minor muscular twitches and nervous tics become more noticeable when the individual is under stress.

10. Skin: Some people have outbreaks of skin problems such as eczema and psoriasis when subjected to abnormal stress.

How the Skin Mirrors Emotions

As the table shows, a substantial number of skin problems are emotionally triggered. Because the skin is part of the immune system's defenses, it's not surprising that stress, fatigue, and other emotional problems that lower the body's resistance show up on its surface.

A study at the University of California, San Francisco, for example, discovered a link between depression, immune system changes, and genital herpes. Blood samples from depressed patients showed a drop in two of the substances that regulate the function of the immune system. Consequently, the depressed patients suffered more herpes recurrences than nondepressed patients.

Condition	Percentage of Cases Where Condition Is Emotionally Triggered	Interval between Stress and Start of Problem
Profuse sweating	100	Seconds
Warts	95	Days
Itching	86	Seconds
Hand eczema	76	2 days
Atopic eczema	70	Seconds for itching
Hives	68	Minutes
Psoriasis	62	Days to 2 weeks
Acne	55	2 days
Herpes	36	Days
Contact eczema	15	2 days

The Three Keys to Surviving Stress

According to Joan Borysenko, Ph.D., author of *Minding the Body, Mending the Mind,* some people can go through tremendous changes in their lives yet remain physically and emotionally well. These are people who've developed "stress hardiness," she says, and they tend to have three characteristic attitudes toward stress that help keep them healthy.

Challenge. Instead of seeing change as a threat, stress-hardy people are willing to view change as challenge and see where it takes them.

Control. Stress-hardy people feel that they are in control rather than helpless. But they also know what things they can't control, and they know when to let go.

Commitment. Stress-hardy people are actively involved in their lives at work and at home.

Stress Hits Home with Baby Boomers

As the chart shows, people between the ages of 30 and 44, the so-called baby boomers, are experiencing more stress today than people of any other age group—including their parents. If science is right, their health will surely suffer for it.

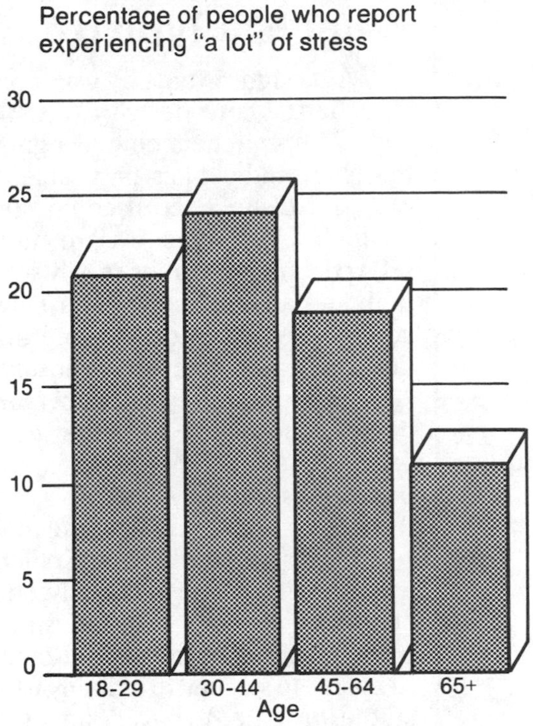

Percentage of people who report experiencing "a lot" of stress

**According to government figures, 84 percent of men and 88 percent of women have experienced stress. Forty percent experience at least a moderate amount of stress during an average week.

Are You a Type A?

Although it usually takes a trained eye to spot all the telltale signs that mark a Type-A personality, the list of traits below can give you a rough idea.

Consider yourself Type A if you habitually:

▼ Eat fast

▼ Move and walk quickly

▼ Speak in quick bursts

▼ Have a loud, jarring voice

▼ Drum your fingers or jiggle your knee

▼ Have a tense posture or facial expression

▼ Play nearly every game to win

▼ Get aggravated waiting in lines or driving

▼ Do two things at once whenever possible

▼ Interrupt others or finish their sentences

▼ Schedule too many things in too little time

▼ Feel guilt when spending time doing nothing

427

What Is a Type B?

Although a Type B was once classified as anyone who wasn't a Type A, researchers now recognize that such individuals have a separate and distinct set of coping behaviors. Thus, Type B's are more relaxed, unhurried, more easily satisfied, and able to use an alternative coping method in daily living that does not lead to competitive hostility.

Experts think Type B's are more likely to succeed because they don't waste time and energy on minor frustrations and petty details, because they listen better, and because their serenity inspires confidence in others.

The most conspicuously successful Type B in recent times may have been former president Ronald Reagan. He seemed to embody what studies of Type B's have found; that is, they work fewer hours than Type A's, but do just as well.

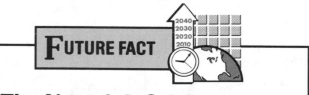

FUTURE FACT

The Next Job Crisis

More than 90 percent of personnel officials responding to a survey said mental health care will become an increasingly important issue in the future. Almost 70 percent believe that mental pressure is such a significant factor at work that companies will someday need to provide "mental health days" as well as vacation days so that workers can unload their stress.

Type-A Behavior: What Really Kills?

For many years, researchers believed aggressive, hurried, competitive people—those designated as having the classic Type-A personality—were working themselves into a heart attack. More recent studies, however, indicate that high levels of hostility and anger are the true killers, not impatience.

In one investigation, Redford B. Williams, Jr., M.D., professor of psychiatry at Duke University Medical Center in Durham, North Carolina, looked at the death rates in a group of 118 attorneys who took a personality test 25 years ago as law students. He found that 20 percent of those who had scored in the highest quarter on the hostility scale had died, compared with 5 percent of those who scored lowest. A similar study of 255 male physicians and a study of 1,877 male workers at Western Electric both found the same link between hostility and death rates.

Such things as talking fast, feeling pressed for time, and working long hours—the traits usually associated with Type-A behavior—apparently have no effect on heart disease.

The "hostile Type A" consists of three personality traits: cynical mistrust of other people's motives, frequent feelings of anger, and aggressive expressions of hostility toward others without regard for their feelings. Dr. Williams says this type of person doesn't simply get annoyed by delays—he gets angry. If he's waiting for an elevator and it's stopped on another floor, the hostile Type A assumes someone is purposely delaying it.

The Cancer Personality

Three long-term personality studies conducted in Europe have uncovered an apparent link between personality and cancer. Researchers found that individuals who tend to repress their emotions in the face of stress are far more likely to die of cancer than others.

The studies, two in Germany and one in Yugoslavia, grouped large numbers of people between the ages of 40 and 65 into four personality types, then recorded premature death rates over the next 10 years. In the Yugoslavian study, summarized in the chart, more than five times as many people classified as Type 1 (emotionally repressed) died of cancer during the ten-year investigation than died of heart disease. The two German studies showed strikingly similar results. In fact, personality type proved more predictive of fatal lung cancer for Type 1's than smoking.

Type 1 individuals are characterized as "underaroused" or "understimulated." They tend to have one valued person or object as their emotional focus, and become strained or depressed if they experience loss, distance, or separation from that person or object. Behavioral therapy administered to 50 Type-1 subjects in one of the German studies starkly reduced cancer deaths in that group, however. None of the 50 receiving therapy died of cancer, while 16 of 50 subjects in a Type-1 control group died of the disease.

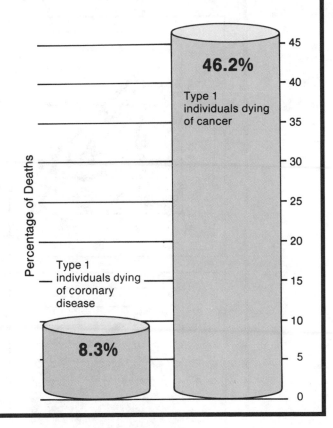

Estimates of Type-A prevalence range from 50 to 80 percent among urban men, with lower rates for women and rural men.

Saved by Their Fighting Spirit

Researchers have found that the will to live is often the most important aspect of survival and that without it, seriously ill patients usually die.

In a study of 57 women with breast cancer, a significant correlation was noted between emotional response three months after a mastectomy and survival rates ten years later. The women's responses were divided into four categories. The "hopeless" group believed that there was nothing further they could do. The "indifferent" group showed no signs of distress. Those in the "denial" group denied they had had cancer and rationalized the operation as a preventive measure. Women in the "fighting spirit" category said, in effect, "I will beat this thing." The four charts summarize the results.

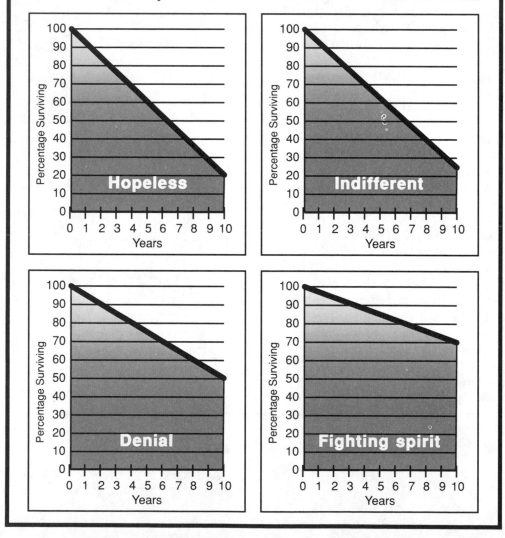

Optimists
Are Healthier

A positive attitude bodes well for good health and longevity. This finding is based on a 35-year followup of Harvard graduates first interviewed in 1946. They've undergone physical examinations every 5 years since then, and those whose interviews suggested an optimistic outlook in their early years have remained healthier than those whose outlook was pessimistic. In other words, their attitude at 25 predicted their health at 65.

Investigators were able to categorize three different types of pessimistic explanatory responses for negative events as follows:

▼ Global: "It will ruin my whole life."

▼ Stable: "It will never go away."

▼ Internal: "It was my fault."

They believe people who explain bad events in any of those three ways may neglect basic health care and become more passive than optimists when faced with illness. The researchers also speculate that pessimism has a negative effect on the immune system.

A pair of psychologists who've kept records of patients referred to them with skin problems find that 75 percent have atopic eczema, while the others are victims of psoriasis, urticaria, and alopecia in roughly equal numbers. About 60 percent are women and 40 percent are men. Fifty percent of all patients show a "stress behavior pattern," defined as a response to stress that leaves them overextended, exhausted, and emotionally upset.

Thoughts and Feelings
That Affect Health

Positive	Negative
Love	Anger
Trust	Suspicion
Friendship	Alienation
Intimacy	Withdrawal
Sense of community	Me against them
Responsible for actions	Victim of circumstance
Confidence	Fear
Optimism	Pessimism
Exaltation	Depression
Stimulation	Boredom
Strong goals	No direction

Hypnotherapy and Kids

Investigators agree that the visualization skills needed to be a good hypnosis subject are generally easier to access in children than in adults. When researchers studied the medical histories of 505 children and adolescents treated by hypnosis for everything from bed-wetting, chronic pain, and asthma to habit disorders, obesity, and anxiety, they found encouraging results (see chart). More than half the children who achieved complete cures did so after only one or two sessions.

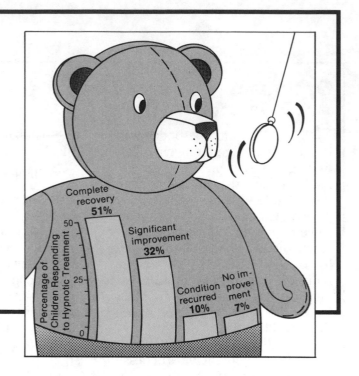

Some Disorders for Which Hypnosis is Useful

As primary treatment:

- ▼ Drooling
- ▼ Bed-wetting
- ▼ Habit control
- ▼ Hypertension
- ▼ Insomnia
- ▼ Migraine headaches
- ▼ Nail biting
- ▼ Pain associated with fractures, burns, injections
- ▼ Sleepwalking
- ▼ Tics

- ▼ Warts

As an adjunctive treatment:

- ▼ Asthma
- ▼ Cerebral palsy
- ▼ Diabetes
- ▼ Drug abuse
- ▼ Malignancies
- ▼ Obesity
- ▼ Phobias
- ▼ Rheumatoid arthritis
- ▼ Seizures

The Healing Power of Pets

As a result of several studies, researchers now believe regular contact with pets can reduce heart rate, blood pressure, and levels of stress. At the University of Maryland, 93 heart-attack patients fared better when they owned a pet. Only 1 of 18 pet owners died, compared to 1 of 3 patients who didn't have pets.

When surveyed, almost half of all responding physicians and psychologists say they now recommend pet interaction for their patients. Among those who do, treatment for loneliness and depression is an almost universally cited reason. But, as the chart shows, pets are being recommended for a number of other health problems as well, both physical and psychological.

Dogs and cats head the list of animals prescribed for pet therapy, favored by 94 percent and 71 percent of therapists, respectively. But birds, fish, gerbils, guinea pigs, and other small animals are prescribed by 15 to 20 percent of the doctors who write pet prescriptions. Notably, 95 percent of the responding doctors who recommend pets to their patients own or have owned a pet.

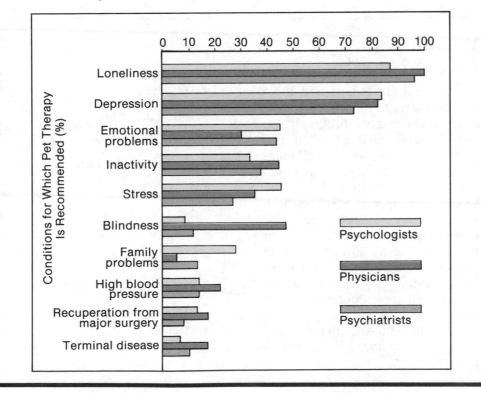

How Pets Work Their Magic

Researchers have discovered nine ways in which pets help increase their owners' health and resistance to disease.

1. They provide companionship.

2. They give us something to care for.

3. They provide pleasurable activity.

4. They are a source of constancy in changing lives.

5. They make us feel safe.

6. They return us to play and laughter.

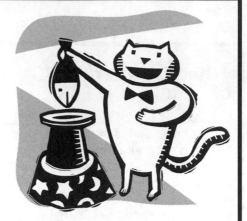

7. They are a stimulus to exercise.

8. They comfort with touch.

9. They are pleasurable to watch.

Visualizing Better Health

One of the easiest and most effective ways to interrupt habitual worry and stress is through a more skillful use of your imagination. The technique known as guided imagery allows you to do just that, imagining yourself in a beautiful, peaceful, serene setting—either somewhere you've been or a fantasy place. By immersing yourself in this pleasant scene for several minutes, imagery proponents say your body will relax and go into a physiologic state in which it can use its energy for repair, restoration, and healing.

Positive guided imagery has been shown to have a beneficial effect on:

▼ Heart rate

▼ Blood pressure

▼ Local blood flow

▼ Gastrointestinal function

▼ Muscle tension

▼ Sexual response

▼ Immune function

▼ Pain control

▼ Recovery from surgery

▼ Weight loss

▼ Habit control

Meditators Have a Health Advantage

Transcendental meditation (TM) practitioners apparently gain a good return on their 40-minute daily investment, not the least of which is better health. As the chart shows, hospital admissions over a five-year stretch were dramatically reduced for meditators in all categories except childbirth. By learning to relax deeply and dissipate stress on a regular basis, meditators appear able to improve physical health and strengthen their immune systems. Other studies have shown that TM practitioners are less likely to smoke, consume alcohol, or use drugs—all habits that detract from health.

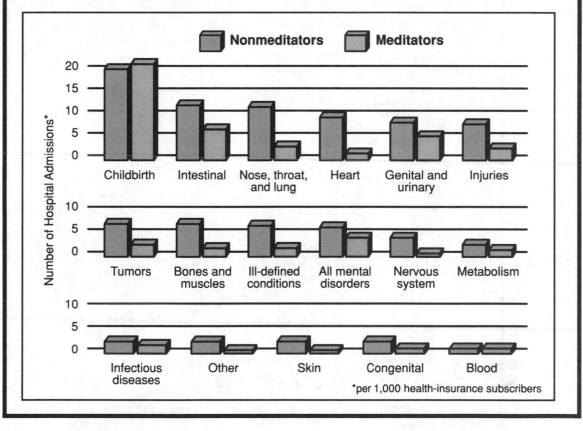

Marriage is Good for Your Health

Data from a National Health Interview Survey of 122,859 Americans reveals that married men and women are less likely than single people to report that chronic health conditions limit their activity or that acute health problems restrict it (see chart).

Married people also report fewer injuries than single or divorced persons, but more than widows or widowers. Divorced women have the highest rate of accidents, according to the survey—nearly twice the rate of married women. Other studies have shown that divorced women have a poorer immune system than happily married women. There are six times as many deaths from pneumonia among separated or divorced women, and they have 30 percent more physician visits for acute illness than do their married counterparts.

Some researchers believe that, in light of such statistics, physicians should routinely inquire about patients' marital status and caution divorced and separated women that they need to pay special attention to their health.

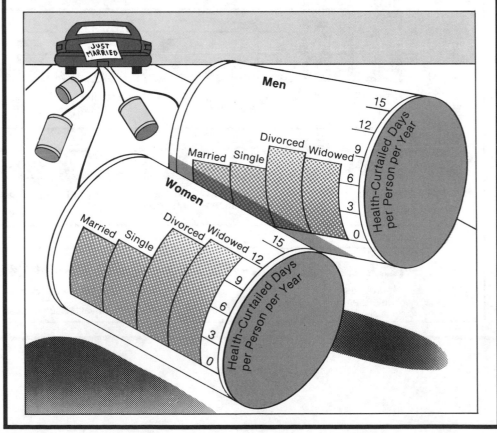

35

MOODS AND EMOTIONS

Moods and emotions are a lot like the weather—with us every day, sometimes very predictable, and yet at other times nearly impossible to forecast. The people around us, our environment—just about everything can affect mood.

We are tuned into emotions almost from the beginning. Three-month-old babies who cannot yet walk or talk, can—to some degree—detect and even mirror the emotional condition of their mothers, studies show.

As adults, we often remain just as impressionable. When mother nature's temperature goes way up, for example, so does mankind's: Violence escalates in hot weather.

And if we work, our moods tend to be up Friday through Sunday and down Monday through Thursday. But the evidence seems overwhelming that we could be a lot happier and healthier by learning how to regularly influence our moods for the better.

While we can't control the weather —or a boss or spouse's sour disposition —we *can* take steps to improve our mood and health.

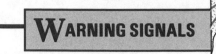

14 Warning Signals for Depression

Almost everybody occasionally feels blue, suffering from a brief low mood.

If the blues come often enough to interfere with the enjoyment of life, you may be undergoing a prolonged mood change. If you have four or more of the symptoms listed here for two or more weeks, you may be suffering from depression, says Priscilla Slagle, M.D., in her book *The Way Up From Down*.

Here's what to look for.

Fatigue. You tire easily and lack ambition for getting things done.

Too much or too little sleep. Your sleeping patterns have been disrupted or you may use sleep as an escape.

Indecision. Even minor decisions become difficult.

Loss of sexual desire. You may completely lose interest and drive.

Changes in eating patterns. You notice you are gaining or—more likely—losing weight.

Anxiety. You feel restless and agitated.

Guilt. You feel remorse or shame over real or imagined events.

Hopelessness. You feel nothing can be done to help you.

Helplessness. You feel unusually dependent on others.

General loss of interest. You feel indifference toward people and activities previously important to you.

Irritability. Trivial things make you feel impatient, annoyed, and jumpy.

Social withdrawal. You prefer to be alone more than usual.

Physical changes. These could include stomach cramps, nausea, chest pains, rapid breathing, sweating, and headache.

Suicidal thoughts. These may range from wishing you were dead to actually contemplating suicide.

IS THAT A FACT?

Big boys don't cry.

Actually, men do cry. But not as easily as women, and part of the reason is a difference in hormones. Women have higher levels of the hormone prolactin, which is found in tears, and their tear glands are anatomically different from men's. Men often only get watery eyes, while women shed tears that spill over the cheek.

What Makes Us Angry or Impatient?

In general, waiting. More specifically . . .

What Makes People Happy?

Asked to name their most uplifting experiences, many people gave down-to-earth answers.

1. Relating well with spouse or lover

2. Relating well with friends

3. Completing a task

4. Feeling healthy

5. Getting enough sleep

6. Eating out

7. Meeting responsibilities

8. Visiting, phoning, or writing someone

9. Spending time with family

10. Taking pride in home

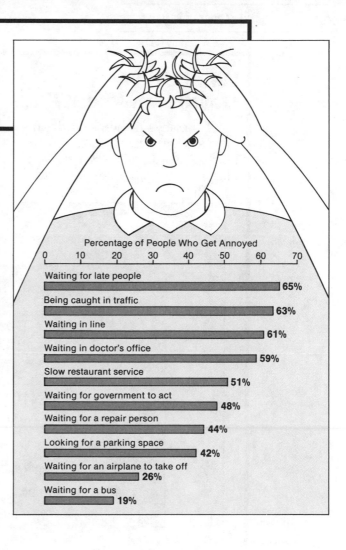

Percentage of People Who Get Annoyed

Waiting for late people	65%
Being caught in traffic	63%
Waiting in line	61%
Waiting in doctor's office	59%
Slow restaurant service	51%
Waiting for government to act	48%
Waiting for a repair person	44%
Looking for a parking space	42%
Waiting for an airplane to take off	26%
Waiting for a bus	19%

Five Emotions That Hinder Thinking

Emotions are strictly emotions and thoughts are strictly thoughts, right? Not really. The two overlap. And certain emotions can really interfere with thinking. Reuven Bar-Levav, M.D., a psychotherapist and author of *Thinking in the Shadow of Feelings*, lists five.

1. Fear

2. Romantic "love"

3. Hate

4. Anger

5. Hurt

439

What Do We Daydream About?

For many Americans, daydreams provide a harmless emotional escape hatch. According to a Roper Organization survey, money and travel are the most frequently turned-to themes. Almost no one fantasizes about being elected to political office.

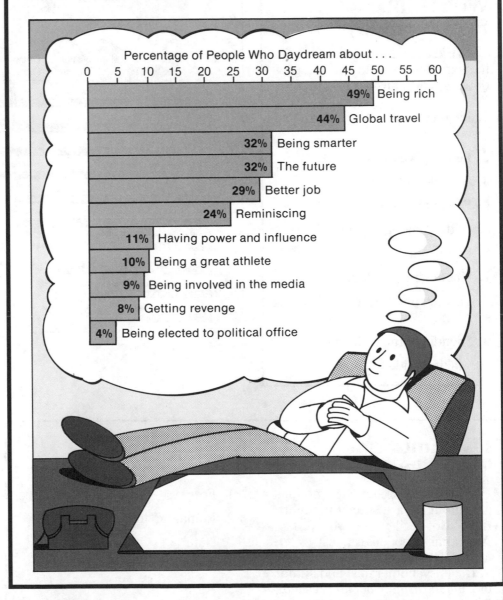

Percentage of People Who Daydream about . . .

49%	Being rich
44%	Global travel
32%	Being smarter
32%	The future
29%	Better job
24%	Reminiscing
11%	Having power and influence
10%	Being a great athlete
9%	Being involved in the media
8%	Getting revenge
4%	Being elected to political office

The Foods That Shape Our Moods

There may be more to that old saying, "You are what you eat," than you realized. Researchers have found that some foods increase brain chemicals that have a stimulating mental effect, while others increase brain chemicals that have a calming effect. In general, low-fat proteins are stimulators while carbohydrates are soothers.

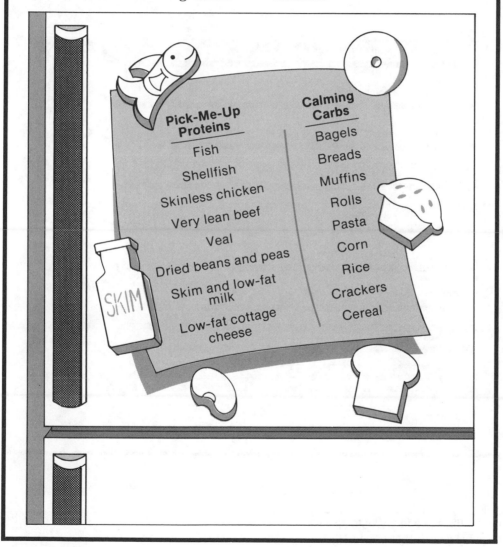

Pick-Me-Up Proteins

Fish

Shellfish

Skinless chicken

Very lean beef

Veal

Dried beans and peas

Skim and low-fat milk

Low-fat cottage cheese

Calming Carbs

Bagels

Breads

Muffins

Rolls

Pasta

Corn

Rice

Crackers

Cereal

Anxiety—
What Causes It?

When Americans were queried about what makes their hearts race and their palms sweat, these were the types of situations that were cited most frequently.

PERCENTAGE
OF
PEOPLE
WHO
WORRY

Situation

Being with a group of strangers	**78.6**
Talking with an authority figure	**78.6**
Giving a speech	**46.4**
Meeting a date's parents	**39.3**
Saying something stupid	**37.5**
Asking for a date	**33.9**
Attending a party	**32.1**
Going on a date	**26.8**
Starting a new job	**25.0**
Going on a job interview	**23.2**

Researchers say women cry five times as often as men. For both sexes, the average cry lasts six minutes. Peak crying time is between 7:00 P.M. and 10:00 P.M., when emotional downers from relationships or television movies are most likely to hit hardest.

In the Mood for Murder

Hot temperatures can make people hot under the collar. Data from field studies over several decades indicate that, on the average, there are more assaults, rapes, and homicides in July and August than in any other months. This chart plots homicide incidence on a month-by-month basis.

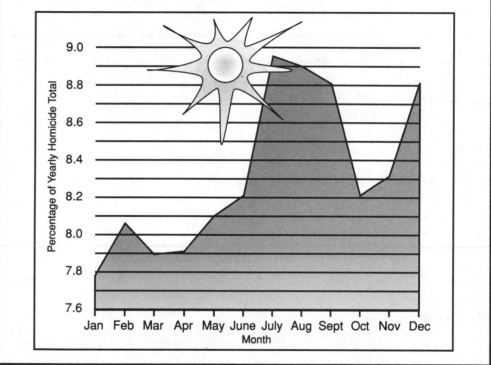

IS THAT A FACT?

Watching violence on TV encourages violent and hostile feelings in children.

Psychological research has shown three clear tendencies in children who view TV violence.

▼ They may become less sensitive to the pain and suffering of others.

▼ They may be more fearful of the world around them.

▼ They may be more likely to behave in harmful or aggressive ways.

How Health Habits Affect Mood

Bad personal health habits can translate into bad feelings like depression. In one study, people with poor habits like smoking cigarettes or skipping breakfast were more likely to be feeling low. Here's the breakdown, habit by habit.

Health Habit	Prevalence of Depression (%)		
	Men	Women	Total
Hours of sleep			
Poor: 6 or less, 9 or more	16.2	24.1	21.1
Good: 7–8	7.1	12.3	10.2
Eat breakfast			
Poor: never, rarely, sometimes	11.4	18.6	15.6
Good: almost daily	8.8	15.2	12.8
Eat between meals			
Poor: almost always	7.2	15.0	11.9
Good: never, rarely, sometimes	11.3	17.4	15.0
Desirable weight for height			
Poor: not within desirable limits	12.5	19.9	17.3
Good: within desirable limits	9.6	14.3	12.4
Engage in active sports			
Poor: never or rarely	11.4	21.3	18.5
Good: sometimes, almost daily	9.6	13.2	11.6
Currently smoke cigarettes			
Poor: yes	10.4	22.8	17.1
Good: no	9.9	14.4	12.8
Number of alcoholic drinks per day			
Poor: 5+	18.8	30.0	21.4
Good: 0 to 4	9.1	16.6	13.8

People who get regular physical exercise report more overall satisfaction with life than those who get little or no exercise, U.S. and Canadian population surveys indicate. This connection is strongest for women and persons aged 40 and older.

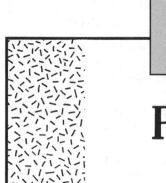

36

PAIN

Everybody has some pain some of the time. But a lot of Americans, about 80 million, have chronic pain. Treating all that pain isn't cheap—each year more than $90 billion is spent on pain relief. In addition, 550 to 600 million workdays are lost.

Not surprisingly, pain is often a companion to diseases such as arthritis and cancer. But everyday stress and tension can also lead to pain.

The hospital would seem to be the one place you could count on to receive relief from pain. But a survey found that 65 percent of hospital patients in pain were undertreated for their pain. Another study found that:

▼ Fifty-eight percent of hospital patients reported experiencing excruciating pain at some point during their stay.

▼ Less than half had been asked by a nurse about their degree of pain.

▼ Patients' degree of pain often was not noted in their medical records.

▼ On average, the doses of analgesics given to the patients were one-fourth of the amount allowed by the physician.

In the United States alone, there are now more than 1,000 pain clinics. Increasingly, doctors and patients are learning that there are many ways to stop pain—at least temporarily.

Mental attitude is also important. Though severe and chronic pain can cause major life changes, the majority of such pain sufferers say they are still satisfied with their lives.

The Two Kinds of Pain

Acute pain is severe here-and-now pain, such as from an injury or appendicitis. It tends to be sharp and last a short time. Typically, once the pain is treated—removing the appendix, for example—the problem is solved. But sometimes acute pain warns of a more difficult-to-discover disorder.

Chronic pain is pain today, tomorrow, and the day after that. It can be constant or recurring, and the intensity may vary. Chronic pain is also more prone to psychological influences, but this isn't to say that chronic pain is usually psychosomatic in origin.

The Mind Can Magnify Distress

The more you concentrate your attention on pain, the worse it tends to be. When dental patients were asked to rate how they felt every five minutes, they reported significantly more pain than when asked to rate their pain just once, at 30 minutes.

Further, the conditions under which pain occurs appear to affect the degree of pain felt. When soldiers wounded in battle during World War II were compared with civilians who had suffered injuries of similar severity, it was found that the majority of soldiers never needed any pain relief. Researchers believe the soldiers had a higher threshold for pain because being wounded was not unexpected, and because it was a somewhat positive event—they survived and were temporarily spared from more combat.

The Path of Pain: Getting to "Ouch!"

A man walking barefoot steps on a piece of glass: "Ouch!" But what actually happens in that instant? A lot. First, cells in the injured tissue emit several chemicals which activate local nerve endings. Then the stimulated nerve endings send an electrochemical impulse through the nerves to the spinal cord. From there the impulse moves to the thalamus region of the brain and on to the cerebral cortex. During this process, the sensation of stepping on a piece of glass is consciously recognized as pain. Depending on the number of nerve endings involved, the pain registers as mild or severe.

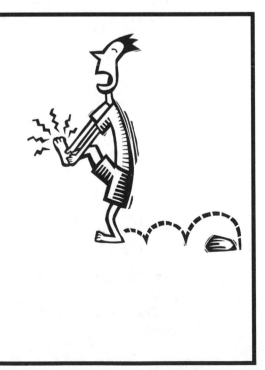

How Pains Compare

Different kinds of pain strike with different levels of intensity. Arthritis and toothache can be very painful, for instance, but apparently not nearly as painful as first-time childbirth.

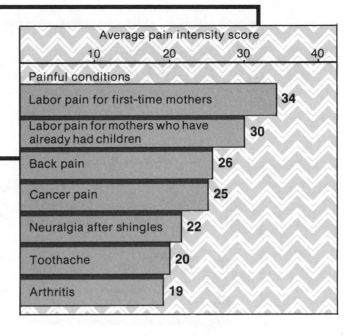

Average pain intensity score

Painful conditions

Labor pain for first-time mothers	34
Labor pain for mothers who have already had children	30
Back pain	26
Cancer pain	25
Neuralgia after shingles	22
Toothache	20
Arthritis	19

Smokers experience twice as much pain as nonsmokers.

Fewer Aches as We Age

In five of six categories studied, people aged 18 to 24 had more pain than those 65 and older; the older people did report more joint pain.

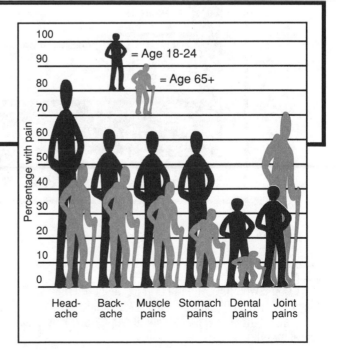

= Age 18-24

= Age 65+

Percentage with pain

Head-ache Back-ache Muscle pains Stomach pains Dental pains Joint pains

Capsaicin, an organic compound found in hot red peppers, is now available in a therapeutic cream used to relieve the painful itch of shingles.

Lost Workdays Due to Pain

Adults employed full-time lose 550 million workdays each year because of pain. Headaches alone claim nearly 157 million workdays. Here is the complete breakdown.

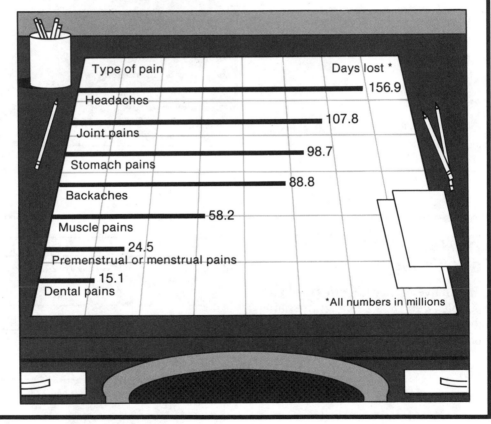

Type of pain	Days lost *
Headaches	156.9
Joint pains	107.8
Stomach pains	98.7
Backaches	88.8
Muscle pains	58.2
Premenstrual or menstrual pains	24.5
Dental pains	15.1

*All numbers in millions

People who have an arm or a leg amputated almost always experience "phantom pain" — a feeling of pain in the missing part. The pain usually disappears slowly over several months.

More Stress Equals More Pain

Most people can't avoid some occasional stress, and some occasional pain. But more stress also seems to translate into more pain. In the Nuprin Pain Report survey, people who said they experienced stress every day were labeled the "high-stress" group. Those who reported stress less often than once a week were labeled the "low-stress" group. When comparing the two groups several differences emerged.

▼ In each of the seven categories of pain used in the study—headache, backache, muscle pain, joint pain, stomach pain, premenstrual and menstrual pain, and dental pain—the high-stress group was more likely to be at least an occasional victim.

▼ In the previous year, 14 percent of the high-stress group had experienced 101 or more days of headaches, compared with just 2 percent of the low-stress group.

▼ In the previous year, 20 percent of the high-stress group had reported 101 or more days of backaches, compared with only 7 percent of the low-stress group.

How Sufferers Rate Their Aches

Persons with various types of recurring pain were asked to rate their pain on a severity scale. The chart indicates the percentage of responses in each category.

Type of Pain	Percentage of People with Each Type of Pain				
	Slight	Moderate	Severe	Unbearable	Not Sure
Backache	16	44	23	14	2
Dental pain	4	38	36	23	—
Headache	22	42	26	9	2
Joint pain	22	41	22	12	2
Muscle pain	34	40	18	5	3
Premenstrual or menstrual pain	20	33	32	14	—
Stomach pain	24	35	28	7	5

Who's Tough Enough to Stand the Pain?

Researchers tested pain tolerance of athletes and nonathletes by asking them to immerse their feet and lower legs into ice-cold water. A time limit of 12 minutes was set for the test; if the participants removed one or both feet from the water, the test was stopped and the immersion time was recorded.

Surprisingly, nonathletes scored better than karate enthusiasts, though far below boxers and football players.

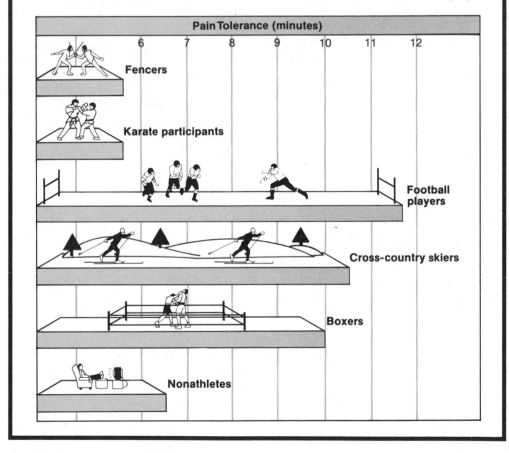

Pain Tolerance (minutes)

Fencers
Karate participants
Football players
Cross-country skiers
Boxers
Nonathletes

In major industrialized countries, acute pain affects about 50 percent of the population; chronic pain affects about 30 percent of the population.

The Pros and Cons of Painkillers

There are two categories of pain relief drugs (analgesics)—narcotics and nonnarcotics. Both have advantages and disadvantages, as this table summarizes.

	Form	How They Work	Benefits	Drawbacks
Nonnarcotics	Aspirin Acetaminophen Ibuprofen Typically taken in tablet form.	Relieve pain by acting on peripheral nerves; they have little effect on the brain.	Can relieve even severe pain for a short time. Studies of patients having wisdom tooth extractions, as well as studies of people with chronic pain, have shown two aspirin tablets to be as potent as 30–60 mg of codeine for relieving pain. And they're not addictive.	Overuse can irritate the stomach. For best results, the drugs should be taken with liquid, and not on an empty stomach.
Narcotics	Morphine and related drugs Given intravenously in hospitals.	Can stop or at least slow pain signals being processed in the central nervous system.	Pack more pain-relieving power and allow many patients to live more satisfying lives. Though they are potentially addictive, few patients become hooked. In a study of more than 11,000 people treated with narcotics, only four had trouble stopping the medication after it was no longer required.	Cause drowsiness, nausea, constipation, and in large doses, semi-consciousness. Over time, they become less effective. After a patient stops taking them, withdrawal symptoms and a short-term increase in pain may occur.

Who Treats Pain?

A medical doctor remains the most popular choice among pain sufferers. Only 3 percent of people surveyed said they had consulted a pain specialist.

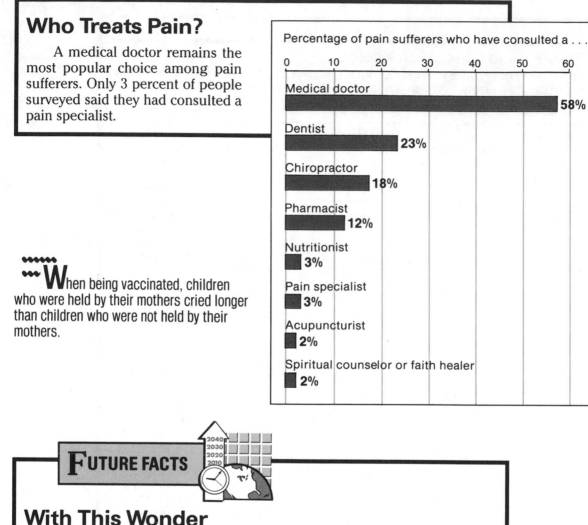

Percentage of pain sufferers who have consulted a . . .

Medical doctor	58%
Dentist	23%
Chiropractor	18%
Pharmacist	12%
Nutritionist	3%
Pain specialist	3%
Acupuncturist	2%
Spiritual counselor or faith healer	2%

When being vaccinated, children who were held by their mothers cried longer than children who were not held by their mothers.

FUTURE FACTS

With This Wonder Drug, We'll Be Feelin' No Pain

Researchers hope to develop a pain-controlling drug as potent as morphine, but without its risk of addiction. One possibility is to develop a strong and safe variant of bradykinin—the powerful pain-producing chemical the body releases when tissue is injured.

Weaker bradykinin stand-ins were first synthesized several years ago. Scientists theorize that a stronger drug could perhaps replace and block natural bradykinin at its source—preventing the nerve cells from firing and stopping even severe pain before it starts.

Five Ways to Find Relief without Drugs

Nondrug treatment methods can effectively control pain—independently or in combination with drugs. Here are five of the most popular and effective methods.

Acupuncture. The Chinese have practiced this healing art for centuries. The insertion of thin needles at precise points on the body has been used to treat chronic pain and as an anesthetic during simple surgery. More recently, laser acupuncture has been used to treat head and neck pain.

Biofeedback. This technique teaches people to control their internal physiological responses, such as heart rate and muscle contractions associated with stress. Biofeedback has proved effective for many kinds of pain, including amputees' "phantom limb" pain and migraine headache.

Hypnosis. Most useful for short-term acute pain, hypnosis works, at least in part, by diverting the patient's attention away from the discomfort. However, hypnosis may also stimulate the release of endorphins —natural painkilling chemicals in the brain.

Relaxation training. The patient simply concentrates on deep breathing, repeats a single word aloud or silently, visualizes a peaceful scene, or progressively tenses and relaxes muscles. Ideally, relaxation training should be practiced once a day.

TENS. TENS stands for transcutaneous electrical nerve stimulation. This method has worked especially well in relieving chronic pain from bursitis and osteoarthritis. Using electrodes, a weak electric current is placed on the skin. TENS may work by stimulating large nerve fibers that repress the transmission of pain signals, or it may simply increase the number of natural opiates.

In a study of chronic pain patients, introverts showed more improvement after acupuncture than extroverts.

Ninety percent of people get some pain relief from placebos—"real"-looking pills that contain no active ingredients.

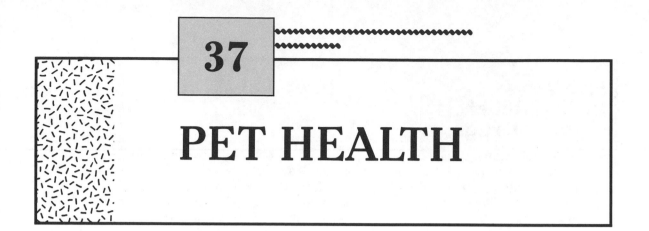

37

PET HEALTH

Americans own an estimated 54.6 million cats, 52.4 million dogs, and 12.9 million birds. And those numbers don't begin to count the millions of fish, rabbits, turtles, lizards, snakes, gerbils, guinea pigs, hamsters, ferrets, and ant farms sharing our homes.

Our pets are important to us—scientists say they make us happier and healthier. And in return for their furry or feathery loyalty, we're spending more to make their lives healthy, comfortable, and safe.

Pet food, for instance, is a $6.3 billion business. Pampered pets can feast on gourmet food. Dogs dine on lamb and rice meat loaf. Cats sup on hand-cut chunks of seafood packed in aspic. Dessert is a scoop of canine ice cream. And in between meals, there are pooch and kitty snacks—a $430 million-a-year segment of the total pet food market. Meanwhile, fat cats and dogs slim down on high-fiber, low-calorie, and low-fat "lite foods."

Today, more than 46,700 veterinarians in the United States treat animals with all the latest in health care, prolonging their health and their important contribution to our lives. The latest health trends for animals include pacemakers, blood banks, high-tech dentistry, cardiopulmonary resuscitation, advanced cancer treatment, behavioral psychology, and high-tech reproductive aids.

How Do You Know Your New Pet Is Healthy?

Start your relationship right—with a healthy animal. Here are some things to look for when choosing your pet. And, after making your choice, have your new friend checked by your veterinarian.

Signs of Health

Dog and Cat
Active
Plays and runs
Wrestles with siblings
Good appetite
Clear, bright eyes
Cool, dry nose
Solid feces
Clean ears
Bright, clean teeth
Shiny fur, no scaly skin

Bird
Eyelids smooth and sharp
No eye discharge
Ear (behind and below the eye) should have no discharge
Balance should be good, not wobbly
Breathing rate should be 30 breaths per minute (large birds) to 100 per minute (small birds) in resting state
No swelling or discharge around nostrils
No white crusts or discharge around mouth
From 25–50 formed droppings per day

When Your Pet Needs Its "Shots"

As a baby, your pet receives natural immunity from its mother. After weaning, the natural immunity fades. Your veterinarian can replace that immunity with a series of vaccinations. Here's a general table of recommended shots and when they should be given.

Pet	Vaccine	Age (Weeks)
Cats*	Panleukopenia (feline distemper)	6–8, 9, 12
	Viral rhinotracheitis	6–8, 9, 12
	Calicivirus	6–8, 9, 12
	Pneumonitis	6–8, 9, 12
	Leukemia	9, 12, 24
	Rabies	16
Dogs†	Distemper	6, 9, 12, 15
	Measles	6
	Parvovirus	6, 9, 12, 15
	Hepatitis	9, 12, 15
	Leptospirosis	9, 12, 15
	Parainfluenza	9, 12, 15
	Rabies	16

*Annual boosters required on vaccinations.

†Annual boosters required on vaccinations except measles. For some animals, including show and working dogs, a booster is necessary every 6 months.

When Should You Call the Vet?

Call for professional help when your pet has any of these signs or conditions.

▼ Injuries from being hit by a car or falling

▼ Suspected broken bone

▼ Bleeding from any part of the body

▼ Eye injury

▼ Pale or purplish-blue gums or mouth

▼ Difficulty breathing

▼ Trembling, shaking, or other discomfort

▼ Collapse (animal seems suddenly weak, loses consciousness)

▼ Vomiting or diarrhea that lasts more than 24 hours

▼ Inability to urinate

▼ Swallows a foreign object, drugs, medications, or poison

When Your Pet Can Make You Sick

Studies show that pets are good for our health. They provide companionship, make us laugh, and encourage us to exercise. Yet, pets can also pass along germs, called zoonoses, to their beloved owners. There are more than 30 zoonotic diseases. The table lists some of the most common ones along with preventive measures.

Illness	Animal Carrier	Prevention
Campylobacter	Dog, cat	Good hygiene
Cat scratch fever	Cat	Avoid scratches and bites; avoid unknown cats
Kawasaki disease	Dog, cat	Get rid of fleas
Intestinal parasites (hookworms, roundworms)	Dog, cat	Good hygiene
Leptospirosis	Dog	Vaccination
Salmonella	Dog, cat, turtle	Good hygiene
Skin diseases (ringworm, fleas, scabies, mites)	Cat, dog	Eliminate pests
Streptococcus	Dog	Have dog tested
Toxoplasmosis	Cat	Good hygiene, wear gloves when changing cat litter; restrict cat's hunting

How Male and Female Dogs Differ

The second most important question—after you've chosen the type of dog you want—is whether to get a male or female. In dogs, gender makes a big difference. Although body size and appearance between the sexes is not strikingly different, behavior varies markedly.

This chart shows some of the differences between male and female dogs. The longer the bar, the more agreement among the experts that one sex exceeds the other in a particular trait.

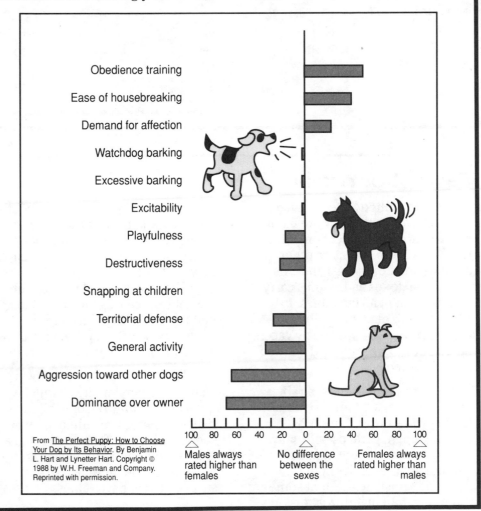

Obedience training
Ease of housebreaking
Demand for affection
Watchdog barking
Excessive barking
Excitability
Playfulness
Destructiveness
Snapping at children
Territorial defense
General activity
Aggression toward other dogs
Dominance over owner

100 80 60 40 20 0 20 40 60 80 100

Males always rated higher than females

No difference between the sexes

Females always rated higher than males

From The Perfect Puppy: How to Choose Your Dog by Its Behavior. By Benjamin L. Hart and Lynetter Hart. Copyright © 1988 by W.H. Freeman and Company. Reprinted with permission.

If Your Dog Were Human, How Old Would It Be?

Dogs age much faster than humans, but it's still possible to make comparisons between them and us. At six months, for example, your puppy is the age equivalent of a human Little Leaguer. Your puppy becomes a teenager just two months later. If your dog lives to the ripe old age of 21, you'll have a centenarian on your hands.

Dog's Age	Human Equivalent (Years)
6 months	10
8 months	13
10 months	14
12 months	15
18 months	20
2 years	24
4	32
6	40
8	48
10	56
12	64
14	72
16	80
18	88
20	96
21	100

Facts about Rabies

▼ In the United States, skunks, raccoons, and bats are more likely to have rabies—an infection of the nervous system—than are other animals, including dogs and cats. In Canada, foxes and skunks carry 74.6 percent of all the rabies. In Mexico, 93.5 percent of rabies is carried by dogs. A previously vaccinated pet will be protected if bitten by an infected animal.

▼ There are two kinds of rabies in cats and dogs. In "dumb rabies," the pet will sit with its mouth hanging open, perhaps with saliva oozing from its mouth, and a peculiar look in its eyes. It might be assumed—mistakenly—that something is caught in its throat or mouth. Don't pry the animal's mouth open to look inside if there is any chance of rabies. You can be infected if you have a cut or scratch on your hand.

The other type of rabies, "furious rabies," causes the animal to hallucinate. A dog will snap at imaginary objects. A cat may scratch for no apparent reason.

▼ Most often, a pet with rabies will show a personality change. A quiet animal may become aggressive. An aggressive animal may be suddenly loving. Take your pet to a veterinarian immediately if it is bitten by a wild animal, or if you suspect it may have rabies.

Where Rabies Strikes

The map shows locations and total number of rabies cases reported during 1986.

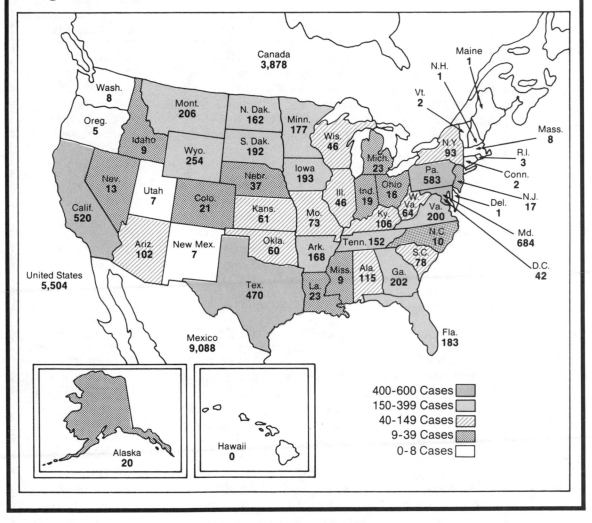

Canada
3,878

Maine
1

N.H.
1

Vt.
2

Wash.
8

Mont.
206

N. Dak.
162

Minn.
177

Mass.
8

Oreg.
5

Idaho
9

Wyo.
254

S. Dak.
192

Wis.
46

N.Y.
93

R.I.
3

Conn.
2

Nev.
13

Utah
7

Colo.
21

Nebr.
37

Iowa
193

Mich.
23

Ill.
46

Ind.
19

Ohio
16

Pa.
583

N.J.
17

Del.
1

Calif.
520

Kans.
61

Mo.
73

Ky.
106

W.
Va.
64

Va.
200

Md.
684

Ariz.
102

New Mex.
7

Okla.
60

Ark.
168

Tenn. 152

N.C.
10

D.C.
42

United States
5,504

S.C.
78

Tex.
470

La.
23

Miss.
9

Ala.
115

Ga.
202

Mexico
9,088

Fla.
183

Alaska
20

Hawaii
0

400-600 Cases
150-399 Cases
40-149 Cases
9-39 Cases
0-8 Cases

You can evaluate your pet's weight by look and feel. A trim dog or cat is lean and firm with a clearly defined waistline behind the ribs. You should be able to feel each rib. If you can't, your pet may need to diet.

Rating the Dog Breeds for Personality

When you're looking for a dog, there are many factors you may want to consider. Some are cute but are snappy with children. Some are easily trained, others aren't. This table lists the best and worst breeds in a number of categories related to temperament.

Watchdog	Playfulness	Affection	Destructiveness
Best-suited	*Most playful*	*Most affectionate*	*Most destructive*
Rottweiler	Standard poodle	Lhasa Apso	West Highland white terrier
German shepherd	Airedale terrier	Boston terrier	Irish setter
Doberman pinscher	Cairn terrier	English springer spaniel	Airedale terrier
Scottish terrier	Miniature schnauzer	Cocker spaniel	German shepherd
West Highland white terrier	English springer spaniel	Toy poodle	Siberian husky
Miniature schnauzer	Irish setter	Miniature poodle	Fox terrier
Least-suited	*Least playful*	*Least affectionate*	*Least destructive*
Bloodhound	Bloodhound	Chow chow	Bloodhound
Newfoundland	Bulldog	Akita	Bulldog
Saint Bernard	Chow chow	Bloodhound	Pekingese
Basset hound	Basset hound	Rottweiler	Golden retriever
Vizsla	Saint Bernard	Basset hound	Newfoundland
Norwegian elkhound	Alaskan malamute	Collie	Akita

Housebreaking	Activity Level	Obedience Training	Behavior around Children
Easiest to train	*Friskiest*	*Easiest to train*	*Most snappish*
Bichon frise	Silky terrier	Miniature poodle	Scottish terrier
Miniature poodle	Chihuahua	German shepherd	Miniature schnauzer
Standard poodle	Miniature schnauzer	Standard poodle	West Highland white terrier
Welsh corgi	Fox terrier	Shetland sheepdog	Chow chow
Australian shepherd	Irish setter	Doberman pinscher	Yorkshire terrier
Doberman pinscher	West Highland white terrier	Australian shepherd	Pomeranian
Hardest to train	*Most lethargic*	*Hardest to train*	*Least snappish*
Basset hound	Basset hound	Chow chow	Golden retriever
Dachshund	Bloodhound	Fox terrier	Labrador retriever
Fox terrier	Bulldog	Afghan hound	Newfoundland
Dalmatian	Newfoundland	Bulldog	Bloodhound
Pekingese	Collie	Basset hound	Basset hound
Beagle	Saint Bernard	Beagle	Collie

Walking the Dog— How Far?

How much exercise does your dog need? That depends on its breed, and the state of its health. This chart shows typical daily mileage needed by some breeds, but that doesn't mean you have to do all the walking, too. If you have a fenced area where your dog can exercise, it may easily cover the distance by itself just running back and forth. Of course, if you do decide to exercise with your dog, you'll both benefit.

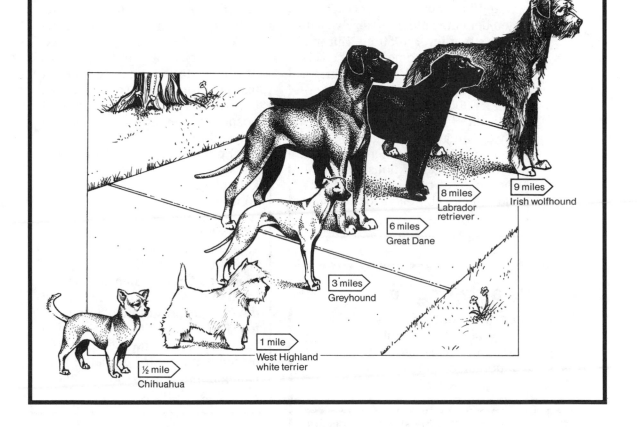

8 miles
Labrador retriever

9 miles
Irish wolfhound

6 miles
Great Dane

3 miles
Greyhound

1 mile
West Highland white terrier

½ mile
Chihuahua

About 20 to 40 percent of people with allergies may react to dogs and cats. Allergy researchers have found no distinctions between breeds. From 40 to 60 percent of owners will develop a sensitivity to hamsters and guinea pigs after long exposure.

When Cats Get Their Dander Up

Cats in well-insulated houses pose a special problem for their owners with allergies. A study at the Allergic Diseases Research Lab of the Mayo Clinic found that in an ordinary house with one cat, there were 17 nanograms (ng) of cat allergen per cubic meter of air. Two cats raised that level to 50 ng. But in a super-insulated home—where cracks were sealed and windows triple glazed for energy efficiency—there were 1,900 ng from two cats. Even with filtering, there was five times the amount of cat allergen in the air of a "tight" house as there was in the normal, unfiltered house. Limiting the range of cats within the house did help limit the allergens, researchers said.

Animal Facts of Life

Some animals produce families once or twice a year. Others double and triple their numbers in less than 30 days—an important consideration for the potential pet owner.

Animal	Gestation (Days)	Litter Size
Mouse	19–21	10–12
Rabbit	31–32	8
Hamster	16–18	6–8
Gerbil	24–25	5
Guinea pig	65–72	3

Is That A Fact?

Cats have nine lives.

That old adage may have at least some basis in fact, says Jared M. Diamond, a professor of physiology at the UCLA School of Medicine.

Why? Because cats can survive falls that would kill most people. That was the conclusion of two New York City veterinarians who studied cats that accidentally fell from heights of 2 to 32 stories and lived. The cat that fell 32 stories landed on concrete, but was released after two days of hospital observation with only a chipped tooth and a small amount of air trapped in his chest. (By comparison, few humans have survived falls of more than 6 stories onto concrete.)

What makes cats so special? According to Dr. Diamond, their relatively small mass reduces impact stress. And they have an inner "gyroscope" that rotates them as they fall so all four feet point downward and the impact is distributed among all four limbs. In addition, cats tend to fall at a relatively slow speed of about 60 miles per hour, compared with falling humans, who travel at about 120 miles per hour.

Before you leave your pet in a kennel, check the references and tour the entire facility, including housing, feeding, and exercise areas. There should be someone on the premises or nearby at all times and a veterinarian should be available.

Selecting a Pet Bird

Do you want a long-term companion, a low-cost tweeter, someone to talk to who will also talk back? Here are some birds to consider.

Type of Bird	Considerations	Life Span (Years)
Finch	Easy care	2–3
Canary	Easy care; males sing, so are usually more expensive	8–10
Budgerigar	Easy care	8–15
Cockatiel	Easy care, easy to train	15–20
Lovebird	Not easy to tame or train	15–20
Amazon	Good talkers, especially double-yellows and yellow-naped; can be screamers	50–60
African grey	Talkers; never scream	50–60
Macaw	Will talk, but not as much as certain Amazons or African greys	50–60

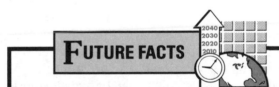

FUTURE FACTS

Spot's Got Insurance (and Other New Toys)

Peer into the future and you'll find pets like Spot and Muffy taking even more important places in the family. Here's what experts predict the decades will bring.

Spot and Muffy carry insurance that pays the doctor bills for a yearly premium of less than $100. When they ride in the car, they have their own seat belts that fit like a vest and buckle into the car's seat-belt system. This gives them the same safety that their tiny masters and mistresses get when buckled into a child's car seat.

If Spot and Muffy wander too far from home (or lose their collars), no problem. The lost pet is simply taken to the local animal shelter where a worker can get its vital information in seconds from an implanted computer chip the size of a grain of rice. That chip, when scanned much like a bar-code scanner, works like an identification card.

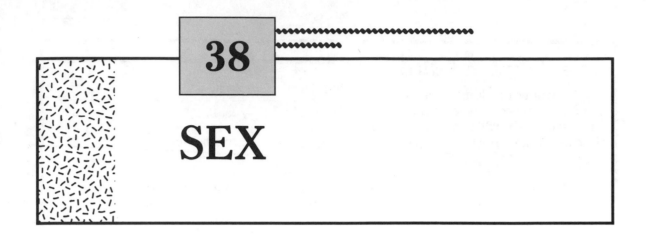

38

SEX

Sex can be healthy, or in this era of AIDS and other sexually-transmitted diseases, sex can be dangerous and even deadly. Yet sex remains inviting— not to mention important—for adults of all ages.

Many older people, despite myths to the contrary, continue to make sex a regular part of their lives. And couples of all ages with "satisfying" sex lives report being happier in their relationships.

Over the last two decades, sex has become a more publicly discussed subject. And to some extent, attitudes have changed. One study found that from 1985 to 1989 the percentage of parents who talked about birth control with their children doubled, climbing to 62 percent. The majority of surveys usually show that most Americans are not offended by the sexual content of novels, movies, and television programs. For better or worse, sex is no longer in the shadows. In fact, one study estimates that children see 60,000 references to sex on television each year.

Still, Americans remain divided in their opinions on the morality of premarital sex, with the vast majority (78 percent) believing extramarital sex to always be wrong. And finally, most say that they don't want to live in a society with even more sexual freedom.

Marital Sex— How Often?

The longer a couple is married, the less often they have sex. Fifteen percent of couples married ten or more years have sex once a month or less.

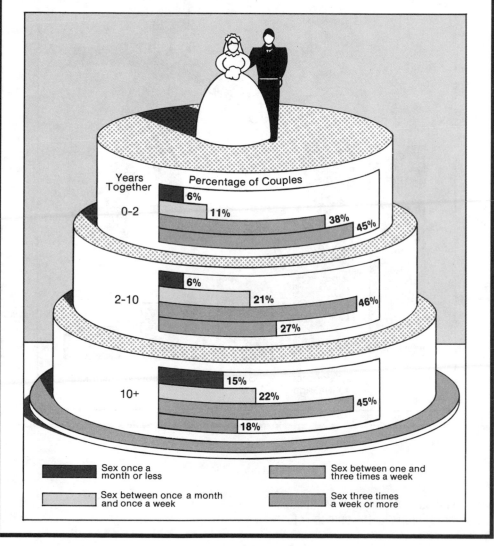

Years Together | Percentage of Couples

0-2
6%
11%
38%
45%

2-10
6%
21%
46%
27%

10+
15%
22%
45%
18%

- Sex once a month or less
- Sex between once a month and once a week
- Sex between one and three times a week
- Sex three times a week or more

Why Couples Argue

Couples argue about a lot of things—sex included—but money is actually the hottest topic. (Answers listed here add to more than 100 percent due to multiple responses.)

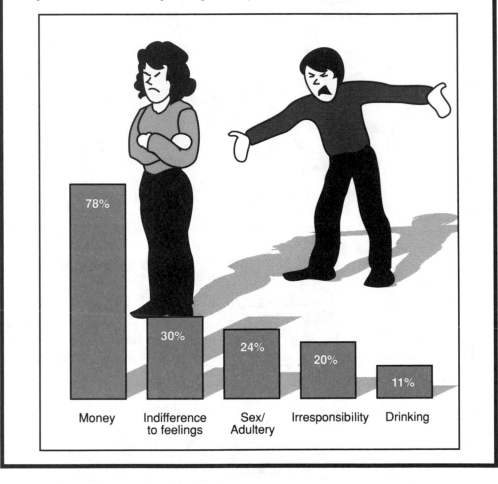

Money	Indifference to feelings	Sex/ Adultery	Irresponsibility	Drinking
78%	30%	24%	20%	11%

In one survey, 66 percent of college men admitted that they've gotten a woman drunk for the purpose of convincing her to have sex.

Happy . . . and Not Interested

It is possible to be "happily married" and not interested in sex. Surveys show this is more true of women than of men.

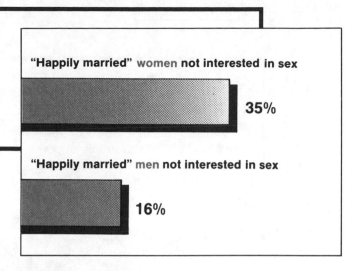

"Happily married" women not interested in sex

35%

"Happily married" men not interested in sex

16%

Sex in the Workplace

The following questions were posed to readers in a survey by *Men's Health* magazine. More than 97 percent of those who responded to the survey were male.

Q. Between two co-workers of the opposite sex who are not romantically involved, what is out of line as far as touching goes?

A. Any physical contact at all: 6.1 percent; a handshake: 1.6 percent; a pat on the back: 11 percent; a touch on the knee: 45.3 percent; a kiss on the cheek: 27.9 percent; none of these is appropriate: 29.3 percent.

Q. Have you ever been the subject of a workplace rumor in which you were falsely accused of having an affair?

A. Yes: 45.9 percent; no: 54.1 percent.

Q. Have you ever been the

subject of such a rumor that was true?

A. Yes: 33.6 percent; no: 66.4 percent.

Q. All other things being equal, would you hire someone of the opposite sex who was sexy over someone who was not?

A. Yes: 60.4 percent; no: 39.6 percent.

Q. Have you ever had sex in your place of work?

A. Yes: 26.1 percent; no: 73.9 percent.

Q. If you could completely eliminate all the sexual undercurrents in your place of work—all the sexual gossip, innuendo, come-ons and flirtations—would you do it?

A. Yes: 30 percent; no: 70 percent.

About as Satisfying as a Good Book

Asked to name three or four things that give them the most personal satisfaction or enjoyment each day, an overwhelming majority of people mentioned their family. Making love tied for fifth place along with reading books, magazines, and newspapers.

1.	Family	70%
2.	Television	46%
3.	Friends	44%
4.	Music	29%
5.	Reading books, magazines, and newspapers	26%
5.	**Making Love**	**26%**
6.	Work	24%
7.	Socializing	20%
8.	House or apartment	17%
8.	Radio	17%
9.	Meals	16%
9.	Car	16%
10.	Hobbies	14%
11.	Exercise	12%
12.	Following sports	10%
13.	Clothes	7%

When Sex Is Wrong: Some Opinions

Survey after survey confirms that Americans believe husbands and wives should take their pledges of fidelity seriously. Given a chance to hedge their answers, most people still said extramarital sex was always wrong.

Opinion varies widely on the question of whether or not premarital sex is wrong. While a substantial number believe premarital sex is always wrong, many believe it is wrong only sometimes or never wrong.

he more money a man makes, the more likely he is to be unfaithful to his wife, according to a *Playboy* magazine survey. Among husbands making $60,000 or more a year, 70 percent had been unfaithful. Of those making $10,000 to $20,000 a year, 31 percent had had an affair.

From age 20 to age 70, the typical person spends 600 hours having sex. This amounts, on average, to 12 hours a year, 1 hour a month or 2 minutes a day.

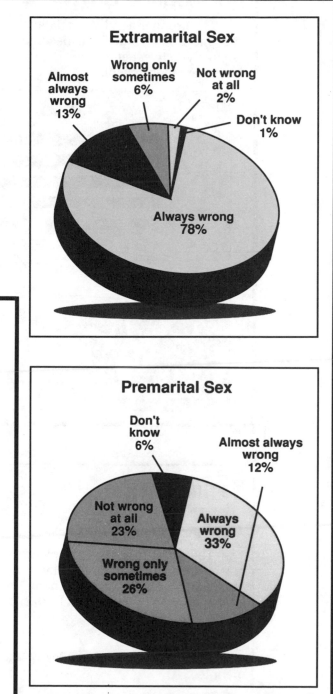

Extramarital Sex

Almost always wrong 13%

Wrong only sometimes 6%

Not wrong at all 2%

Don't know 1%

Always wrong 78%

Premarital Sex

Don't know 6%

Almost always wrong 12%

Not wrong at all 23%

Always wrong 33%

Wrong only sometimes 26%

Sexual Activity of Teenage Girls

The sooner a girl starts dating, the more likely she is to become sexually active before she graduates from high school.

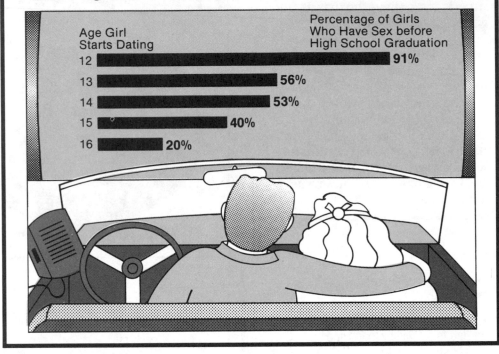

Age Girl Starts Dating	Percentage of Girls Who Have Sex before High School Graduation
12	91%
13	56%
14	53%
15	40%
16	20%

I S THAT A FACT?

Older people cannot have sex.

The truth is that many older people lead sexually fulfilling lives; they simply may need to give themselves more time to complete the lovemaking process.

Sex isn't as enjoyable for older people.

The fact is that many older people report sex in their later years to be the best of their lives, because they feel more secure and know better how to please one another.

Men over 70 can't have erections.

The truth is that unless a man has a physical or psychological disorder, getting an erection should be no problem—though it may take a little longer than it used to.

Contraception Methods

The woman most often takes responsibility for birth control. The two most popular methods are the pill and female sterilization.

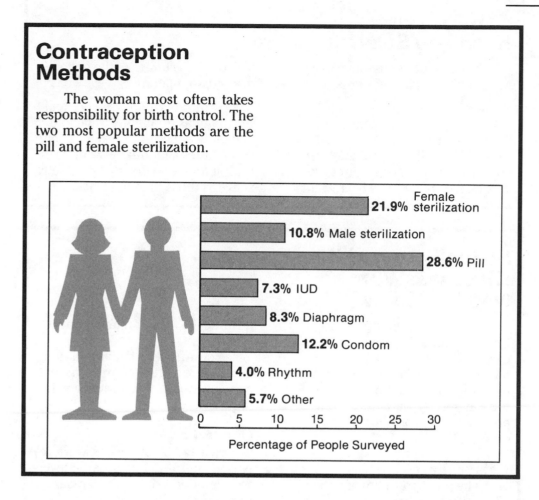

21.9% Female sterilization
10.8% Male sterilization
28.6% Pill
7.3% IUD
8.3% Diaphragm
12.2% Condom
4.0% Rhythm
5.7% Other

Percentage of People Surveyed

Six Physical Causes of Impotence

Impotence may be caused by psychological factors, but many studies suggest that more often than not impotence has a physical cause. And if the cause is physical, these are the most likely culprits.

1. Diabetes: 40 percent

2. Vascular disease: 30 percent

3. Rectal surgery for bladder, rectal, and prostate cancer: 13 percent

4. Spinal cord injuries, pelvic fractures, and other injuries: 8 percent

5. Endocrine disorders (other than diabetes): 6 percent

6. Multiple sclerosis: 3 percent

Can Exercise Keep You Sexy?

A study of competitive swimmers indicates the answer is yes:

▼ Ninety-seven percent of those in their forties and 92 percent of those in their sixties said they were sexually active. Those figures are very high compared to what research has found in studies of the general over-40 population.

▼ Swimmers in their forties had sex about as frequently as people in their twenties and thirties—about seven times a month. Swimmers in their sixties were nearly as sexually active as those in their forties.

Sexually Transmitted Diseases: What You Need to Know

Syphilis and gonorrhea are not the only sexually transmitted diseases (STDs). Chlamydia and genital herpes are also major STDs, and, of course, AIDs has forever changed the way society views sex. (For facts and statistics about AIDS, see chapter 3.)

Chlamydia

The most prevalent of all sexually transmitted diseases in the United States, it affects 3 to 4 million people each year.

Symptoms: In men, painful urination and possibly discharge. In women, yellow discharge—there may be no other symptoms.

Action: Get an examination, avoid sex until infection is cured, and use condoms to prevent further infection.

Genital Herpes

More than 700,000 new cases are reported each year.

Symptoms: One or more lesions on genitalia. Pain possible. Lesions form scabs, which shed between outbreaks.

Action: Get an examination, avoid sex when symptoms are present, and use condoms when they're not.

Gonorrhea

Nearly 800,000 cases were reported in 1987, and it is believed several hundred thousand cases go unreported each year.

Symptoms: In men, frequent urination, burning during urination, and some discharge. In women, discharge and painful urination.

Action: Get an examination, take antibiotic as prescribed, and avoid sex until infection is cured. Use condoms to prevent recurrence of infection.

Syphilis

After many years of decline, reported cases are on the rise.

Symptoms: Lesion, chancre, or rash without pain.

Action: Same as for gonorrhea.

Syphilis, Gonorrhea Trends

After several years of decline, cases of syphilis have increased. Gonorrhea increased dramatically from 1950 to 1980 before entering a decline.

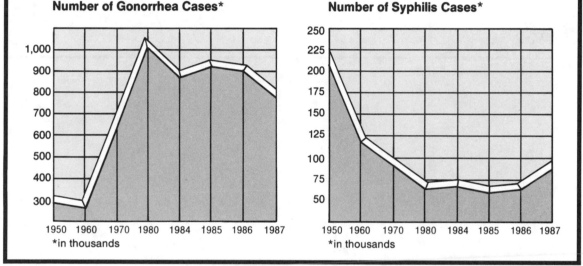

Number of Gonorrhea Cases*

1,000
900
800
700
600
500
400
300

1950 1960 1970 1980 1984 1985 1986 1987
*in thousands

Number of Syphilis Cases*

250
225
200
175
150
125
100
75
50

1950 1960 1970 1980 1984 1985 1986 1987
*in thousands

Sexual Side Effects

Unfortunately, drugs that may work wonders on high blood pressure or depression may also leave the patient wondering what's wrong with his or her sex life. Many drugs carry sexual side effects—at least for some people some of the time.

Antidepressants. These drugs influence moods and emotions and in turn can influence sex drive and arousal. Brand names include Aventyl, Elavil, Norpramin, Sinequan, and Tofranil.

Tranquilizers. These can delay and prevent orgasm. Brand names include Compazine, Mellaril, Prolixin, Stelazine, and Thorazine.

High blood pressure medicines. Antihypertensives may inhibit desire, erection, and ejaculation. Brand names include Aldoril, Catapres, Esimil, Eutron, Regroton, and Sandril.

Social and street drugs. Such drugs are often reputed to be aphrodisiacs. In reality, they are dangerous and more likely to cause sexual problems. They include alcohol, cocaine, marijuana, and opiates.

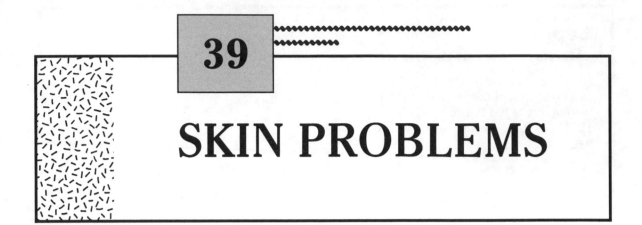

39

SKIN PROBLEMS

Sometime during your life, you'll probably have a skin problem. Nearly everyone does—some babies are born with birthmarks, teenagers get acne, homemakers, up to their elbows in dishwater, fight dermatitis, weekend hikers step into poison ivy, and retirees discover that the price of years spent in the sun can be skin cancer.

Your skin plays an important role in your health and well-being. It carries your blood vessels, supports your nerve endings, and houses your sweat glands. Your skin protects you from the harsh extremes and sharp edges of environment, controls your temperature, and shields you against a loss of fluids. When necessary, it thickens by forming calluses at places where it gets the most wear and tear. And it fends off bacteria, serving as your most extensive shield against disease.

No wonder the skin runs into more than its share of difficulties. One survey shows 7 million Americans see their doctors each year because of skin problems. Skin diseases account for 3 million lost workdays annually and up to 50 percent of claims filed with Worker's Compensation.

Common Skin Problems and Solutions

We can't all be perfect—and our skin shows it. Here are some frequently encountered problems that can mar our surface.

Condition	Symptoms and Cause	Treatment
Acne	Blackheads, whiteheads, pimples, and boil-like lesions on face, back, chest, shoulders, neck are caused by rising hormone levels that enlarge sebaceous (oil) glands. Oil is invaded by bacteria.	Wash with soap and warm water twice a day thoroughly enough to clean, but gently enough to avoid irritation. Shampoo frequently and keep hair away from face. Men should shave as seldom as possible and shave lightly to avoid nicking pimples. Avoid foods that seen to worsen acne. Try medicated makeups. Use water-based cosmetics. Consult your doctor about medications.
Bruising	Black-and-blue marks can stem from loss of fat and connective tissue. Support is weakened around blood vessels, causing them to break more easily. Sometimes bruising is caused by medications, clotting problems, or internal disease.	See your doctor.
Dry skin	Itchy, flaking skin can be caused by aging, weather, and frequent bathing.	Smear on petroleum jelly. Use moisturizers containing urea, lactic acid, lanolin, and ammonium lactate.
Cherry angiomas	Red spots are formed from loops of dilated blood vessels. They occur in 85% of middle-aged and older people.	Not usually treated.
Chapped lips	Dry, cracked, and sore lips are caused by sun, cold weather, dry air, and repeated moistening with the tongue.	Lip balms, lip sunscreens.
Contact dermatitis	Itchy, flaking skin or dense blisters on swollen skin; can be caused by cosmetics, soap or dry-cleaning chemicals left in clothing, nail polish, cigarette smoke, or contact with rubber or jewelry and other metal objects.	Avoid contact with materials that cause rash.
Heat rash	Rash caused when perspiration oversaturates the skin. The skin then swells up, closing over the sweat glands, locking bacteria and other germs inside.	Wear light, loose, absorbent clothing to help sweat evaporate. Use an absorbent powder and an alchohol-based astringent on trouble spots.

(continued)

Common Skin Problems and Solutions—*Continued*

Condition	Symptoms and Cause	Treatment
Hives (urticaria)	Red or pale bumps caused by blood plasma leaking into the skin through tiny gaps between the cell linings of small blood vessels. Histamine, a natural chemical released by an allergic reaction, causes the gaps to open. The reaction may be caused by food, drugs, emotional stress, or physical stress.	Find cause of allergic reaction and eliminate. Use antihistamines on a regular schedule.
Liver spots	Flat brown spots on face, hands, back, and feet are caused by sun exposure as we age.	Spots will not respond to "fading" creams. No treatment necessary.
Seborrheic dermatitis	This flaky, itchy skin problem may be caused by hormonally induced sebaceous gland activity. It can also be indicative of Parkinson's disease or other diseases of the nervous system. It can also be caused by stress.	May subside with no treatment. Rub cortisone preparations on affected areas. Shampoo frequently with products containing zinc pyrithione, selenium sulfide, sulfur, tar, or salicylic acid.
Shingles (herpes zoster)	Painful blisters that run in bands, typically around the chest or belly, down arms or legs, across the scalp, forehead, or eyelids. They are caused by a virus closely associated with chicken pox.	Ease mild case with cool compresses or lotion on the blisters. See a dermatologist if you suspect shingles.
Spider veins	These are tiny but visible treelike veins that appear on the nose, cheeks, or legs. They may run in families, and can be caused by some diseases. Estrogen may account for development of spider veins in puberty, in women taking birth control pills, or in those who are pregnant.	Injection therapy (sclero-therapy) results in 50–80% improvement in treated vessels.
Varicose veins	Enlarged, riverlike veins that become swollen and twisted in older people. Can be caused by prolonged standing.	Avoid standing for long periods, elevate feet when possible, wear support hose or elastic bandages. Surgery or injections may help.
Warts	Bumps made of extra layers of skin are caused by a viral infection (human papilloma virus) of the skin's layer. Varieties include hand wart, food wart, flat wart, and genital wart. Can be passed from person to person.	Warts sometimes disappear by themselves within several months or years. Other treatments include painting with salicylic acid or cantharidin, then cutting; cryotherapy (freezing); electrosurgery (burning); laser therapy; or peeling.

Hives: Things That Go Bump in Your Life

About one person in five will develop the itchy bumps called hives at some point in life. On any given day, 11 men and 14 women out of every 1,000 people will have hives. Many cases are caused by an allergic reaction to something in the environment. If your hives are occasional and last a short time, then you have a good chance of tracking the culprit and eliminating it from your life. This chart shows some of the foods, drugs, and infections that can sometimes make the body bumpy.

Foods	Drugs	Infections
Peanuts	Aspirin	Chicken pox
Eggs	Penicillin	Upper respiratory viral infections
Nuts	Sulfa drugs	Mononucleosis
Beans	Tetracyclines	Serum hepatitis
Chocolate	Codeine	Rheumatic fever
Strawberries		
Tomatoes		
Seasonings (mustard, ketchup, mayonnaise, spices)		
Fresh fruits (especially citrus)		
Corn		
Fish		
Pork		
Food additives and preservatives such as yellow dye #5 and monosodium glutamate (MSG)		

Burns: A Matter of Degree

If you get burned, you may be able to minimize the damage with the right reaction. This table shows the different types of burns and what can be done for each.

Depth	Appearance	First Aid
First degree	Light to dark pink. Swelling, weeping, peeling may occur. Painful.	Rinse with cool water and soap. Keep clean and dry. Wash 4 times a day with soap and water.
Second degree	Mottled pink or red to dull white or tan. Blisters may be present or area may feel dry to touch. Painful.	Immerse in cool, soapy water for short periods. Cover with clean cloth and see doctor. Do not break blisters.
Third degree	White, tan, black, brown, or deep red. Pain usually absent initially.	Wrap in clean cloth and find medical help immediately.

Cosmetic Reactions

Contact dermatitis—redness, swelling, hives, some skin weeping—can be as close as your moisturizer. Or the eye shadow you paint on. Or even your hair coloring. These charts show the cosmetics that most often cause reactions and the ingredients that are usually at fault.

Type of Cosmetic	Percentage of Cases
Skin-care products	28
Hair preparations	24
Facial makeup	11
Nail preparations	8
Fragrance products	7
Personal cleanliness products	6
Shaving preparations	4
Eye makeup	4
Suntan, sunscreens	3

Cosmetic Ingredient	Percentage of Cases
Fragrance ingredients	30
Preservatives (antibacterial)	28
p-Phenylenediamine	8
Lanolin and derivatives	5
Glyceryl monothioglycolate	5
Propylene glycol	5
Toluenesulfonamide/ formaldehyde resin	4
Ultraviolet absorbers in sunscreens	3
Acrylate or methacrylate	2
Others	10

Skin Cancer Facts

▼ The sun causes at least 90 percent of all skin cancers.

▼ Skin cancer is the most common of all cancers.

▼ In the United States, more than 500,000 new cases of skin cancer are found each year.

▼ One in every seven Americans gets skin cancer.

▼ One in every three cancers is skin cancer.

▼ Most skin cancers are basal cell carcinomas or squamous cell carcinomas. The difference depends on the type of skin cells that form the tumor.

▼ Skin cancer is completely curable if treated in its earliest stages.

An Anti-Aging Cream That Really Helps

Tretinoin cream, a vitamin-A derivative known as Retin-A, may be a fountain of youth for some sun-damaged and aged skin. In one study, 30 people, ranging in age from 35 to 70, applied tretinoin on the fore-arms daily for 16 weeks. All showed "significant improvement" in rough-ness and wrinkling. And 14 of 15 who used the cream on their faces noticed a dramatic reduction in fine wrinkles. Liver spots lightened and solar freckles disappeared. Tretinoin may also reverse precancerous changes in skin cells. Desired effects from the cream take six to nine months. Tretinoin is available by prescription.

The illustrations show what skin looks like before and after treatment with tretinoin.

The illustration on the left shows what happens when skin is overex-posed to the sun (photoaged). The outer layer or corneum becomes thick, making the skin rough and wrinkled. Melanocytes, the pigment-producing cells that live in the germ layer below the corneum, deposit melanin, causing age spots.

The illustration on the right shows skin treated with tretinoin, which thickens the germ layer while smoothing the corneum. New blood vessels form under the epi-dermis, giving skin a more youthful appearance.

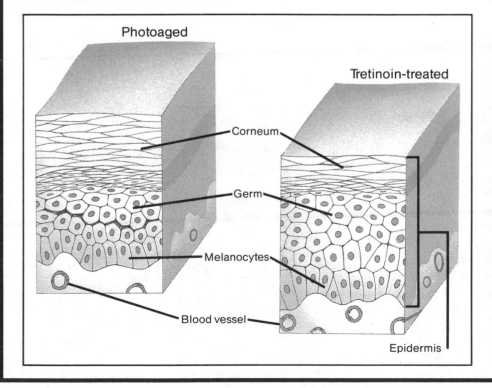

Photoaged — Tretinoin-treated

Corneum
Germ
Melanocytes
Blood vessel
Epidermis

How to Pick the Right Sunscreen

One way to combat the sun's damage to your skin is to wear a sunscreen containing chemicals that absorb and filter the sun's ultraviolet radiation. The higher the SPF (sun protection factor) number of the product, the more it blocks. If your unprotected skin takes 20 minutes to become red in the sun, a sunscreen with an SPF number of 10 will allow you to stay in the sun 10 times longer, or 3 hours and 20 minutes. Use this chart to find the right sunscreen for your skin type.

Complexion	Skin Response	SPF To Use
Very fair	Always burns easily; never tans	15 and up
Fair	Always burns easily; tans minimally	8-15
Light	Burns moderately; tans gradually to light brown	6-8
Medium	Burns minimally; always tans gradually to a moderate brown	4-6
Dark	Rarely burns; tans profusely to dark brown	2-4
Black	Never burns; is deeply pigmented	—

Moles That May Be Dangerous

Everyone has moles. But some moles become more than just brown or black bumps on the skin. They turn into the potentially deadly type of skin cancer known as malignant melanoma. Check your own moles periodically with these danger signs of melanoma in mind.

Asymmetry—One half of mole is unlike the other half.

Irregular border—Edges are scalloped or poorly defined.

Color variations—Hues change from one part to another, including shades of tan and brown, black, and sometimes white, red, or blue.

Size—The diameter is greater than 6 mm (about the same size as a pencil eraser).

Reversing the Skin's Signs of Aging

No one can stop aging entirely, although there are ways to slow the process. Facial plastic surgery can reverse some of the effects.

This table lists some of the signs of aging and some of the cosmetic surgery that can repair the ravages of time.

To test a cosmetic for possible skin reaction, apply a small amount on the inside of your elbow and cover with a bandage. Repeat the test twice a day for four days. If a rash appears, don't use the product.

When the Ozone Is Bygone

Experts say smog and pollution are eating a hole in the atmosphere's natural ultraviolet sunlight filter, the ozone layer. The more pollution, the larger the hole grows and the greater the risk of sun damage to our skin. The trend in deadly melanoma incidence is particularly dramatic and dangerous, with cases doubling every 10 to 15 years. In 1930, one person in 1,500 was affected. By the year 2000, one person in every 90 is expected to be at risk.

Age	Signs	Surgery
30	Eyes: Upper eyelids become hooded; lower eyelids become prominent; wrinkling begins	Eyelid surgery; collagen injections
	Forehead: Frown lines	Collagen injections; face sanding
	Mouth: Wrinkling at corners	Collagen injections; face sanding, chemical peel
40	Eyes: Upper and lower eyelids sag; crow's feet	Eyelid surgery
	Forehead: Deeper frown lines; horizontal wrinkles	Collagen injections; face sanding
	Mouth: Vertical lines around lips; more wrinkling	Chemical peel; collagen injections
50	Cheeks: Pouches from fluid in upper cheek area	Upper face-lift; eyelid surgery
	Chin: Fat creates double chin	Chin surgery
	Eyes: Eyebrows sag	Eyebrow lift; upper face-lift
	Forehead: Forehead sags	Forehead lift
	Jawline: Jawline sags, looking like jowls	Lower face-lift
	Nose: Tip droops	Nasal surgery
60+	Eyes: Lids sag more, giving hooded appearance	Eyelid surgery
	Face: Skin sags as it loses elasticity	Full face-lift
	Forehead: Lines deepen	Forehead lift
	Mouth: Vertical wrinkling around lips	Chemical peel
	Neck: Skin drops in folds; cords form turkey gobbler look	Lower face-lift; neck-lift

"Should I Have Cosmetic Surgery?"

Only you and your doctor can answer that question. But if you're wondering how you might look when the surgery is over, there are some ways to predict the outcome. Ethnic background, general health, age, skin quality, healing history, and degree of surgical correction all influence the end result. Each of the seven basic skin types is affected in different ways. This table can help you evaluate your own chances of satisfaction.

Skin Type	Facial Surgery (scar and lesion removal, face-lift)	Nasal Surgery (reshaping the nose)	Eyebrow Lift	Dermabrasion (sanding, chemical peeling)
Type 1: Fair, thin-skinned, Anglo-Saxon	*Pro:* Scars usually thin. Skin drapes well for face-lift. *Con:* Fine, deep wrinkling around mouth and eyes may be difficult to remove. Signs of age appear early.	*Pro:* Thin skin allows more chiseled look. Swelling and oiliness minimal. *Con:* Cartilage or bone irregularity is more obvious.	*Pro:* Rarely heavy scars. *Con:* Bruising is obvious. Crepe wrinkles a problem.	*Pro:* Scars thin. Slight pigmentation. *Con:* None.
Type 2: Fair, blue-eyed, blond, northern European	*Pro:* Scars thin, become almost invisible. Heals well. *Con:* Deep wrinkling difficult to remove around mouth, eyes. Signs of age appear early.	*Pro:* Same as type 1. *Con:* Slightly thicker skin; irregularities might show.	*Pro:* Scars very fine; heavy scars rare. *Con:* Bruising is obvious. Fine wrinkles a problem to remove.	*Pro:* Same as type 1. *Con:* None.
Type 3: Ruddy, freckled, redhead	*Pro:* Fine scars. Signs of age appear later. *Con:* Scar quality less predictable. Possibility of postoperative pigmentation.	*Pro:* Bone and cartilage structure usually good. *Con:* Some postoperative oiliness; may bruise easily; longer postoperative swelling.	*Pro:* Fine scar lines. *Con:* Heavier scarring may occur. Fine, white scar will contrast with peachy skin.	*Pro:* Scars fine and thin. *Con:* Scars heavier than with types 1 and 2. Possibility of postoperative pigmentation. Skin cancer most common in this group.

Skin diseases affect nearly 7 percent of the U.S. military population, where they are the fourth largest cause of total disability.

Skin Type	Facial Surgery (scar and lesion removal, face-lift)	Nasal Surgery (reshaping the nose)	Eyebrow Lift	Dermabrasion (sanding, chemical peeling)
Type 4: Darker, oily, brunette, southern European	*Pro:* Fine scars. Small wrinkles less common. Signs of age appear later. *Con:* Darker scarring common, may be heavier in front of and behind ears.	*Pro:* Bone and cartilage structure adequate. *Con:* Not as likely to look fine or chiseled. Longer postoperative swelling.	*Pro:* Fine scars. Wrinkling less likely. *Con:* Scars may be thicker; bruising longer.	*Pro:* Skin cancer less common. *Con:* Dark or heavy scarring more common.
Type 5: Oily, olive, dark, Greek, Turkish	*Pro:* Signs of age appear later. *Con:* Heavy, darker scars common.	*Pro:* Bone and cartilage structure adequate. *Con:* Drooping cartilage resists change. Postoperative swelling and oiliness.	*Pro:* Baggy eyelids less obvious. *Con:* Thicker scars. Bruise pigment may last.	*Pro:* Skin cancer rare. *Con:* Dark or heavy scarring more obvious and common.
Type 6: Black	*Pro:* Signs of age appear later. No tiny wrinkles. *Con:* Excess tissue scarring (keloids) and dark or light pigmentation changes possible.	*Pro:* Similar to type 5. *Con:* Cartilage structure prevents easy reconstruction.	*Pro:* Baggy lids less common. *Con:* Keloids.	*Pro:* Skin cancer rare. *Con:* Keloids. Dark or light pigmentation changes.
Type 7: Far Eastern, Oriental	*Pro:* Signs of age appear later. No fine wrinkles. *Con:* Same as type 4.	*Pro:* Similar to type 4. *Con:* Low nasal bridge may cause problem.	*Pro:* Symmetry permanence of new eyelid creases. *Con:* Additional surgery needed for eyelid crease.	*Pro:* Similar to type 4. *Con:* Similar to type 4.

Apply a paste of baking soda and water to mosquito or other bug bites. The alkaline moisture alleviates itching.

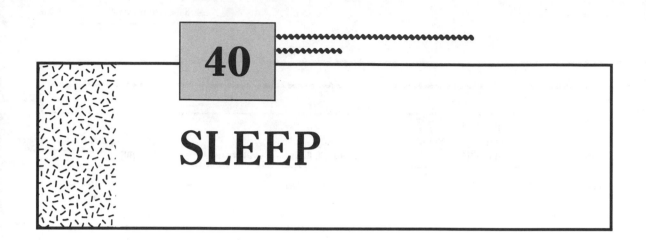

40

SLEEP

Science has patiently probed the dark kingdom of sleep for many years, yet many mysteries remain—not the least of which is why we sleep at all.

Though we know that animals do it, no one knows why the sloth needs 20 hours of sleep a day and the horse only 2. Some scientists believe we sleep in order to replenish brain cells and body tissues worn down while awake. Others say sleep is a device all living creatures use to keep quiet and stay out of trouble—that is, out of the mouths of hungry predators. If that's true, sleep may be something humans eventually learn to do without as our natural predators disappear.

And why not? After all, some 100 million Americans experience sleeping problems of one sort or another, even though most of us will spend about 220,000 hours—that's 25 years—doing it by the time we reach 70. Wasted time? Not for the part of your brain that gets to play Hollywood producer, conjuring up new plots, characters, and special effects in the form of nightly dreams. Just giving your mind such free rein may make sleep worth all the time you invest in it.

For whatever purpose it serves, all of us ultimately sleep for one simple reason—we must. There is no force as inevitable, save death itself.

The Patterns of Sleep

The newborn spends two-thirds of its time asleep (represented by shaded areas in chart), waking at intervals of 2 to 6 hours. Its sleep is distributed almost evenly over a 24-hour period, which quickly wears down new parents, accustomed as they are to an adult sleep pattern. Thankfully, the infant's sporadic sleep/wake cycle doesn't last too long. By one year of age, most babies restrict daytime sleeping to a mid-morning and midafternoon nap, with the majority of sleep coming at night.

The amount of time spent sleeping during the day steadily decreases during a child's early years. Though most preschoolers still take an afternoon nap, they begin staying awake all day once they reach school age. The multiphase sleep pattern of infancy has changed into the single-phase pattern of adulthood.

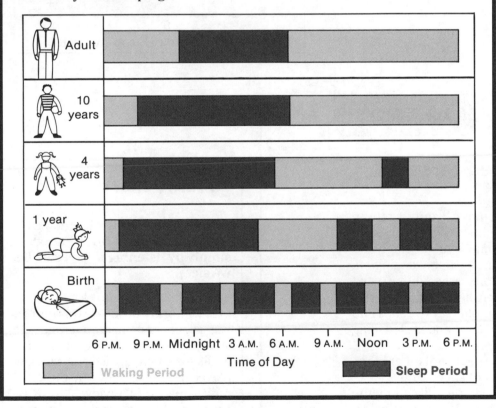

		6 P.M.	9 P.M.	Midnight	3 A.M.	6 A.M.	9 A.M.	Noon	3 P.M.	6 P.M.

Time of Day

Waking Period · Sleep Period

On average, we have 1,825 dreams a year, or 127,750 by the time we reach 70.

How Long We Sleep

A poll of 800,000 Americans over the age of 30 reveals that most of us (42 percent) sleep between 8 and 9 hours per night, while another one-third sleep between 7 and 8 hours. Only 1 person in 1,000 sleeps less than 4 hours a night, while 4 in 1,000 sleep between 4 and 5 hours nightly. At the other end of the scale, 16 people per 1,000 sleep more than 10 hours.

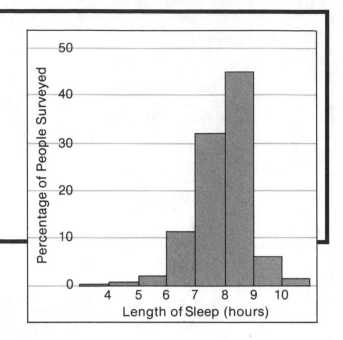

How the Stars Doze Off

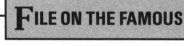

Do you have trouble falling asleep sometimes? You're in good company—many stars of stage and screen also have trouble dozing off. When someone asked them what they do about it, here's what they said:

Burt Reynolds says he slips into a hot tub, "the most underrated thing in the world."

Dolly Parton counts "her blessings," instead of sheep.

Suzanne Somers likes to write poetry, "especially love poetry," when she can't doze off.

Ricardo Montalban reads "as dull a book as I can find," noting that he's sure to be snoozing somewhere in the middle of it.

IS THAT A FACT?

We can learn foreign languages and other types of information simply by listening to tapes while we sleep.

False. Most claims for that type of learning are based on reports of a Russian experiment in which a whole village had its learning of English facilitated when English phrases were played all night long on the state radio. But careful review of the Russian literature revealed numerous flaws in that study, while carefully-controlled experiments in the United States have shown that such techniques have virtually no effect on learning.

Neither a Long nor a Short Sleeper Be

Although sleep has been associated with good health since ancient times, that assumption remained untested until the middle of this century. Then, beginning in the early 1960s, a six-year-long survey of over a million adults revealed a surprising connection between length of sleep and mortality.

The mortality rate was 2½ times higher for short sleepers than for those people who sleep 7 to 8 hours per night. Even more surprising, the death rate was between 1½ and 2 times higher for those who slept more than 10 hours nightly.

What killed the short and long sleepers? Heart disease, cancer, and suicide, to name three—as well as just about every other major cause of death you can think of. All causes were more prevalent in long and short sleepers alike.

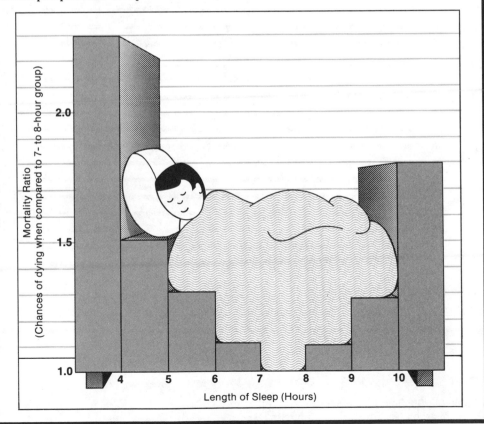

The 25-Hour Day

Our subjective, "internal" clock contains 25 hours instead of 24. This chart shows what typically happens to us when we are isolated from daylight and all external information about time is withheld.

When a clock is available (days 1 through 3 in the chart), we typically sleep and wake to its rigid, externally imposed schedule. When our own clock is allowed to take over and no external forces tell us when to sleep (beginning with day 4), we go to bed 40 minutes later. During each succeeding day we continue to go to bed later than the day before. After 12 days without a clock, we start going to bed in the morning and waking in the evening.

If our isolation is allowed to continue for 25 days, we will have slept and awakened only 24 times.

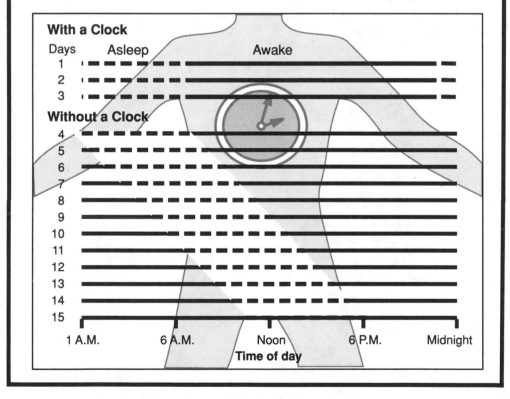

In a 7-hour sleep period, a healthy senior citizen will awaken 153 times, on average. By comparison, a healthy 25-year-old wakes 10 times.

The Sleep/Dream Cycle

Our current concept of dreaming began with the discovery that periods of rapid-eye-movement (REM) sleep occur throughout the night. Scientists noticed that if they woke sleeping volunteers during these times, most would report they'd been dreaming, and they could usually give a vivid account of their dream. Scientists also noticed that brain wave activity during REM sleep was similar to that of wakefulness. During non-REM (quiet) sleep, brain waves are similar to those of a comatose patient.

We now know that sleep consists of two alternating, distinctly different states. The sleep period begins with a long period of non-REM sleep, followed by a period of REM sleep. These periods alternate throughout the night, with about 90 minutes of deep sleep between each dreaming period.

The length of dreams is roughly the same as the length of time spent in REM sleep, meaning that a long period of REM sleep will result in a long dream that's filled with detail and plenty of plot twists.

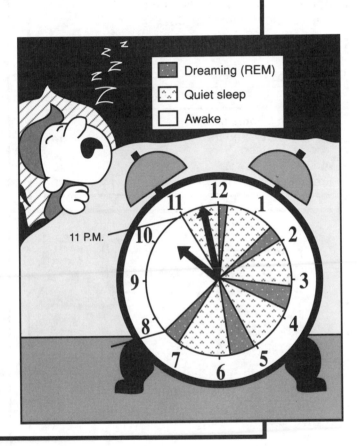

Dreaming (REM)

Quiet sleep

Awake

11 P.M.

 Scientists have shown that a hot bath taken 30 minutes before bedtime warms the brain and increases the amount of deep sleep you experience. Somewhat more surprisingly, an inflatable hair-dryer hood may do the same thing.

The Four Biggest Sleep Complaints

There are four basic sleep complaints that make up the insomniac syndrome and, to a greater or lesser degree, disturb the sleep of teenagers and senior citizens alike.

Complaint	Percentage of People Reporting, by Age		
	15-25	35-45	55-65
Less than 5 hours' sleep	5	7	14
Longer than 1½ hours to get to sleep	2	4	14
Awake before 5 A.M.	1	3	10
Frequently wake up	5	14	23

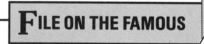

FILE ON THE FAMOUS

Well-Known Insomniacs

Sleep, or the lack thereof, knows no social boundary. Insomnia has plagued the well-known and little-known alike. Among the better known:

Charles Dickens

Ben Franklin

Cary Grant

Rudyard Kipling ("Oh pity us! We wakeful.")

Vincent van Gogh

The Meaning of Dreams

In classic Freudian theory, dreams were believed to express some hidden fear or desire. Falling, for example, might symbolize the fear of losing love, which might stem from childhood anxiety and anger toward parents who were unfeeling or remote.

But a new breed of dream scientists has questioned whether our dreams, regardless of content, really mean anything at all. These researchers believe dreams are simply the by-products of the brain's routine nighttime activity, not long-buried hidden impulses.

In this more recent view of dreaming, certain cells in the primitive brainstem are jostled by electrical activity during REM sleep, sending random electrical messages to the parts of the brain that control vision, hearing, and movement. The higher part of the brain notices that the cells for perception and movement have been switched on, so it flips through scenes and characters stored in memory and fits them into the activity already taking place. The result is what we experience as a dream.

What We Dream About

Are dreams simply the result of cells bumping in the night, or do they hold deeper meaning about our lives? The debate is far from settled. In the meantime, the chart shows how 1,000 people responded to a survey about their dreams.

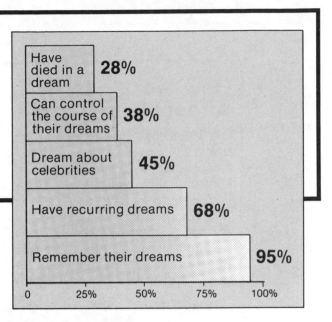

Have died in a dream	28%
Can control the course of their dreams	38%
Dream about celebrities	45%
Have recurring dreams	68%
Remember their dreams	95%

0   25%   50%   75%   100%

Sleepwalking— Strolling in Harm's Way

Some 10 to 20 percent of people questioned can recall one or more sleepwalking episodes, making these mysterious night strolls rather common occurrences. Though its cause is unknown, sleepwalking tends to run in families and may be an inherited tendency. It usually peaks in early adolescence; only 2.5 percent of adults sleepwalk regularly.

In a sleepwalking episode, the possibility of harm coming to the individual is strong. Sleepwalkers have fallen out of windows after mistaking them for doors. For that reason, doors and windows should be locked shut when sleepwalking is persistent. Within an episode, a sleepwalker can usually be guided back to bed and can certainly be awakened. He will likely be confused, however, and may need some gentle reassurance.

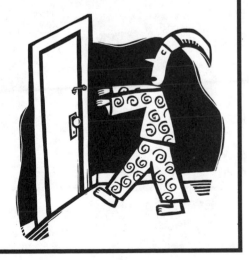

How Sleeping Pills Affect Sleep Quality

Ironically, regular sleeping pill users often end up sleeping less and complaining more about sleep problems after taking pills than they do before starting medication.

The chart shows a fairly typical scenario leading to what's known as "rebound insomnia." After more than three weeks without a good night's sleep, the restless insomniac pro-filed here decides to get a prescription for sleeping pills. She takes these as instructed and reports better sleep for about the next month. But, when the prescription runs out, real trouble begins. Her sleep is dramatically reduced for the next several nights, and it takes several weeks before her quality of sleep even returns to its former subpar level.

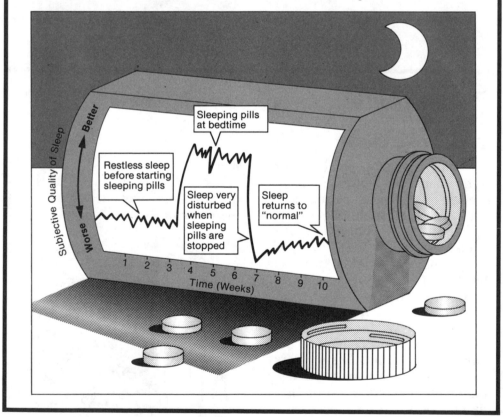

Age Brings Less Sleep, Fewer Dreams

Few physiological processes change more throughout your lifetime than sleep. A newborn may spend close to 18 hours asleep each day. By age ten, a child may require only half that much. By adulthood, 7 or 8 hours of sleep may be enough, while 6 hours may suffice in old age.

But more than sleep quantity changes with age—quality is affected as well. From infancy to adulthood, necessary REM (dream) sleep dwindles to one-fourth of a night's sleep. By age 65, REM sleep shrinks to about one-fifth of total sleep time.

In old age, sleep often becomes more fragmented, and the number of nighttime arousals has more of an effect on daytime alertness than the number of hours slept. This holds true even if the wakenings are so brief they aren't even remembered.

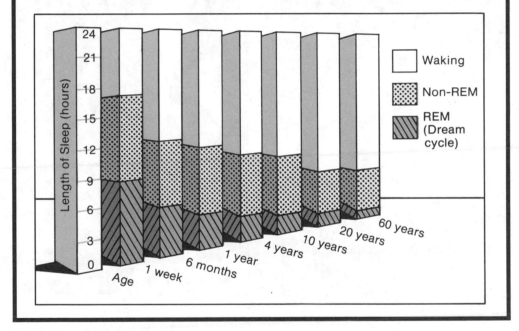

How do dolphins, which depend on air to breath, keep from drowning in their sleep? Probably by allowing only half their brain to fall asleep at any one time. After 30 to 60 minutes, the halves reverse roles so that the sleeping side wakes as the other side dozes. Simultaneous sleep in both halves of a dolphin's brain has almost never been observed.

Sleep Positions: What They Mean

Do you sleep scrunched up like a snail in its shell? Flat on your back? Flat on your stomach? Ever give it much thought? Neither do most people, but some researchers say sleep positions are intimately related to your waking behavior patterns. Here's what it all means.

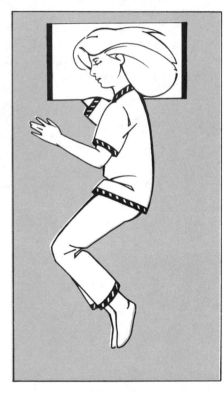

Semifetal. Sixty percent of all sleepers feel best in this position, a sign of a well-balanced person.

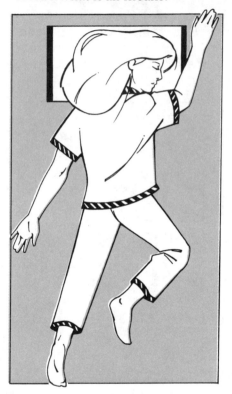

Prone. Preferred by 25% of all sleepers, this position signals a fussy and domineering personality.

The most efficient sleepers of all are preteens, who can fall asleep within 5 or 10 minutes and spend 95 percent of their time in solid, continuous deep sleep.

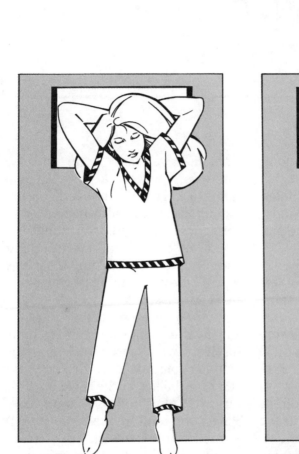

Royal. Self-reliant and assured, the royal position is favored by 7.5% of sleepers.

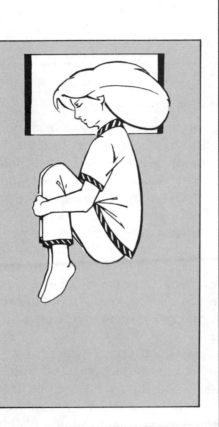

Full fetal. Also favored by 7.5% of sleepers, this position indicates insecurity and inhibition.

Most people think a mattress is good for 15 years, but the Better Sleep Council recommends changing your bedding sooner, especially if it shows the following signs: lumps or sags where you lie, an uneven surface on the box spring, or tears, wear, or stained mattress ticking.

41

STROKES

Cerebrovascular disease, commonly known as stroke, is the third leading cause of death in the United States. Although its incidence in this country has declined by nearly half in the past two decades, stroke still strikes 500,000 Americans every year. Some of its victims fully recover. But many others suffer lifelong debilitation. And some die: Stroke disease claimed 147,800 lives in 1986. It kills one out of every 20 Americans between the ages of 55 and 74.

A stroke occurs when a part of the brain is suddenly cut off from its vital blood supply. Nerve cells in the brain control most bodily movements as well as sensation, communication, and other mental faculties. When these cells are deprived of a continuous blood supply for as few as four to ten minutes they will die, taking many of those faculties with them.

Blood clots are a major cause of blood flow obstruction. One common type of stroke called cerebral thrombosis occurs when a blood clot called a thrombus forms in an artery to the brain. When a blood clot called an embolus travels to the brain from elsewhere in the body, a type of stroke called a cerebral embolism occurs. Blood vessels can also become dangerously constricted by the long-term effects of high blood pressure and atherosclerosis. A bursting blood vessel called a cerebral hemorrhage can also cause a stroke.

Strokes are a source of major and long-lasting handicaps among many survivors who must undergo a slow fight to regain speech, movement, and other capabilities. Of the 2 million stroke survivors alive today in the United States, one-tenth require total care in a nursing home, hospital, or at home. One study of survivors seven years after their strokes revealed that a full 71 percent remained impaired in their abilities to perform their jobs, 31 percent needed assistance in self-care tasks such as bathing and cooking, and 20 percent required help just getting around. Strokes cost Americans $13.5 billion in 1989, a figure that included medical services, medications, and lost productivity.

The Most Likely Stroke Victim

Though often sudden in their onset, strokes are usually the culmination of progressive disease over many years. Certain factors, some unavoidable, others controllable, have been found to significantly increase the risk. The person most likely to have a stroke:

▼ Is an elderly man. Overall, more men than women have strokes.

▼ Is black. Both male and female blacks have nearly twice the risk of stroke as their white counterparts, possibly because of a greater incidence of high blood pressure and diabetes among blacks.

▼ Has high blood pressure. About two-thirds of those suffering a first stroke had blood pressures of 160/95 mm Hg or above, a study showed.

▼ Is diabetic.

▼ Has a family history of stroke.

▼ Has had a previous stroke or small strokes.

▼ Has a high blood cholesterol level.

▼ Has atherosclerosis or heart disease.

▼ Smokes cigarettes.

▼ Is a heavy drinker.

▼ Is overweight.

▼ Gets no regular exercise.

▼ Suffers from chronic stress.

Stroke Deaths on the Decline

Since 1976, stroke mortality in the United States has declined by more than 40 percent. Improvements in the detection and control of high blood pressure, one of the biggest risk factors in the disease, have probably contributed to this decline.

Your chances of surviving a stroke with no handicap: 1 in 3.

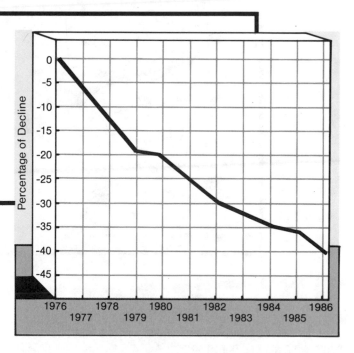

Where Stroke Deaths Strike

Death rates from strokes are higher in southern states than elsewhere in the United States, according to the National Center for Health Statistics. Nine of the ten states with the highest stroke death rates for white men and women aged 55 to 74 are in the South. The fewest men died from strokes in the western states of Montana, Idaho, Utah, Colorado, Arizona, and New Mexico, and the eastern states of Maine, Vermont, Connecticut, and Rhode Island. The lowest rates of stroke death among women occurred in Rhode Island, Maryland, Colorado, and Connecticut. Differences across the country in blood pressure levels, medical care, and socioeconomic factors may contribute to the variation in stroke death rates, medical experts theorize.

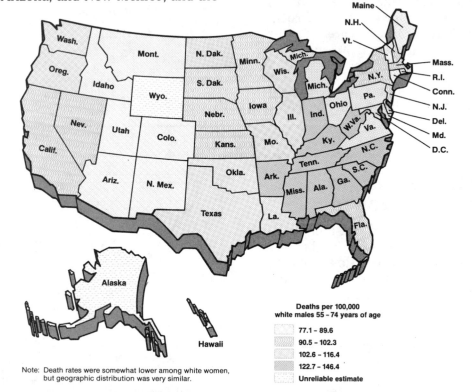

Deaths per 100,000 white males 55 – 74 years of age

77.1 – 89.6
90.5 – 102.3
102.6 – 116.4
122.7 – 146.4
Unreliable estimate

Note: Death rates were somewhat lower among white women, but geographic distribution was very similar.

Chances that a person who survived a first stroke will have a second one: 1 in 4.

Stroke Risk— An Ethnic Mix

Could race or ethnic group affect your risk of stroke? Perhaps. Black Americans have the most strokes. Filipino-Americans have one-fifth as many. A look at the incidence of stroke death in Los Angeles revealed these additional variations.

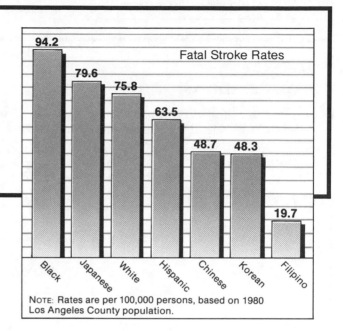

Fatal Stroke Rates

Black	Japanese	White	Hispanic	Chinese	Korean	Filipino
94.2	79.6	75.8	63.5	48.7	48.3	19.7

NOTE: Rates are per 100,000 persons, based on 1980 Los Angeles County population.

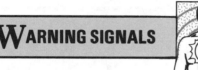

WARNING SIGNALS

Warning Signs of a Stroke

Strokes often occur suddenly, but sometimes advance symptoms give you invaluable time to head for help.

What appear to be signs of an impending major stroke are actually mini-strokes or TIAs (transient ischemic attack), which occur when a blood clot is lodged temporarily in an artery to your brain. TIA symptoms will usually pass within a few minutes or, at the longest, after 24 hours. Slight though their impact may seem, don't ignore them.

Seek immediate medical help if you or someone you know experiences:

▼ Sudden, temporary weakness of the face, hand, arm, or leg on one side of the body

▼ Temporary difficulty speaking or loss of speech altogether, or trouble understanding someone speaking

▼ Double vision or sudden, temporary dimness of vision or loss of vision, particularly in one eye

▼ Unexplained headaches, or a change in the pattern of headaches

▼ Temporary dizziness, unsteadiness, or sudden falls

▼ Slight clumsiness of a limb, which might come across as a change in handwriting

Strokes around the Globe

The rate of death from strokes in Bulgaria is almost four times as high as it is in America, according to the World Health Organization, which compiled these statistics from member nations throughout the world.

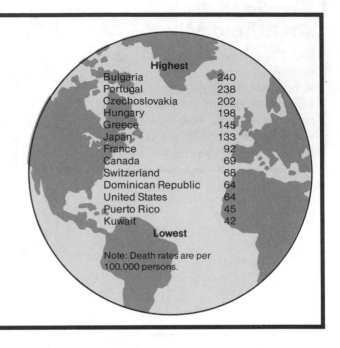

Highest

Bulgaria	240
Portugal	238
Czechoslovakia	202
Hungary	198
Greece	145
Japan	133
France	92
Canada	69
Switzerland	68
Dominican Republic	64
United States	64
Puerto Rico	45
Kuwait	42

Lowest

Note: Death rates are per 100,000 persons.

Six Ways to Prevent a Stroke

True, you can't change certain inherited factors that appear to contribute to the risk of stroke, but other factors may be within your control. Practicing the following healthy habits may make a difference in avoiding stroke.

1. Control your high blood pressure.

2. Don't smoke.

3. Don't drink heavily.

4. Eat a low-fat diet.

5. Get your exercise.

6. Reduce stress.

Lower Your Blood Pressure, Lower Your Stroke Risk

Keeping your blood pressure under control appears to directly decrease your risk of having a stroke, according to a great deal of scientific research. In one long-term study, blood pressure control and incidence of stroke were examined among the residents of Rochester, Minnesota, over a 29-year period. Stroke incidence among women residents declined evenly and steadily as blood pressure control increased. Among men, stroke incidence also fell, though not until several years after blood pressure was brought under control.

The Damage Diagrammed

Brain cells injured in a stroke cannot heal or regenerate. The damage may be slight or severe, temporary or permanent, depending on which brain cells in particular are affected (see illustration below) and how severely they are damaged.

The usual result is hemiparesis, or paralysis of one side of the body. A person with right hemiplegia is paralyzed on the right side of his body. This is due to damage on the *left* side of his brain, which controls movement on his right side. In the case of someone with left hemiplegia, the opposite applies. The right and left brain hemispheres are also specialized in other functions, as the illustration at right shows. The ability to speak or to understand the speech of others, for instance, is controlled by the left brain. Loss of this ability is called aphasia.

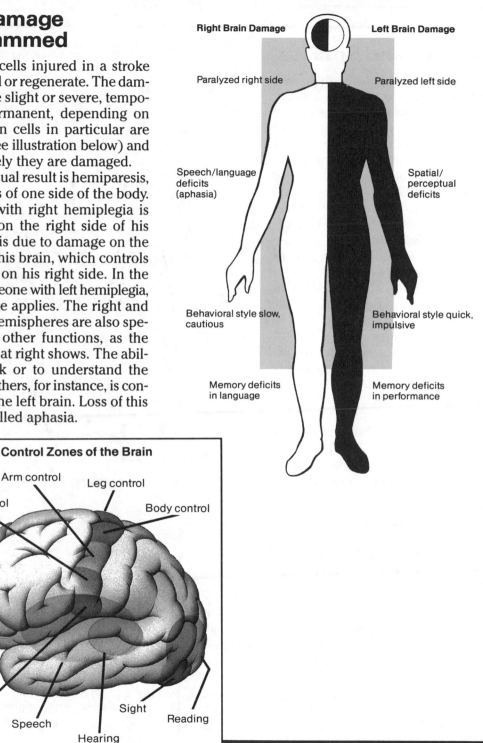

Right Brain Damage

Paralyzed right side

Speech/language deficits (aphasia)

Behavioral style slow, cautious

Memory deficits in language

Left Brain Damage

Paralyzed left side

Spatial/perceptual deficits

Behavioral style quick, impulsive

Memory deficits in performance

Control Zones of the Brain

Arm control

Leg control

Hand control

Body control

Front

Face control

Speech

Hearing

Sight

Reading

Strokes and Smokes

Smoking cigarettes substantially increases your risk of having a stroke, research has shown. The habit may cause blood vessels of the brain to harden and constrict. Some studies have shown that in long-term smokers considerably less blood reaches the brain than in nonsmokers.

In one long-term study of 4,255 men and women, smokers had significantly more strokes than nonsmokers. And the more cigarettes per day, the higher the risk: Heavy smokers (those who puffed 40 or more cigarettes a day) had twice the risk of stroke as light smokers (10 cigarettes a day).

But there's good news for ex-smokers. The long-term study showed that the risk of an ex-smoker having a stroke decreased significantly two years after he stopped. And after five years, his risk was reduced to the same level as that of a person who had never smoked.

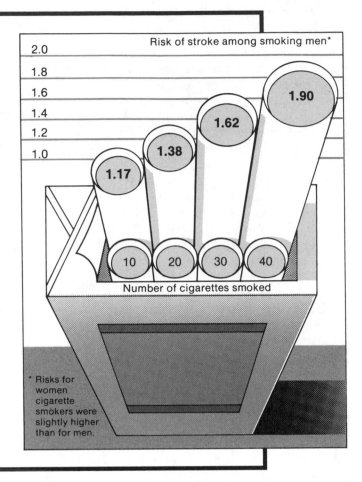

Risk of stroke among smoking men*

2.0
1.8
1.6 1.90
1.4 1.62
1.2 1.38
1.0 1.17

10   20   30   40

Number of cigarettes smoked

* Risks for women cigarette smokers were slightly higher than for men.

Fight Strokes with Fitness

Physical fitness may protect you from a stroke. In a study sponsored by the National Institutes of Health, 3,000 men were rated for their fitness. Those with the lowest ratings had a 3.4 times greater risk of dying of a stroke than men with the highest fitness ratings. In fact, the unfit men had a risk of stroke even greater than that of cigarette smokers.

Estrogen replacement therapy may cut in half a woman's risk of dying from a stroke, according to a study of nearly 5,000 elderly women. Estrogen may reduce blood cholesterol levels or help to lower blood pressure.

Excess Alcohol, Excess Risk

Heavy alcohol consumption may be a factor in strokes among men, according to a British study. In examining the drinking habits of 230 stroke patients, researchers found a high proportion of heavy drinkers among them. Three of the patients, in fact, had been binge drinking just before their strokes.

Among male heavy drinkers—those whose consumption averaged four or more drinks daily—the risk of stroke was four times higher than in nondrinkers. (It is uncertain whether women who drink heavily also have increased risks, the researchers noted, since few women in their study reported heavy drinking, possibly because they were unwilling to report real intake.) Alcohol may contribute to strokes by affecting blood pressure, blood flow, or clot formation, the researchers theorize.

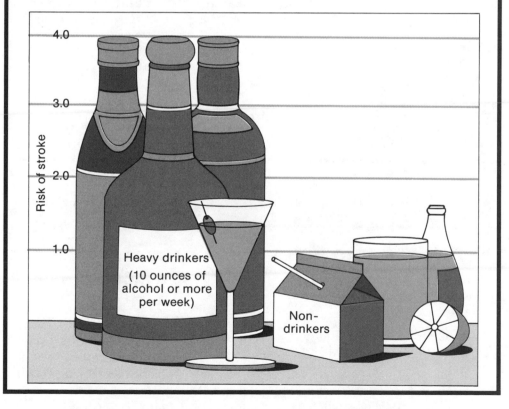

De-Stroke Your Diet

Eating more vegetables and fresh fruit may help protect against stroke. One study found that eating as little as one additional serving a day of these foods might cut the risk of fatal stroke by as much as 40 percent. The mechanism for this improvement is believed to be potassium. This mineral is known to help control high blood pressure, the greatest risk factor for stroke. Yet potassium may have a stroke-protective effect independent of its effect on blood pressure, at least one study has suggested.

Foods high in potassium include:

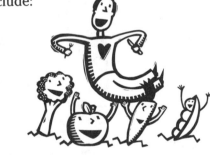

Food	Portion	Potassium (mg)
Avocado	1	1,204
Potato, baked	1 med.	844
Cantaloupe	½	825
Prunes, dried	½ cup	600
Watermelon	1 slice	560
Raisins	½ cup	545
Orange juice	1 cup	496
Broccoli, raw	1 med. stalk	490
Lima beans, large, boiled	½ cup	478
Banana	1	451
Apricots, dried	¼ cup	448
Squash, winter, baked	½ cup	445
Skim milk	1 cup	406
Sweet potato, baked	1 med.	397
Whole milk	1 cup	370
Sardines, Atlantic	1 can	365
Kidney beans, boiled	½ cup	355
Sunflower seeds, dried	⅓ cup	331
Apricots, fresh	3	313
Flounder, baked	3 oz.	292
Tomato, raw	1 med.	254
Peach	1	171
Green pepper	1 large	144

Risk Rises with Age

Number of men per 10,000 persons under the age of 45 who will have a stroke: 2.

Number of men per 10,000 between 45 and 64 who will have a stroke: 60.

Number of men per 10,000 between 65 and 84 who will have a stroke: 288.

IS THAT A FACT?

Only adults have strokes.

Not true. While it doesn't happen very often, children can suffer strokes, too. Strokes in newborn infants, in fact, are a major cause of cerebral palsy, a serious muscle disorder.

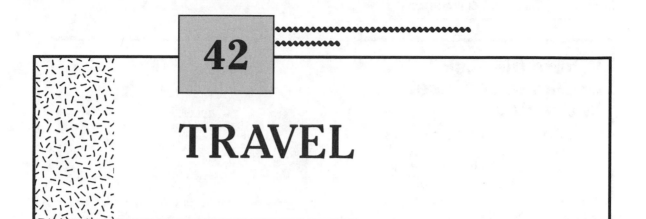

42

TRAVEL

Diarrhea, disease, disaster. From sailing the Mayflower to flying in jumbo jets, travel and health risks have been, and continue to be, occasional companions.

The volume of travelers makes this relationship inevitable. Consider that in 1987 scheduled airlines in the United States carried some 420 million passengers. Intercity buses were busy as well, transporting 324 million people.

And despite a rise in the fear of flying and concern over international terrorism—from 1985 through 1988 there were at least ten terrorist or criminal actions resulting in explosions on commercial passenger airplanes, including two bombings and two hijackings of U.S. carriers—more than 40 million Americans travel abroad each year.

The risk of a disaster while traveling remains small. However, surveys indicate that 25 to 75 percent of all travelers suffer one or more symptoms of an illness while traveling; most travelers endure some minor health problems some of the time.

But for most people, the rewards of travel continue to outweigh the risks. One study found the majority of people to be more satisfied with their lives immediately after a vacation than immediately before a vacation.

Bon voyage.

Where the Risk of Digestive Upset Is Greatest

Gastrointestinal upset strikes as many as 50 percent of all travelers to certain areas of the world. Contaminated food and water containing bacteria, viruses, or parasites are usually responsible.

Highest Risk
Latin America
Africa (North and East)
Middle East
Asia

Moderate Risk
Southern Europe
Some Caribbean islands

Lowest Risk
Northern Europe
Canada
Australia
New Zealand
United States

Can Traveler's Diarrhea Be Prevented?

The answer appears to be a qualified "yes." In a study conducted by researchers from the University of Texas Health Science Center, U.S. students attending summer classes in Mexico were given tablets containing a high dose of bismuth subsalicylate (the key ingredient in Pepto-Bismol), a low dose, or none at all (a placebo). Results of the study, which lasted 21 days, are summarized here.

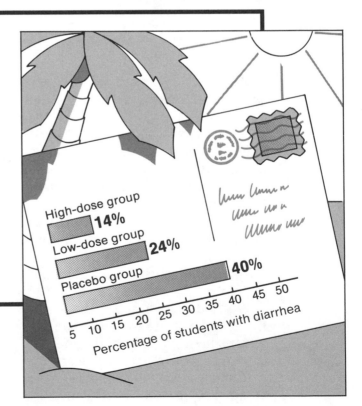

High-dose group **14%**
Low-dose group **24%**
Placebo group **40%**

5   10   15   20   25   30   35   40   45   50
Percentage of students with diarrhea

The Dos and Don'ts of Drinking the Water

In the United States, tap water can almost always be considered safe to drink. Making that assumption in other countries (even including much of Europe) is risky business. When in doubt, remember these rules.

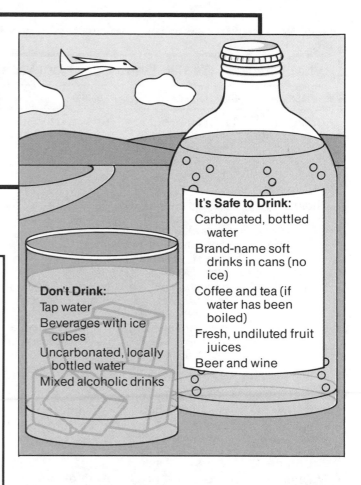

Don't Drink:
Tap water
Beverages with ice cubes
Uncarbonated, locally bottled water
Mixed alcoholic drinks

It's Safe to Drink:
Carbonated, bottled water
Brand-name soft drinks in cans (no ice)
Coffee and tea (if water has been boiled)
Fresh, undiluted fruit juices
Beer and wine

Staying in the Plane without the Pain

Sometimes an earache or head cold can make flying so painful that exiting before landing—even without a parachute—doesn't seem like such a bad idea. But one needn't go that far. The following might help.

1. Use a decongestant spray to keep nasal passages open during descent, when cabin pressure increases.

2. Pinch nostrils shut, and gently blow into nose. This forces air into the inner ear.

3. Stay seated upright to help depressurize the inner ears.

4. Drink a glass of water or fruit juice each hour to keep hydrated.

5. For an earache, hold over each ear a Styrofoam cup into which a paper towel soaked in warm water has been placed. It looks crazy, but it works.

"I Need a Doctor"

Easily said in English in Chicago, but what if you're in Madrid or Moscow? Here's some help.

Spanish: *Necesito un medico.*

French: *J'ai besoin d'un medecin.*

Italian: *Ho bisogno di un medico.*

German: *Ich brauche einen Artzt.*

Russian: *Mue nuzhen vrach.*

What You Don't Want to Bring Back from Vacation

Disease	Description	Location	Risk	Precautions
African sleeping sickness	Transmitted by the bite of the tsetse fly; symptoms include fever, rash, confusion	Confined to parts of tropical Africa	Low	Avoid heavily infested areas; don't wear dark, contrasting colors; they appear to attract the tsetse fly
Cholera	Acute intestinal infection usually acquired by drinking contaminated water or eating contaminated food	Parts of Africa and Asia	Very low	Vaccination is available but not recommended for most travelers; follow safe eating and drinking habits
Dengue fever	Transmitted by mosquitoes and characterized by sudden onset of high fever, headache, rash, and joint and muscle pain	South Pacific, tropical Asia, most of Caribbean, Mexico, Central America, and parts of South America and Africa	Predicted increase in the Americas over next few years	Use mosquito repellent; cover arms and legs
Hepatitis, viral, Type A	Transmitted by contaminated food and water, direct person-to person contact; brings flu-like symptoms	Mainly developing countries	Relative to sanitation conditions	Get injection of immune globulin before travel; follow safe eating and drinking habits
Malaria	Transmitted by mosquitoes (occasionally by blood transfusion); brings flulike symptoms; can cause coma or death	Parts of Africa, Central and South America, Asia, and Oceania	Appears greatest in sub-Saharan Africa	Get preventive drug 1–2 weeks before travel; use insect repellents; avoid outdoors from dusk to dawn
Plague	A disease of rats and other rodents usually spread to humans by fleas	Western third of United States, parts of South America and Africa, Southeast Asia, and USSR	Generally low; increased risk in mountainous or upland areas	Vaccination is available but generally not recommended; avoid rodent-dense areas
Yellow fever	Transmitted by mosquitoes; characterized by fever and jaundice	Parts of Africa and South America	Fatal cases have occurred in unvaccinated tourists visiting rural areas	Vaccination required by some countries in Africa and South America

Think First, Eat Second

While enjoying a foreign country it's easy to forget discretion. After all, isn't buying food from a street vendor just part of the "when in Rome" mentality?

But food from street vendors, food kept standing on buffet tables, and any other food that is less than hot are all to be avoided if you want to play it safe. In fact, it might be wise to go by the old adage: "If you can't peel it, cook it, or boil it, forget it."

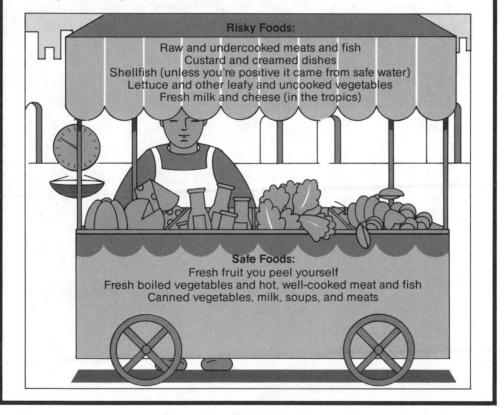

Risky Foods:
Raw and undercooked meats and fish
Custard and creamed dishes
Shellfish (unless you're positive it came from safe water)
Lettuce and other leafy and uncooked vegetables
Fresh milk and cheese (in the tropics)

Safe Foods:
Fresh fruit you peel yourself
Fresh boiled vegetables and hot, well-cooked meat and fish
Canned vegetables, milk, soups, and meats

People who crave new experiences (such as travel), tend to have lower levels of the brain chemical norepinephrine. New experiences, however, seem to increase norepinephrine levels.

Don't Leave Home without These

A camping vacation or really roughing it in the wilderness for a few days can be great fun and a real adventure. But experts recommend that you be prepared by taking along the following items in your safety kit.

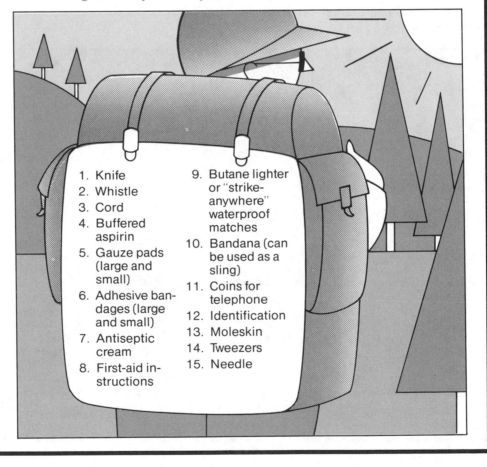

1. Knife
2. Whistle
3. Cord
4. Buffered aspirin
5. Gauze pads (large and small)
6. Adhesive bandages (large and small)
7. Antiseptic cream
8. First-aid instructions
9. Butane lighter or "strike-anywhere" waterproof matches
10. Bandana (can be used as a sling)
11. Coins for telephone
12. Identification
13. Moleskin
14. Tweezers
15. Needle

Trekkers, take note: Aerobic capacity drops about 4 percent per 1,000 feet above the 4,000-foot level in a sedentary person, but only half that in an aerobically fit person.

Off the Beaten Path: Where Lyme Disease Lurks

Also called Lyme arthritis, this disease was first reported in the United States in the mid-1970s in Old Lyme, Connecticut. The disease is spread by the deer tick (a tiny bloodsucker no bigger than a pinhead) and often is carried by deer and other animals, including dogs, birds, horses, and rodents. If your vacation plans include the great outdoors, be aware that frequenting wooded and grassy areas increases the risk of contracting Lyme disease. The map below shows the number of cases annually (per 100,000 persons) in different areas of the country.

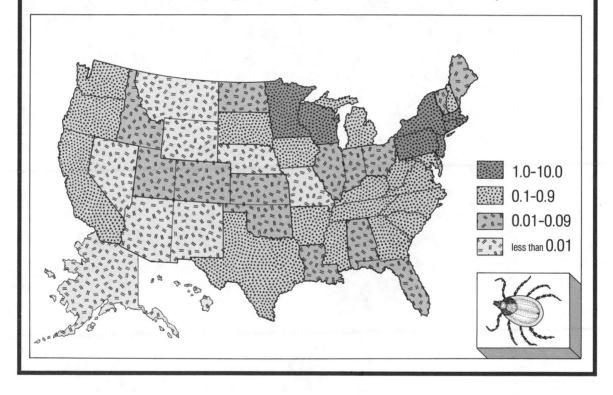

▨	1.0-10.0
▦	0.1-0.9
▨	0.01-0.09
▨	less than 0.01

When traveling to areas where mosquitoes are known to transmit diseases such as malaria, leave the perfume and cologne behind. Fragrances can attract mosquitoes.

Medical Emergencies Can Keep You Grounded

A year-long survey of medical emergencies at the Seattle-Tacoma International Airport showed that medical emergencies involving com- mercial air travelers were three times more likely to occur on the ground in the airport terminal than during a flight.

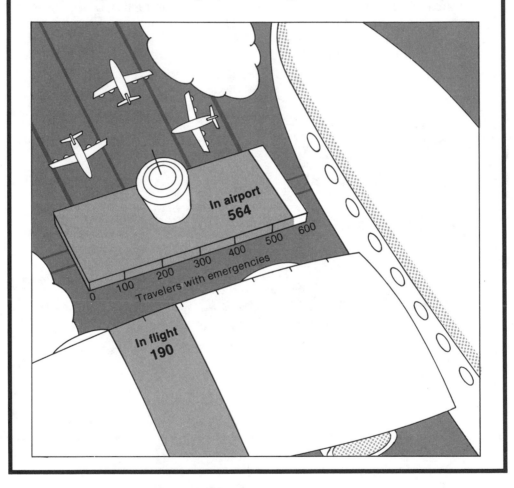

If your aircraft's cabin pressure is lost at 40,000 feet, you'll only have about 15 seconds to put on the oxygen mask before the drop in pressure will begin to affect you.

Fear of Flying Soars to New Heights

According to a survey in 1980, only one out of every ten air travelers was afraid to fly. But just three years later, another survey found that 33 percent of the American public was at least occasionally afraid. Then in 1989, 44 percent of adults polled in a telephone survey reported some fear of flying; 10 percent said they were *always* afraid.

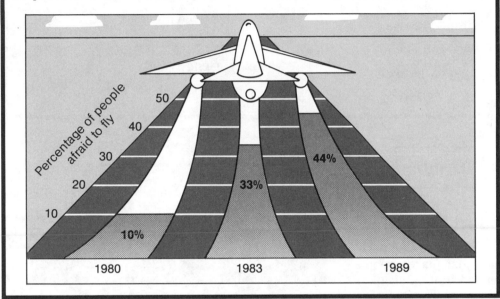

Percentage of people afraid to fly

50
40
30
20
10

10%

33%

44%

1980   1983   1989

When research subjects were asked, "What is the worst thing you can imagine happening to you?" people who liked to travel gave a variety of answers. But people who considered themselves "homebodies" most frequently answered, "An auto accident," thus suggesting anxiety about travel.

Stow It—Carefully

Stowing carry-on luggage in overhead compartments is probably a lot more dangerous than the typical African safari. To avoid back injuries, plant your feet firmly, shoulder width apart. Then unlock your knees and bend them slightly. Tighten stomach muscles and lift slowly—first to your waist, then shoulders, then overhead.

They Prefer Terra Firma

If you're afraid to fly, you're not alone. In fact, you're among pretty select company. Famous people who were, or are, afraid to fly, include:

Ronald Reagan

Muhammad Ali

Glenda Jackson

Jackie Gleason

Maureen Stapleton

Phil Rizzuto

Ray Bradbury

Aretha Franklin

John Madden

Gene Shalit

Bob Newhart

FUTURE FACTS

Sickness in Space

In a car, on a boat, in a plane . . . those are the usual places people have experienced motion sickness . . . until now. But guess what? The first tourists to book a charter to the moon will problaby have to remember to take along some Dramamine, or something stronger. Even astronauts (most of them, at least) get motion sickness (or more precisely, what NASA calls zero motion sickness), once they leave Earth's gravity behind.

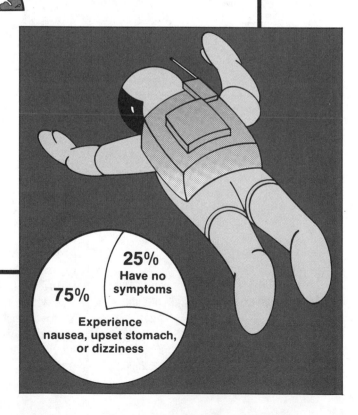

25% Have no symptoms

75% Experience nausea, upset stomach, or dizziness

Hop on the Bus, Gus

People argue about whether it's safer to travel by car or airplane, but the fact is neither is as safe as traveling by bus. From 1978 through 1987, the death rate for intercity and school bus passengers has not exceeded 0.05 deaths per 100,000,000 passenger miles. In contrast, the death rate for scheduled airlines has been as high as 0.17 deaths per 100,000,000 passenger miles, and the death rate for automobiles has been as high as 1.29 deaths per 100,000,000 passenger miles.

Year	Passenger Cars & Taxis		Buses		Scheduled Airlines	
	Deaths	Rate*	Deaths	Rate*	Deaths	Rate*
1978	28,035	1.26	28	0.03	175	0.09
1979	27,713	1.28	28	0.03	371	0.17
1980	27,339	1.29	42	0.05	28	0.01
1981	26,410	1.25	41	0.05	22	0.01
1982	22,859	1.02	32	0.04	218	0.10
1983	22,739	0.98	49	0.05	17	0.01
1984	23,373	0.98	37	0.03	39	0.02
1985	22,983	0.96	47	0.04	202	0.07
1986	24,704	1.00	36	0.03	3	0.001
1987	23,587	0.92	36	0.03	252	0.07

*Deaths per 100,000,000 passenger miles.

43

VISION PROBLEMS

Nearly 500,000 people in the United States are legally blind. And each year, an estimated 47,000 people become blind—that's one person every 11 minutes.

Another 11.4 million people are visually impaired. Of these, 1.4 million have a severe vision impairment—they can't read standard newsprint even with the help of glasses.

Glaucoma, macular degeneration, senile cataract, optic nerve atrophy, diabetic retinopathy, and retinitis pigmentosa are the leading causes of blindness, accounting for 51 percent of all cases. Cataracts are responsible for nearly one-third of all visual impairment.

While more than 80 million Americans suffer some kind of eye disease, it's estimated that one-third of them seek help too late to prevent serious vision loss. When people do seek help in time, the results are often very good.

More than 770,000 eye operations are performed each year. Cataract surgery has more than a 90 percent success rate. Corneal transplantion has also proven to be highly successful, becoming the most common form of organ transplantation practiced in the United States.

Eight Simple Steps for Clearer Vision

1. Take occasional breaks when spending long periods of time on close work (using a computer, sewing, or reading).

2. Always make sure you have good lighting.

3. Watch television from a distance about five times the width of the television screen.

4. Clean your eyewear daily.

5. Wear sunglasses that block 75 to 90 percent of visible light and provide a high degree of ultraviolet radiation protection.

6. When traveling, always carry a spare pair of glasses or contacts.

7. If you perform hazardous work such as operating a power saw, or play a sport such as racquetball or squash, wear eye-protective equipment.

8. Get a complete vision examination every one to two years.

Extended use of a video camera in bright light can cause temporary vision problems. While sighting with one eye, tightly closing the other eye for clearer focus and to block the sun apparently can deform the surface of the cornea, resulting in temporary double images.

WARNING SIGNALS

Warning Signs of Endangered Sight

Medical advances have made it possible for millions of people to retain sight that otherwise would have been lost forever. But early diagnosis is critical. So look closely at these ten early warning signs of possible vision problems.

▼ Dizziness, headaches, or nausea following close eye work

▼ Difficulty adjusting to darkness (night blindness)

▼ Severe pain in and around the eyes

▼ Cloudy, blurred, or diminished vision

▼ Double vision, spots, or a reddish tint over the visual field

▼ Dark shadows, blank spots, or other defects in the field of vision

▼ Rainbow-colored rings around lights

▼ Colors, particularly blues, appear faded

▼ Vertical lines appear bent or distorted

▼ Excessive tearing or discharge, swelling or other noticeable changes in the appearance of the eye

A Guide to Common Vision Problems

Most people who require eyeglasses or contact lenses to see sharply have one or more of these conditions.

Condition	What It Is	Who Has It	Symptoms	Treatment
Nearsightedness (myopia)	Seeing things clearly up close usually isn't a problem, but seeing clearly at a distance is difficult. This condition typically begins fairly early in life and levels off by the early 20s.	About 30% of Americans are nearsighted to some extent.	Squinting to see more clearly. Many nearsighted people find themselves struggling to read road signs. Some may notice a decline in their ability to play sports, or to watch them from a distance.	Prescription glasses or contact lenses will usually allow the nearsighted person to see more clearly. But until the condition stops progressing, frequent lens changes may be required.
Farsightedness (hyperopia)	Generally, farsighted people see more clearly at a distance than up close. But they may have some trouble focusing on distant objects as well.	To some degree, 60% of Americans are farsighted.	Squinting when doing close work or reading. A pattern of eye fatigue and headaches after working on a computer.	Prescription lenses should make vision clear and crisp again, although many slightly farsighted people function well without glasses or contacts.
Astigmatism	This condition is usually the result of an irregularly shaped cornea and may develop at any age.	As many as 70% of Americans have astigmatism to some extent.	Blurred and distorted vision, squinting, eye fatigue, headaches.	Prescription glasses and contacts solve this problem for most sufferers; some people not as adversely affected do not wear glasses or contacts.
Presbyopia	Sometimes confused with farsightedness, this condition is marked by a slow decline in the eyes' ability to focus on near objects, particularly those at reading distance.	The effects usually aren't apparent until a person is past 40. By age 50, nearly everyone has presbyopia to some degree.	Blurred vision at reading distance. Headaches and eye fatigue associated with computer work.	Prescription glasses and contact lenses can help, but finding the right prescription is difficult because this condition complicates nearsightedness, farsightedness, and astigmatism. As the condition worsens, prescriptions usually must be altered.

Are Nearsighted People Smarter?

Maybe so. An Israeli study of more than 157,000 male military recruits aged 17 to 19 found a connection between nearsightedness, years of education, and high IQ's. Here are the results.

27.3%
8.0%

Percentage of Nearsighted People

25
20
15
10
5
0

IQ of 80 or below | IQ of 128 or higher

19.7%
7.5%

Percentage of Nearsighted People

25
20
15
10
5
0

8 or less years of education | 12 or more years of education

IS THAT A FACT?

If you have 20/20 vision, your eyesight is perfect.

A lot of people think that's what 20/20 means, but they're wrong. Actually, 20/20 means being able to see clearly at 20 feet what a "normal" eye can see clearly at 20 feet. But 20/20 is not the ultimate in sharpness. Some people can see even better than 20/20—20/15, for example. With their eagle eyes, they can view objects from 20 feet away with the same sharpness that a normal-sighted person would have to move in to 15 feet to achieve.

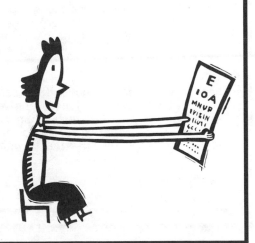

Contact Lenses Compared

It's no longer simply a choice between hard and soft lenses. Today's contact lens wearer has a lot of options to consider.

Type	Advantages	Disadvantages
Soft	Generally comfortable and relatively easy to adapt to. Because these lenses hang over the cornea, they're less likely to fall out during sports and recreational activities. Glare from the sun is less bothersome than with hard lenses.	Fragile and vulnerable to tearing, these lenses have a life expectancy of just 9–12 months. They also need to be cleaned more often than hard or gas-permeable lenses. In addition, it may be harder to get a perfect fit with soft lenses, and vision may not be as clear.
Extended-wear soft	Very convenient. These lenses can be worn 24 hours a day, 7 days a week. They only need to be removed once a week for cleaning.	If cleaning and disinfecting is done carelessly, the risk of infection is much greater than with regular soft lenses because of the amount of time between cleanings. A short life span—about 6 months.
Hard	These still give the best acuity, and they are durable, with a life span of 9–12 years with proper care. Hard lenses, which rest on the cornea, can correct a wide variety of visual imperfections.	Considered the least comfortable of lenses. They can be worn a maximum of 12–16 hours a day. Some people may experience a fair amount of pain and swelling of the cornea. This means many wearers will need glasses as well. When switching to glasses, wearers may suffer some distorted vision.
Rigid gas-permeable	Not as abusive to the cornea, and can be worn longer than the traditional hard lenses. Good life span of 1½–4 years.	Take some getting used to; as long as a month for some people. Initial cost may be higher than for soft lenses. Also, they don't protect against dust as well as soft lenses do.
Disposable	Convenience is the big appeal. Wear the lenses for a week and then throw them away. There's no care or cleaning, or the costs that go with them.	Currently, only effective for people with minor to moderate nearsightedness. And the start-up costs are higher (these lenses come in multipacks) than for other lenses. The long-term effects these lenses may or may not have on vision are unknown.

Five Myths about Sunglasses

Let's start with the most basic: **Sunglasses are really just for looks.** That, of course, is not true. Bright sunlight can damage the cornea, the lens, and the retina of the eye. And while squinting and the natural constriction of the eye's pupil do a lot to filter out sunlight, *good* sunglasses can do a lot more. Other myths:

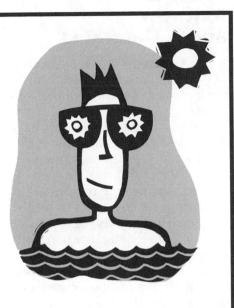

▼ **All sunglasses are essentially the same.** Actually, some glasses offer little added protection. Make sure any pair of sunglasses you buy screens out at least 80 percent of the sun's harmful ultraviolet rays—the label should state the level of protection. The best glasses screen out 95 percent.

▼ **If the sunglasses are expensive, they must be good.** Price and protection are not necessarily related. Don't assume anything, read the label.

▼ **Lens color isn't important to safety.** Yellow or blue-colored lenses may make a fashion statement, but they distort colors and are not good choices for driving. Also, if you can still easily see your eyes in a mirror, the lenses probably aren't giving you much protection from ultraviolet light.

▼ **Lens material and type don't matter.** That depends on what you're doing. The Food and Drug Administration requires all sunglasses to be "impact resistant," but that doesn't mean glass lenses won't shatter. For sports and active work, go with plastic lenses. In addition, polarized lenses are a plus around water and snow because they reduce reflection and glare. Gradient lenses are good for driving because they are darker at the top and lighter at the bottom, giving you a better look at the road ahead.

Approximately 100 million Americans either wear, or need, glasses.

What You Need to Know about Cataracts

A cataract, which is a clouding of the eye's lens, blocks or changes the passage of light required for vision.

What causes it? Scientists don't know exactly what causes the changes in the chemical composition of the eye that accompany a cataract. But the most common form of cataract—senile cataract—is related to aging. Heredity also can be a factor: Sometimes babies are born with congenital cataracts or develop them during the early years of their lives. Cataracts may also be associated with diabetes and other diseases, drugs, and eye injuries.

How many people are affected by cataracts? About 3.6 million Americans suffer some visual impairment due to cataracts. Each year nearly 700,000 new cases of cataracts occur; most of these are senile cataracts. More than 41 million Americans over the age of 40 have senile cataracts. Senile cataracts are responsible for 1 out of every 12 cases of blindness.

What are the signs of a cataract? Symptoms include fuzzy, blurred, or double vision; the need for frequent changes in eyeglass prescriptions; a feeling of having a film over the eyes; changes in the color of the pupil, which is normally black; and problems finding the right amount of light for reading or other close work. It should also be noted that cataracts develop slowly, and without pain, redness, or tearing in the eye.

What can be done for a cataract? Surgical removal of the clouded lens has proven to be both safe and effective. Typically, a cataract is removed when it has progressed to the point where it interferes with daily living. During or after surgery, the natural lens must be replaced. There are three choices: special eyeglasses, special contact lenses, and intraocular lenses. The last are clear plastic lenses that are implanted in the eye during the cataract operation.

How Cataract Surgery Helps

Cataract surgery has proven quite effective, as shown by these results from a study of more than 290 elderly patients who underwent cataract operations with intraocular lens implantation. On average, the amount of visual impairment was reduced by more than 50 percent.

	Presurgery	Postsurgery
Visual acuity in affected eye	20/100	20/40
Percentage of visual impairment	46.5	21.1

Eye Injuries Are Part of the Game

The games people play sometimes can be dangerous to their eyes. In 1988, Americans were treated for an estimated 31,808 eye injuries during sports and recreational activities. Baseball was the most hazardous sport for 5- to 14-year-olds, basketball was the most dangerous for 15- to 24-year-olds, and racquet and court sports accounted for the most eye injuries in the 25 to 64 age group.

Activity	Estimated Eye Injuries (1988)	
	Number	Percent
Basketball	5,492	17.3
Baseball	4,755	14.9
Racquet and court sports*	3,416	10.7
Swimming and pool sports	3,220	10.1
Football	2,090	6.6
Ball sports (unspecifed)	1,290	4.0
Soccer	892	2.8
Golf	491	1.5
Hockey (all types)	330	1.1
Wrestling, boxing, and martial arts	308	1.0
Total selected sports	22,284	70.0
Other sports and recreational activities	9,524	30.0

*Includes racquetball, tennis, squash, paddleball, badminton, handball, and volleyball

Facts about Glaucoma

▼ Glaucoma is a progressive disease typically associated with too much pressure within the eye. The pressure decreases the blood supply to the retina, continually destroying nerve cells.

▼ The cause of glaucoma is unknown, but the disease occurs four times more frequently among persons who have blood relatives with glaucoma. Other people at high risk: diabetics, persons with recently controlled high blood pressure, blacks (their glaucoma rate is eight times higher than that of nonblacks), victims of eye injury, and people 65 and older.

▼ Nearly 2 million Americans aged 35 and older are affected.

▼ Unfortunately, any sight glaucoma has taken cannot be restored. But treatment sometimes can control glaucoma. Any one of a variety of drugs, taken as eyedrops or pills, is usually tried first. If medication proves unsuccessful, conventional or laser surgery to relieve pressure within the eye is an option.

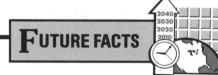

FUTURE FACTS

The Next Century Will Be a Blur for Many

As the older population grows, so, too, should the number of people with eye diseases. By the year 2020, for example, more than 15 million Americans 65 and older are expected to be living with a cataract, and 7.5 million are expected to have macular degeneration.

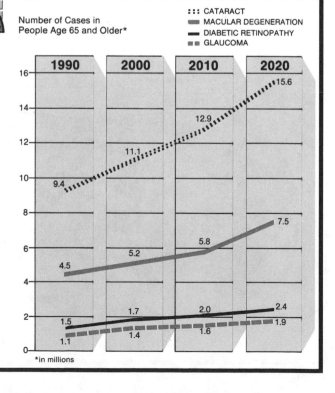

Number of Cases in People Age 65 and Older*

::: CATARACT
■■ MACULAR DEGENERATION
■ DIABETIC RETINOPATHY
■■ GLAUCOMA

	1990	2000	2010	2020
Cataract	9.4	11.1	12.9	15.6
Macular Degeneration	4.5	5.2	5.8	7.5
Diabetic Retinopathy	1.5	1.7	2.0	2.4
Glaucoma	1.1	1.4	1.6	1.9

*in millions

44

VITAMINS AND MINERALS

Vitamins are divided into two groups based on how the body stores them. The fat-soluble vitamins—A, D, E, and K—are stored in moderate quantities, and those reserves can be drawn upon in a pinch. Fat-soluble vitamins are found in foods that contain fats and oils, and they are absorbed right along with the dietary fats. Water-soluble vitamins—the B-complex and C vitamins—are not stored in the body. Excesses are excreted, so these nutrients need to be replenished daily to maintain normal body functions.

There are two ways to get all the essential nutrients—by eating a well-balanced diet and by taking supplements. In a Louis Harris survey for *Prevention* magazine, 59 percent of American adults polled said they try to get an adequate intake of vitamins and minerals. To that end, 52 percent use supplements, with 41 percent reporting daily use.

More women than men take vitamin and mineral supplements, according to data from the first National Health and Nutrition Examination Survey. And people over age 65 take more supplements than people who are younger, except for vitamin E, which is consumed more often by those in their middle years, and iron, which is taken most often by the young. All in all, Americans spend $3.1 billion on vitamins, minerals, and nutritional supplements each year.

Your Recommended Dietary Allowance

How much of each vitamin and mineral do you need each day? Recommended Dietary Allowances (RDAs), the amounts of each nutrient necessary to keep your body in running order, were first established in 1943 by the Food and Nutrition Board of the National Academy of Sciences. Those amounts have been updated periodically as scientific knowledge grows. Here are the latest guidelines, released in October 1989.

Vitamins

Group	Age (years) or Condition	Weight (lb.)	Height (in.)	Protein (g)	Vitamin A I.U.	Vitamin D I.U.	Vitamin E (mg)	Vitamin K (mcg)	Vitamin C (mg)	Thiamine (mg)	Riboflavin (mg)	Niacin (mg)	Vitamin B_6 (mg)	Folate (mcg)	Vitamin B_{12} (mcg)
Infants	0.0–0.5	13	24	13	1,875	300	3	5	30	0.3	0.4	5	0.3	25	0.3
	0.5–1.0	20	28	14	1,875	400	4	10	35	0.4	0.5	6	0.6	35	0.5
Children	1–3	29	35	16	2,000	400	6	15	40	0.7	0.8	9	1.0	50	0.7
	4–6	44	44	24	2,500	400	7	20	45	0.9	1.1	12	1.1	75	1.0
	7–10	62	52	28	3,500	400	7	30	45	1.0	1.2	13	1.4	100	1.4
Men	11–14	99	62	45	5,000	400	10	45	50	1.3	1.5	17	1.7	150	2.0
	15–18	145	69	59	5,000	400	10	65	60	1.5	1.8	20	2.0	200	2.0
	19–24	160	70	58	5,000	400	10	70	60	1.5	1.7	19	2.0	200	2.0
	25–50	174	70	63	5,000	200	10	80	60	1.5	1.7	19	2.0	200	2.0
	51+	170	68	63	5,000	200	10	80	60	1.2	1.4	15	2.0	200	2.0
Women	11–14	101	62	46	4,000	400	8	45	50	1.1	1.3	15	1.4	150	2.0
	15–18	120	64	44	4,000	400	8	55	60	1.1	1.3	15	1.5	180	2.0
	19–24	128	65	46	4,000	400	8	60	60	1.1	1.3	15	1.6	180	2.0
	25–50	138	64	50	4,000	200	8	65	60	1.1	1.3	15	1.6	180	2.0
	51+	143	63	50	4,000	200	8	65	60	1.0	1.2	13	1.6	180	2.0
Pregnant				60	4,000	400	10	65	70	1.5	1.6	17	2.2	400	2.2
Lactating	1st 6 months			65	6,500	400	12	65	95	1.6	1.8	20	2.1	280	2.6
	2nd 6 months			62	6,000	400	11	65	90	1.6	1.7	20	2.1	260	2.6

Boron: A New Essential Mineral?

Boron is a little-known trace mineral that may play a big role in strong and healthy bone development.

What it does: Interacts with cholecalciferol (vitamin D_3). Could influence bone growth. Possibly helps bone use calcium and phosphorus. May prevent calcium loss and bone demineralization. May be a factor in preventing osteoporosis.

Amount needed: 1 to 2 milligrams daily.

Food sources: Fruits, leafy vegetables, and nuts. Meat and fish are poor sources.

Highest levels: In prunes, raisins, almonds, peanuts, hazelnuts, dates, and honey.

					Minerals					
Group	Age (years) or Condition	Weight (lb.)	Height (in.)	Calcium (mg)	Phosphorus (mg)	Magnesium (mg)	Iron (mg)	Zinc (mg)	Iodine (mcg)	Selenium (mcg)
Infants	0.0–0.5	13	24	400	300	40	6	5	40	10
	0.5–1.0	20	28	600	500	60	10	5	50	15
Children	1–3	29	35	800	800	80	10	10	70	20
	4–6	44	44	800	800	120	10	10	90	20
	7–10	62	52	800	800	170	10	10	120	30
Men	11–14	99	62	1,200	1,200	270	12	15	150	40
	15–18	145	69	1,200	1,200	400	12	15	150	50
	19–24	160	70	1,200	1,200	350	10	15	150	70
	25–50	174	70	800	800	350	10	15	150	70
	51+	170	68	800	800	350	10	15	150	70
Women	11–14	101	62	1,200	1,200	280	15	12	150	45
	15–18	120	64	1,200	1,200	300	15	12	150	50
	19–24	128	65	1,200	1,200	280	15	12	150	55
	25–50	138	64	800	800	280	15	12	150	55
	51+	143	63	800	800	280	10	12	150	55
Pregnant				1,200	1,200	300	30	15	175	65
Lactating	1st 6 months			1,200	1,200	355	15	19	200	75
	2nd 6 months			1,200	1,200	340	15	16	200	75

Surveys show that 84 percent of U.S. Olympians and 72 percent of other athletes take vitamin supplements, compared with about 50 percent of the general public.

IS THAT A FACT?

Vitamin tablets keep their potency best when stored in the refrigerator.

Not really. When you open the chilled bottle to remove a tablet, moisture condenses in the bottle. And moisture can reduce a vitamin's potency. For long life, keep your vitamins away from moisture, heat, and sunlight. A cool, dark cabinet is best.

What Vitamins and Minerals Do for Us

Vitamins and minerals play many important roles inside our bodies—that's why they've come to be labeled essential nutrients. This table summarizes their main functions and possible protective roles.

Nutrient	What It Does	How It Protects
Vitamin A	Helps form and maintain healthy eyes, hair, teeth, gums, mucous membranes; involved in fat metabolism.	Stimulates immune system, reduces risk of some tumors, including lung, colorectal, prostate and breast cancers. Prevents stress ulcers related to major burns or injury. May lessen oral cancer; may help reduce stress in chemotherapy patients.
Thiamine (vitamin B_1)	Promotes metabolism of sugars, starches; promotes normal appetite and digestion; necessary for brain and nerve function.	May stop foot pain in diabetics. Muscular endurance enhanced for short time in athletes.
Riboflavin (vitamin B_2)	Helps body use carbohydrates, proteins, fats; maintains good vision; maintains mucous membranes; important for brain function.	May help protect against esophageal cancer.
Niacin	Helps appetite and digestion; helps change food to energy; needed for nervous system.	Reduces post-heart-attack risk. Reduces cholesterol and triglyceride levels.
Vitamin B_6 (pyridoxine)	Plays role in protein and fat metabolism; helps form red blood cells; works for nervous system and brain cells; important for mental health.	May be useful for premenstrual syndrome. May improve schizophrenia and seizures, boost stamina. Reduces swelling in carpal tunnel syndrome.
Vitamin B_{12} (cobalamin)	Helps build genetic material for cell nuclei; forms red blood cells; essential for function of all body cells; important for mental health.	May halt some brain disorders. May prevent some rare birth defects.
Folate (folic acid)	Helps form body proteins and genetic materials for cell nuclei; helps build red blood cells.	Lowers risk of neural-tube birth defects; may deter cleft palate; fights spontaneous abortion. Used in treatment of cervical dysplasia. Helps stop periodontal disease. May improve interaction of retarded children (with Fragile X syndrome) with outside world.
Vitamin C	Binds cells together; strengthens blood vessel walls; needed for healthy gums; helps resist infection; promotes healing of wounds and cuts.	May help protect against cancer of esophagus, stomach, larynx, cervix. May slow kidney and eye problems in diabetics. May help asthma patients breathe easier during exercise. May help combat cardiovascular disease. Coun-

Nutrient	What It Does	How It Protects
		teracts the stress of high temperatures. Restores fertility to men with sperm clumping.
Vitamin D	Helps body absorb calcium, phosphorus.	Helps prevent osteoporosis, osteomalacia. May help prevent breast and colon cancer. May prevent some kinds of deafness. May help control diabetes in older people.
Vitamin E	Helps form red blood cells, muscles, tissues.	May prevent dangerous blood clots. Protects against breast cancer; inhibits growth of some cancer cells and neutralizes nitrosamines.
Vitamin K	Needed for normal blood clotting and normal bone metabolism.	Undetermined.
Calcium	Builds strong bones, teeth; helps blood to clot; helps nerves and muscles to function; helps change food to energy.	Helps lower blood pressure. May help protect against colon cancer. Helps protect against osteoporosis.
Iodine	Controls metabolism; necessary for normal functioning of thyroid gland.	May relieve pain and soreness in fibrocystic breast disease.
Iron	Makes hemoglobin that carries oxygen from lungs to cells and makes myoglobin that stores oxygen in muscles.	Boosts resistance to cold temperatures. Improves attention span and cooperativeness in children.
Magnesium	Activates enzymes to transfer and release energy in body.	Strong link between magnesium levels and diabetic retinopathy. Lowers blood pressure. Prevents life-threatening blood clots and reduces risk of stroke. May relieve migraines. Helps control epilepsy.
Phosphorus	Builds strong bones, teeth; helps change food to energy.	Undetermined.
Potassium	Needed for nerve conduction and muscle contraction.	May help prevent high blood pressure. Protects against fatal strokes.
Selenium	Helps prevent breakdown of fats and body chemicals.	May help protect against breast, lung, and colon cancer.
Zinc	Works with red blood cells to move carbon dioxide from tissues to lungs.	May prevent some birth defects. Heals cold sores, and may prevent herpes virus from multiplying. Speeds wound healing.

Some Additional Nutrients: Safe and Adequate Amounts

Scientists know that additional nutrients are necessary for keeping your body in working order, but no RDAs have yet been established for them. Instead, there are estimated "safe and adequate" daily intake ranges recommended for these vitamins and minerals.

	Age (years)	Vitamins		Trace Elements*					Electrolytes		
		Biotin (mcg)	Pantothenic Acid (mg)	Copper (mg)	Manganese (mg)	Fluoride (mg)	Chromium (mcg)	Molybdenum (mcg)	Sodium (mg)	Potassium (mg)	Chloride (mg)
Infants	0–0.5	10	2	0.4–0.6	0.3–0.6	0.1–0.5	10–40	15–30	120	500	180
	0.5–1	15	3	0.6–0.7	0.6–1.0	0.2–1.0	20–60	20–40	200	700	300
Children and Adolescents	1–3	20	3	0.7–1.0	1.0–1.5	0.5–1.5	20–80	25–50	225	1,000	350
	4–6	25	3–4	1.0–1.5	1.5–2.0	1.0–2.5	30–120	30–75	300	1,400	500
	7–10	30	4–5	1.0–2.0	2.0–3.0	1.5–2.5	50–200	50–150	400	1,600	600
	11+	30–100	4–7	1.5–2.5	2.0–3.0	1.5–2.5	50–200	75–250	500	2,000	750
Adults		30–100	4–7	1.5–3.0	2.0–3.0	1.5–4.0	50–200	75–250	500	2,000	750

*Since the toxic levels for many trace elements may be only several times usual intakes, the upper levels for the trace elements given in this table should not be habitually exceeded.

Factors That Boost Absorption

Even if you eat carefully and take supplements, you may not be getting all the benefits you could—unless you pay attention to factors like these that affect nutrient absorption.

▼ Supplements are absorbed best when taken with food.

▼ Take the fat-soluble vitamins (A, D, and E) with foods that contain fat. A low-fat diet containing 15 to 20 percent of calories from fat is still sufficient.

▼ Take vitamin C in small doses spread throughout the day.

▼ Vitamin C enhances iron absorption. Adding 60 milligrams of vitamin C at mealtime, for instance, will triple iron absorption from rice.

▼ Vitamin D enhances calcium absorption.

▼ Take small doses of calcium. If you take 1,000 milligrams each day, for instance, take it in three or four divided doses. One of those should come at bedtime, to give your body something to "chew on" besides your bones during the night.

The Classic Deficiency Diseases

The importance of many nutrients was discovered quite by accident, when dietary shortages led to physical symptoms. In the days of the Roman Empire, for instance, soldiers stationed along the Rhine River suffered from loose teeth and bleeding gums when they ate the local fare. But then they discovered an herb—now believed to be sorrel—that would cure their gum trouble. Centuries later, British sailors suffered from the same symptoms, until oranges and lemons were added to their shipboard staples. It wasn't until much later that scientists recognized that vitamin C was the substance responsible for halting these symptoms of scurvy. The essentiality of most vitamins and minerals was discovered in this way. First, people became sick with a deficiency disease. Then someone discovered an ingredient in food that would cure the disease. Here are some of the classic deficiency diseases and their symptoms.

Disease	Deficient Nutrient	Symptoms	Occurrence
Beriberi	Thiamine	Peripheral paralysis, heart failure, edema	Common in southeast Asian populations whose diet consists primarily of polished white rice
Goiter	Iodine	Enlarged thyroid	Found among some South American Indian tribes and in other areas where soil is deficient in iodine
Pellagra	Niacin	Reddish rash that turns rough and dark, mental problems	Found in poor and undernourished people in the Deep South in early 1900s
Rickets	Vitamin D	Softening of bones that can produce deformities	Affected children in northern European cities in early 1900s
Scurvy	Vitamin C	Bleeding gums, loose teeth, multiple bruises, rough skin, loss of appetite	Common among sailors between 1500s and mid-1700s

A teaspoon of sugar (about 10 grams) taken along with a calcium supplement will help your body absorb the mineral better, according to the U.S. Department of Agriculture's Human Nutrition Research Center on Aging.

Get Your Vitamins and Minerals Here

The best way to get the vitamins and minerals to fuel your body is to eat foods high in those essential nutrients. Here are some of the top food sources.

Nutrient	Food	Portion	Amount
Vitamin A	Beef liver, braised	3 oz.	30,327 I.U.
	Sweet potato, baked	1	24,877* I.U.
	Carrot, raw	1	20,253* I.U.
	Spinach, cooked	½ cup	7,371* I.U.
	Cantaloupe	¼	4,304* I.U.
	Broccoli, cooked	1 spear	2,537* I.U.
Thiamine (vitamin B_1)	Pork, center loin, roasted	3 oz.	0.77 mg
	Cured ham, roasted	3 oz.	0.70 mg
	Pork shoulder, braised	3 oz.	0.46 mg
	Peanuts, dry roasted	½ cup	0.32 mg
	Soy flour, full fat, raw	½ cup	0.24 mg
	Black beans, boiled	½ cup	0.21 mg
	Split peas, boiled	½ cup	0.19 mg
Riboflavin (vitamin B_2)	Beef liver, braised	3 oz.	3.49 mg
	Beef kidneys, simmered	3 oz.	3.45 mg
	Chicken liver, simmered	3 oz.	1.49 mg
	Malted milk	1 cup	1.15 mg
	Ice milk, soft-serve vanilla	1 cup	0.54 mg
	Yogurt, low-fat	1 cup	0.49 mg
	Milk, whole	1 cup	0.40 mg
	Brewer's yeast	1 Tbsp.	0.34 mg
	Roquefort cheese	2 oz.	0.34 mg
	Brie cheese	2 oz.	0.30 mg
Niacin	Chicken, light meat	3 oz.	10.6 mg
	Swordfish, baked	3 oz.	10.0 mg
	Beef liver, braised	3 oz.	9.1 mg
	Halibut, baked	3 oz.	6.0 mg
	Salmon, pink, canned	3 oz.	5.5 mg
	Peanuts, dry roasted	¼ cup	4.9 mg
Vitamin B_6 (pyridoxine)	Beef liver, braised	3 oz.	0.77 mg
	Banana	1 med.	0.66 mg
	Avocado	1 med.	0.56 mg
	Carrot juice, canned	1 cup	0.53 mg
	Chicken, light meat	3 oz.	0.51 mg
	Hummus	½ cup	0.49 mg
	Sunflower seeds	¼ cup	0.45 mg

*Beta-carotene sources of vitamin A

Nutrient	Food	Portion	Amount
Vitamin B₁₂ (cobalamin)	Clams, mixed species, canned, drained	3 oz.	84.05 mcg
	Beef liver, braised	3 oz.	60.35 mcg
	Beef kidneys, simmered	3 oz.	43.61 mcg
	Tuna, bluefin, fresh, cooked	3 oz.	9.25 mcg
	Beef tongue, simmered	3 oz.	5.02 mcg
	Sockeye salmon, baked	3 oz.	4.93 mcg
Folate (folic acid)	Brewer's yeast	1 Tbsp.	313 mcg
	Chicken livers, cooked	1 oz.	217 mcg
	Beef liver, braised	3 oz.	185 mcg
	Lentils, cooked	½ cup	179 mcg
	Black-eyed peas, cooked	½ cup	179 mcg
	Broccoli, cooked	1 spear	123 mcg
	Red kidney beans	½ cup	114 mcg
	Orange juice	1 cup	109 mcg
Vitamin C	Orange juice, freshly squeezed	1 cup	124 mg
	Grapefruit juice, freshly squeezed	1 cup	94 mg
	Papaya	½ med.	94 mg
	Guava	½ med.	83 mg
	Kiwifruit	1 med.	75 mg
	Orange	1	70 mg
	Brussels sprouts, raw	4	65 mg
	Green peppers, raw, chopped	½ cup	64 mg
Vitamin D	Herring, raw	3.5 oz.	900 I.U.
	Atlantic salmon, canned	3.5 oz.	500 I.U.
	Sardines, canned in oil	3.5 oz.	300 I.U.
	Fortified milk	1 cup	100 I.U.
	Edam cheese	3.5 oz.	84 I.U.
Vitamin E	Wheat germ oil	1 Tbsp.	36.3 I.U.
	Sunflower seeds	¼ cup	26.8 I.U.
	Almonds, dried	¼ cup	15.2 I.U.
	Wheat germ, raw	½ cup	12.8 I.U.
	Sunflower oil	1 Tbsp.	10.9 I.U.
Calcium	Swiss cheese, low-sodium	2 oz.	544 mg
	Provolone cheese	2 oz.	428 mg
	Monterey Jack cheese	2 oz.	424 mg

(continued)

Get Your Vitamins and Minerals Here—*Continued*

Nutrient	Food	Portion	Amount
	Yogurt, low-fat	1 cup	415 mg
	Muenster cheese	2 oz.	406 mg
	Colby cheese	2 oz.	388 mg
	Brick cheese	2 oz.	382 mg
	Sardines, Atlantic, drained	3 oz.	322 mg
	American Cheese	2 oz.	348 mg
Iron	Fortified breakfast cereal	1 cup	21 mg
	Clams	3½ oz.	11.9 mg
	Tofu, raw	¼ block	6.22 mg
	Peaches, dried	10 halves	5.28 mg
	Sirloin, lean, broiled	6 oz.	5.12 mg
	Oysters	3½ oz.	4.34 mg
	Raisins	1 cup	3.43 mg
Magnesium	Pumpkin seeds	½ cup	369 mg
	Toasted wheat germ	1 cup	362 mg
	Sunflower seeds	½ cup	255 mg
	Sesame seeds	½ cup	253 mg
	Tofu, raw, firm	½ cup	236 mg
	Peanut butter, chunky	½ cup	205 mg
Selenium	Tortilla chips	1 oz.	284 mcg
	Potato chips	1 oz.	275 mcg
	Pork kidneys, braised	3½ oz.	207 mcg
	Corn chips	1 oz.	182 mcg
	Tuna, canned	3½ oz.	115 mcg
	Salmon, canned	3½ oz.	75 mcg
	Cracked wheat bread	3 slices	67 mcg
Zinc	Oysters, eastern, steamed	4 med.	50.92 mg
	Pot roast, lean, braised	3 oz.	8.73 mg
	Beef liver, braised	3 oz.	5.16 mg
	Beef, ground lean, broiled	3 oz.	4.56 mg
	Lamb, lean, cooked	3 oz.	4.48 mg
	Pumpkin, squash seeds, roasted	¼ cup	4.22 mg
	Clams, steamed	6 med.	4.12 mg
	Beef, round, lean, broiled	3 oz.	3.98 mg
	Turkey, dark meat, cooked	3 oz.	3.80 mg
	Swiss cheese	2 oz.	2.22 mg

How Vitamins Are Lost

Drying, canning, freezing, peeling, cooking, and all the other steps involved in storing and preparing vegetables take their toll on vitamin content. This chart shows how vitamin C levels shrink depending on a pea's path from pod to plate.

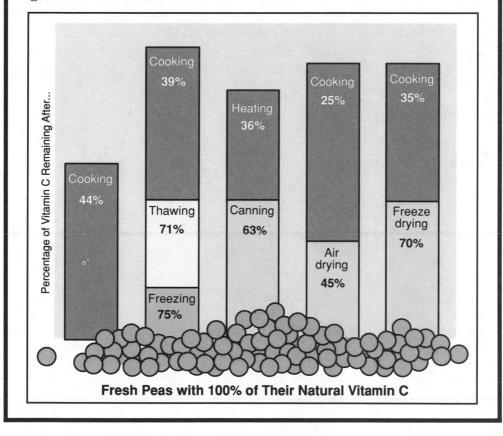

Microwave thawing of frozen food preserves vitamins better than thawing at room temperature or in the refrigerator.

Microwave versus Conventional Cooking

Food scientists were originally concerned that microwave cooking might cause increased destruction of vitamins. But studies have shown that foods blanched, cooked, or reheated in a microwave oven generally retain about the same amount of nutrients (or in some cases even more) as those cooked by conventional methods of heating.

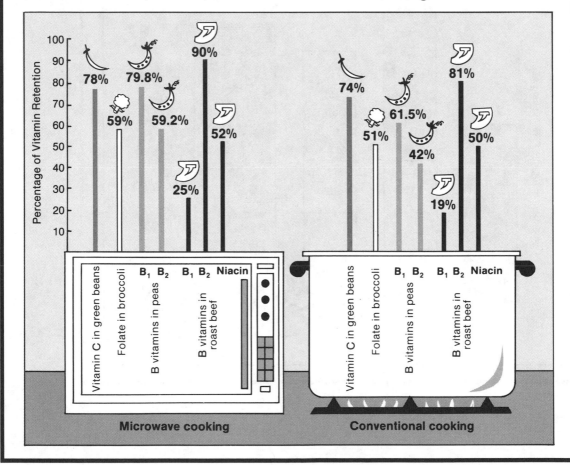

Percentage of Vitamin Retention

Microwave cooking

78% — Vitamin C in green beans
59% — Folate in broccoli
79.8% B_1 — B vitamins in peas
59.2% B_2 — B vitamins in peas
25% B_1 — B vitamins in roast beef
90% B_2 — B vitamins in roast beef
52% — Niacin

Conventional cooking

74% — Vitamin C in green beans
51% — Folate in broccoli
61.5% B_1 — B vitamins in peas
42% B_2 — B vitamins in peas
19% B_1 — B vitamins in roast beef
81% B_2 — B vitamins in roast beef
50% — Niacin

Special Nutrient Needs

Do you have diabetes or arthritis? Do you smoke cigarettes or drink soft water? There can be dozens of factors in your life or lifestyle that rob your body of important nutrients or require that you get extra amounts of certain vitamins or minerals. Are you on this list?

Group	Vitamin A	Vitamin B6	Vitamin B12	Folate	Vitamin C	Vitamin E	Calcium	Copper	Iron	Magnesium	Pantothenate	Selenium	Zinc
Dieter		X					X		X	X			X
Elderly	X			X	X		X						X
Kidney disease	X			X		X							
Smoker	X				X	X							
Alcoholic	X												X
Diabetes						X							
Arthritis					X							X	
Drink soft water										X			
Liver disease						X	X						
Coffee/caffeine drinker							X						
Surgical patient													X
Postmenopausal woman					X								
Pregnant woman	X			X			X	X			X		
Adolescent female	X	X		X			X			X			
Chronic exerciser							X		X	X			
Vegetarian			X										X

How Much Do You Really Get?

Not all the nutrients in the foods we eat or the supplements we swallow are fully absorbed. Under ideal conditions, here's how well your body can be expected to use some nutrients.

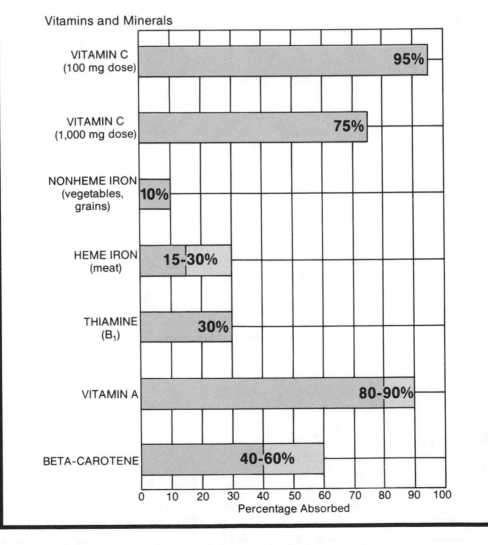

Vitamins and Minerals

	Percentage Absorbed
VITAMIN C (100 mg dose)	95%
VITAMIN C (1,000 mg dose)	75%
NONHEME IRON (vegetables, grains)	10%
HEME IRON (meat)	15-30%
THIAMINE (B₁)	30%
VITAMIN A	80-90%
BETA-CAROTENE	40-60%

The Most Common Deficiencies

Most people fall short of achieving the recommended levels for at least some vitamins and minerals. The chart shows which nutrients are most likely to be lacking. Meanwhile, certain other nutrients, including iodine and sodium, may actually exceed the recommended levels.

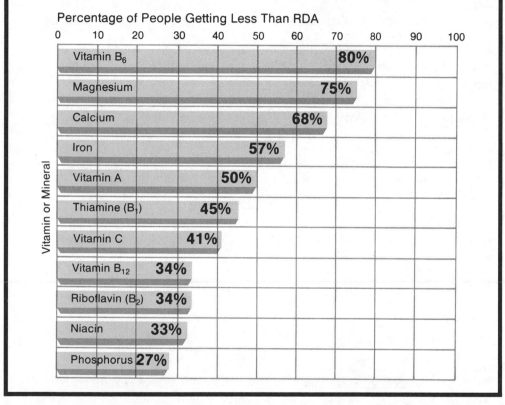

Percentage of People Getting Less Than RDA

Vitamin or Mineral	Percentage
Vitamin B$_6$	80%
Magnesium	75%
Calcium	68%
Iron	57%
Vitamin A	50%
Thiamine (B$_1$)	45%
Vitamin C	41%
Vitamin B$_{12}$	34%
Riboflavin (B$_2$)	34%
Niacin	33%
Phosphorus	27%

Why Do You Take Vitamins?

Here are the most common reasons why people rely on supplements. Incidentally, 97 percent *disagree* with the statement, "It's okay to skip meals as long as you take a vitamin supplement."

Reason	Percentage of Adults
To stay healthy	45
When feeling run-down	45
When there's not enough time for proper meals	41
During illness	40
When exposed to cold/flu	38
While on diet	33
Under stress/worry	20
With heavy work schedule	17
Smoke heavily	13

Nutrients That Disappear with Drugs

Some drugs can affect the way your body absorbs vitamins and minerals, possibly causing a deficiency. Compare your medication use with this chart, and check with your doctor.

Drug	Nutrient Affected	Comments
Antacids		
Aluminum and magnesium hydroxides	Phosphate	May need more phosphate for absorption
Magnesium trisilicate	Thiamine	Beriberi possible with high doses
Sodium bicarbonate	Folate	Interferes with folate absorption
Anticoagulants		
Coumarin, warfarin	Vitamin K	Inhibits vitamin K recycling
Heparin	Vitamin D	Osteopenia (thin bones) may result from long-term use
Anticonvulsants		
Phenobarbital, phenytoin, primidone, diphenylhydantoin	Calcium, vitamin D	Accelerates changing of vitamin D and other metabolites to simpler compounds; interferes with calcium absorption
Anti-inflammatories		
Aspirin	Iron, vitamin C, folate	May require additional supplementation
Antibiotics (internal)		
Neomycin	Vitamins K and B_{12}, iron, calcium	Leads to malabsorption
Contraceptives (oral)		
Estrogen/progestin	Vitamins B_6 and A, folate	B_6 and folate depletion; vitamin A levels may rise
Diuretics		
Benzothiadiazides	Potassium	Enhance potassium excretion
Triamterene	Folate	May require additional supplementation
Glucocorticoids		
Prednisone	Calcium	Interferes with calcium transportation
Hypocholesterolemic agents		
Cholestyramine	Vitamins A, K, B_{12}, and D, iron	Binds bile acids with nutrients so malabsorption results
Hypoglycemic agents		
Biguanides (metformin, phenformin)	Vitamin B_{12}	Inhibits vitamin B_{12} absorption
Laxatives		
Mineral oil	Carotene, vitamins A, D, K	Nutrients dissolve in oil and are lost
Phenolphthalein	Vitamin D, calcium	Inhibits vitamin D and calcium absorption

Signs of Deficiency

You don't have to get beriberi or rickets to be low in the necessary vitamins and minerals. Sometimes we get enough nutrients to stave off serious deficiency disease, but not enough to prevent other symptoms. Here's a listing of some signs to watch for.

Nutrient	Possible Deficiency Symptoms
Vitamin A	Night blindness; abnormal dryness of the eyeballs; dry, rough, itchy skin; susceptibility to respiratory infection, sensitivity to glare
Thiamine (B_1)	Confusion; weakness of eye muscles; loss of appetite; uncoordinated walk; poor memory; inability to concentrate; muscle pain, tenderness, loss of reflexes
Riboflavin (B_2)	Discolored tongue; anemia; cracks at corners of mouth; scaly skin; burning, itchy eyes; sensitivity to light; bleeding gums
Niacin	Dermatitis; insomnia; headache; diarrhea; dementia; pigmentation changes; raw tongue; disorientation
Vitamin B_6 (pyridoxine)	Depression; skin lesions; extreme nervousness; water retention; lethargy; anemia
Vitamin B_{12}	Anemia, accompanied by symptoms such as heart palpitations, sore tongue, general weakness; weight loss; diarrhea
Folate	Anemia; dizziness; fatigue; intestinal disorders; diarrhea; shortness of breath

Nutrient	Possible Deficiency Symptoms
Vitamin C (ascorbic acid)	Easy bruising; spongy, bleeding gums; dental problems; slow wound healing; fatigue; listlessness, rough skin; joint pain
Vitamin D	Softening of bones (osteomalacia); bone pain or tenderness, susceptibility to bone fracture (osteoporosis); excessive tooth decay; muscle wasting
Vitamin E	Muscle degeneration; anemia; nerve dysfunction
Vitamin K	Bruising
Calcium	Softening of bones (osteomalacia); susceptibility to bone fracture (osteoporosis); periodontal disease
Iron	Anemia, accompanied by symptoms such as weakness, fatigue, headache, heart palpitations, mouth soreness, spooning of nails
Magnesium	Foot and leg cramps; muscle weakness; irregular pulse; nervousness
Zinc	Slow wound healing; hair problems; poor resistance to infection; scaling skin; night blindness

Women who feel cold may get too little iron. One study showed that healthy women had lower body temperatures when they were on a low-iron diet than when they were on a high-iron diet.

A Link between Sunshine, Vitamin D, and Cancer?

Because intestinal and breast cancer death rates are highest in areas with the least sunlight, some researchers theorize that lack of vitamin D might be responsible. (We depend on sunlight falling on the skin to trigger vitamin D production.) Death rates are highest in cities in the Northeast and other sites where exposure to the sun is diminished by pollution and indoor lifestyles, and lowest in the South and Hawaii.

Intestinal cancer hot spots

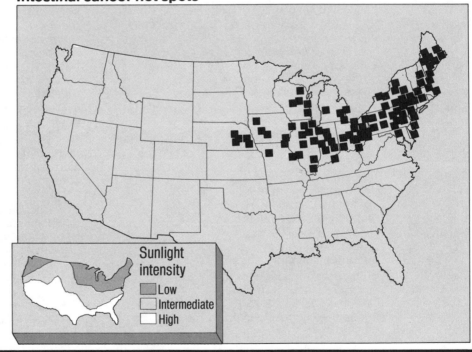

Sunlight intensity
- Low
- Intermediate
- High

If you live in Boston, Minneapolis, or other northern cities, studies suggest you can sit in the sun for 4 or 5 hours on any day between November and March without your skin producing a bit of vitamin D.

Breast cancer hot spots

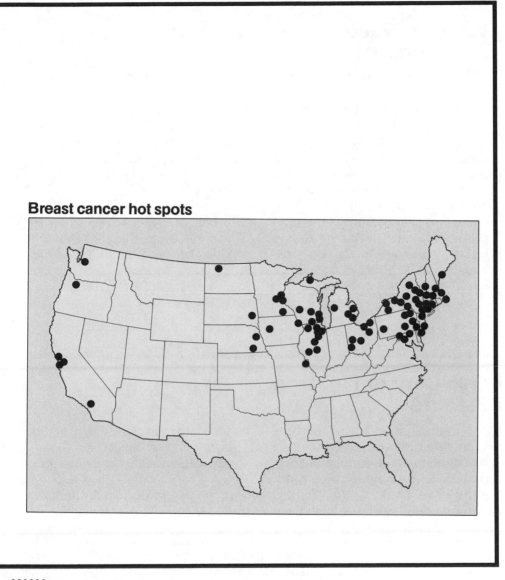

Black, Asian, and white people have the capacity to produce vitamin D from the sun, but because of extra melanin (pigmentation) in the skin of blacks and Asians, they require more time in the sun to produce the same amount of the vitamin as whites do. The skin's ability to manufacture vitamin D from sunlight also decreases with age.

Significantly fewer black people than white people consume vitamin supplements regularly.

Why We Need Antioxidants

Many scientists theorize that aging on the inside of the body—internal wear—is often caused by "free radicals." These are errant molecules with unpaired electrons that bump around looking for something to latch onto. That process is called oxidation, and if it were happening on the outside, you'd call it rust. Oxidation occurs mostly in fats. So cell membranes, which are rich in fat molecules, are the targets. Free radicals attack cells, kill them, or leave them vulnerable to cancer and other diseases.

Free radicals may contribute to aging, cancer, atherosclerosis, high blood pressure, Alzheimer's disease, osteoarthritis, and immune deficiency.

Antioxidants—vitamins A, C, and E, beta-carotene, and selenium—pair with the loose electrons in the free radicals, rendering them harmless.

Five Cancer-Fighting Factors

Preliminary studies show three vitamins and two minerals may have special potential in combating precancerous conditions. Those nutrients—vitamins A, C, and E, plus selenium and calcium—have been shown to reduce the risk of prostate, bladder, breast, lung, colon, stomach, cervical, and intestinal cancers.

These foods deliver two or more of the five protective nutrients.

Food	Portion	Vitamin A (I.U.)	Vitamin C (mg)	Vitamin E (I.U.)	Selenium (mcg)	Calcium (mg)
All-bran cereal	½ cup	1,878	23	4	13	—
Broccoli	1 cup	1,356	82	—	—	42
Brussels sprouts	1 cup	1,122	97	1	—	56
Cantaloupe	1 cup	5,158	67.5	—	—	—
Papaya, fresh	1 cup	2,819	86.5	—	—	—
Skim milk	1 cup	500	—	—	—	302
Sweet potato	4 oz.	24,880	28	5.2	—	32

Questions and Answers about Vitamins

Q. What is the difference between vitamin A and beta-carotene?

A. Animal foods contain only vitamin A, not beta-carotene. Plant sources contain only beta-carotene. In the body, about 10 percent of the beta-carotene (and other carotenoids) converts to vitamin A, depending on the body's needs.

Q. What is the difference between the RDAs and the USRDAs?

A. The U.S. Recommended Daily Allowances (USRDAs) were formulated by the U.S. Food and Drug Administration in 1974, to be used specifically for the labeling of products that have added nutrients or make nutritional claims. They generally reflect the highest recommendations for any age or sex group in the then-prevailing 1968 Recommended Dietary Allowance (RDA) tables of the Food and Nutrition Board. The RDA for iron at that time, for instance, was 10 milligrams daily for adult men, 18 milligrams for adult women. The USRDA was set at the highest value, or 18 milligrams. The USRDAs are used primarily in connection with legal labeling requirements for foods and vitamin preparations.

Q. Why are there so many different names for niacin? Are they different vitamins?

A. Some vitamins come in several forms—niacin is one of them. The two "niacins" that are important to remember are nicotinic acid and niacinamide. Both nicotinic acid and niacinamide act like niacin inside the body, but nicotinic acid in high doses dilates blood vessels, causing a hot "flushing" reaction. Niacinamide doesn't have this side effect.

Q. Is my personal need for a specific vitamin exactly the same as the Recommended Dietary Allowance for that vitamin?

A. Some experts say your personal requirement for a certain vitamin is the minimum intake needed to prevent the symptoms of deficiency. Others argue that it is the amount needed not just to prevent disease, but to ensure *optimal* health. In some cases, your needs may actually be lower than the RDA, because the RDAs are set higher than average requirements. On the other hand, your requirements might be higher—depending on your condition and habits. (See "Special Nutrient Needs" earlier in this chapter.)

Q. Is there an easy way to swallow vitamins?

A. Try washing tablets down with milk or juice instead of water. If you're having trouble swallowing capsules, take a sip and bend forward at the waist instead of throwing your head back. The capsule's buoyancy will help it float toward your throat. Or try a chewable tablet. They're as potent as regular capsules or tablets, but obviously easier to swallow.

45

WEIGHT LOSS

The United States is one of the most affluent countries in the world. Not surprisingly, then, it is also one of the chubbiest: 64 percent of the populace is overweight, according to a 1988 Harris poll conducted for *Prevention* magazine. While some of us need to lose just a few pounds, more than a third of us tip the scales at 10 percent or more above our ideal weight. For a woman who should weigh 120, for example, that's at least 12 pounds of excess fat. Or 16 extra pounds in a man who should weigh in at 160. And despite the many diet and fitness regimens in the news, Americans are growing pudgier every year.

Who are more overweight, men or women? If you guessed women, guess again. More women than men *believe* they are overweight, but more men actually *are* overweight—71 percent overweight compared to 58 percent. Yet women are more likely than men to be on a diet.

Overweight varies between social groups, too. People who work in blue-collar jobs and those who earn middle-class incomes are more likely to carry around extra pounds than professionals who pull in salaries over $50,000.

Excess weight isn't evenly spread across the country. Although about a quarter of all Americans maintain the weight that's right for their height and build, people in some parts of the country are plumper—or leaner—than in others. Among urban areas surveyed in the *Prevention* poll, Philadelphia has the portliest populace, with only 18 percent falling within a normal weight range. Squeezing in for a tight second are Chicagoans, among whom a slim 19 percent maintain proper weight. At the opposite end of the scale are residents of Los Angeles, where 27 percent keep their weight in line. But if the rest of us had to look good in a bathing suit ten months out of the year, we'd probably try harder to stay trim, too.

Seven Ways Excess Weight Can Be Hazardous to Your Health

Pudgy people are taking fat chances with their health, medical experts warn. Being just 10 percent overweight decreases a man's life expectancy by 11 percent and a woman's by 7 percent. Being 20 percent or more overweight can drop one's life expectancy even more. Medical conditions related to obesity that can impinge on your health in a big way include:

1. Increased risk of high blood pressure.

2. Increased risk of heart enlargement due to high blood pressure.

3. Higher blood cholesterol levels.

4. Increased risk of heart attacks.

5. Diabetes, a disease which, though probably inherited, can often be delayed or averted by weight control.

6. Increased incidence of colon and prostate cancers in men, and breast and uterine cancers in women.

7. Increased risk of osteoarthritis, which can be triggered by excess stress on weight-bearing joints.

Compared with normal-weight people of the same age, overweight people aged 45 to 74 are twice as likely to have high blood pressure. And overweight people aged 20 to 44 are *five* times more likely to have pressure problems.

Is That A Fact?

Excess weight doesn't always mean excess fat.

True. A person can be overweight according to ordinary standards without being obese. It is the presence of excess body fat rather than weight per se that determines obesity. A 250-pound football player, for instance, who is technically overweight for his six-foot height may be mostly muscle, with a below-average amount of body fat. On the other hand, a smaller person whose weight falls within a normal range may actually be obese if an inactive lifestyle had led to small muscle mass and excess fat.

And You Think *You* Gain Weight Quickly

The heaviest man in medical history, Jon Brower Minnoch (1941–1983) of Bainbridge Island, Washington, was estimated to have weighed more than 1,400 pounds, according to the *Guinness Book of World Records*. After spending two years on a hospital diet, he was discharged at 476 pounds. He had to be readmitted, however, *having reportedly gained 200 pounds in seven days.*

How the States Rank in Weight Control

Of the 21 most populated states in the United States, Minnesota is in the best shape weight-wise, while Missouri fares the worst. The numbers shown on the map indicate the percentage of each state's population that maintains proper weight. The list summarizes the relative rankings for each state. (Some states share ranks because equal percentages of their populations maintain proper weight.)

1. Minnesota
2. Georgia
3. Tennessee
4. California
4. Massachusetts
4. Texas
5. Florida
5. Virginia
5. Wisconsin
6. Indiana
6. New Jersey
6. New York
6. North Carolina
6. Ohio
7. Louisiana
7. Maryland
7. Michigan
7. Pennsylvania
7. Washington
8. Illinois
9. Missouri

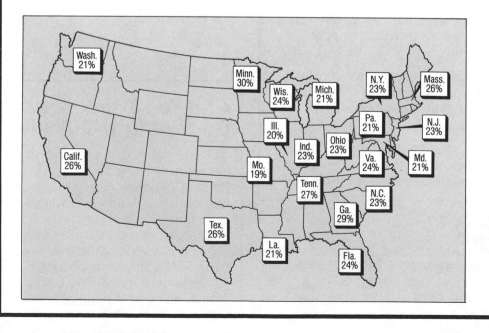

The Ideal Fertility Weight

A svelte figure may slim a would-be mother's chances of becoming pregnant, says G. William Bates, M.D., former professor of obstetrics and gynecology at the Medical University of South Carolina. Fashionably slender women seem to have a disproportionately high incidence of unexplained infertility, says Dr. Bates. In his studies, women who reached their ideal weight range —some by losing weight, many by gaining it—increased their pregnancy success rates. For best results, he advises a woman to weigh within the ideal range shown on this table for six to nine months before attempting to become pregnant.

Height*	Ideal Weight†
4'10"	109–121
4'11"	111–123
5'0"	113–126
5'1"	115–129
5'2"	118–132
5'3"	121–135
5'4"	124–138
5'5"	127–141
5'6"	130–144
5'7"	133–147
5'8"	136–150
5'9"	139–153
5'10"	142–156
5'11"	145–159
6'0"	148–162

*With 1" heels
†Includes 3 lb. for clothes

Prejudice by the Pound

Overweight people are the victims of many forms of social discrimination. Studies have shown, for instance, that:

▼ Children as young as six years old who are shown silhouettes of obese children describe them as lazy, dirty, stupid, ugly, and dishonest.

▼ Obese high school students have lower acceptance rates into prestigious colleges compared with normal-weight students, even when they have the same academic qualifications.

▼ Employers rate overweight people as less desirable employees than normal-weight people, even when they believe the two groups have the same abilities. In one survey, 16 percent of employers said they would not hire obese women under any condition, and an additional 44 percent said they would not hire them under certain circumstances.

▼ Being overweight can lead to being underpaid. In one study of MBA graduates, overweight men's starting salaries averaged more than $2,000 less than those of their counterparts.

▼ The armed services and police and fire departments will not enlist severely overweight people, and often reprimand or discharge people who fail to maintain an acceptable weight.

The Dieting Years

To everything, there is a season. Including, it appears, waging war against excess weight. The likelihood of dieting increases after one's teens and mid-twenties, and peaks in the 50 to 59 age range, according to a national survey conducted by the Calorie Control Council. Most dieters—61 percent—are women.

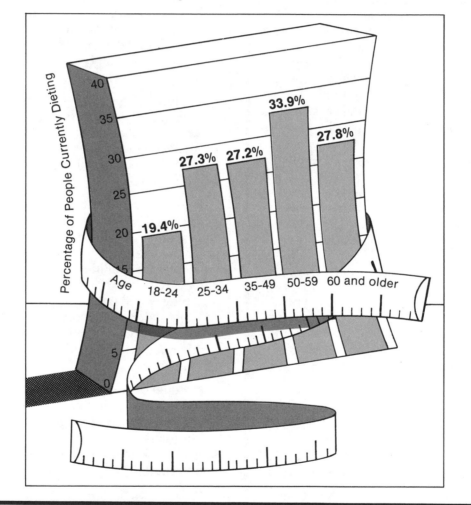

At any given time, an estimated 20 percent of the American population is taking part in some kind of commercial weight-loss program.

Great (and Not So Great) Moments in Weight-Loss History

Late 1700s For the first time, obesity becomes common in Europe, first in elite social groups and then in the rest of society.

Late 1800s Chubby children in the United States are considered to be among the healthiest children in the world.

1879 Saccharin, the first sugar substitute, is discovered. Later it will find favor as an artificial sweetener, especially during the sugar shortages of World Wars I and II.

1880–1920 Major weight-loss fads in the United States include fasting, thyroid medications to "speed up" metabolism, and "Fletcherism," which requires slowly chewing each bite of food many times.

Around 1900 The first "obesity tablets" come on the market. One of them, Phytolacca, contains arsenic and strychnine, among other ingredients. Various reducing soaps, ointments, powders, pastes, oils, and juices promise to sweep fat from the outside of the body.

1930s The bathroom scale arrives in America, and soon every affluent and middle-income household has one.

1937 The noncaloric sweetener cyclamate is discovered.

1938 A diet drug called dinitrophenol, which speeds up the metabolism, is taken off the market after having sped several dieters to their deaths.

1950–early 1970s Amphetamines, which hasten the metabolism and suppress appetite but which later prove unhealthy and addictive, are widely prescribed for weight loss. Pharmacists dispense as many as 2 billion amphetamine pills to U.S. dieters in 1970.

1950s Physicians begin to perform intestinal bypass surgery on the morbidly obese as an aid to weight loss.

1970 After being used widely as an artifical sweetener through the 1960s, cyclamate is banned in the United States after rats fed large doses of the substance developed bladder tumors.

1970s Liquid protein diets are introduced and subsequently cause the death of at least 17 dieters, according to the Centers for Disease Control.

1982 Liposuction, the surgical removal of excess fat deposits, makes its debut and quickly becomes one of the most popular forms of plastic surgery in America.

When Dieters Should See a Doctor

Losing a lot of weight can cause its own set of health problems. If you're more than 30 percent overweight, be sure to check in with your doctor for a complete physical before going on a diet. A check-up is also important *after* you've lost a lot of weight. See a doctor, too, if you're taking medications for high blood pressure, diabetes, or other health problems while you diet. They may require an adjustment in dosage as the pounds come off.

Who Wins at Losing?

Joining a diet program like Weight Watchers is one thing, succeeding at it quite another. Some participants, studies have shown, do better than others.

▼ Married women lose more weight than single women.

▼ Women over 30 lose more weight than women under 30.

▼ Women who attend a group regularly and adhere to the diet strictly lose more weight than those who don't.

▼ Women with higher initial weights and those who have not previously belonged to a group do best.

▼ Participants who reach their recommended weight maintain their losses better than those who do not reach their goal.

A Growing Appetite

The average American teenager eats 1,817 pounds of food in a single year. This is equivalent in weight to a total of 474 Big Macs, 349 Whoppers with cheese, 286 frozen pizzas, 726 hot dogs, 210 peanut-butter-and-jelly sandwiches, 159 banana splits, 600 doughnuts, 200 boxes of Cap'n Crunch cereal, 1,271 chocolate sandwich cookies, 340 Twinkies, 188 packages of M&M's, 690 Hershey bars, 129 Fudgsicles, 47 gallons of chocolate ice cream, 1,178 Reese's peanut butter cups, and one serving of home-cooked meat loaf, mashed potatoes, and spinach.

Total number of editorial pages that eight of the leading American women's magazines in America devoted in 1989 to the subject of weight loss: 437.

Total number of pages in the same magazines devoted to the subject of food: 2,356.

The Facts about Diet Pills

▼ People who rely on diet pills for weight loss usually gain the weight back as soon as they stop taking the pills.

▼ The more of any diet pill you take, the more you risk side effects, which can include high blood pressure, headaches, seizures, nausea, irritability, sleep disturbances, and a feeling of being crazed.

▼ Amphetamines have long comprised one major category of prescription-only diet drugs. They suppress the appetite but are not effective over a long period of time and have serious side effects, including addiction. Doctors today are more likely to prescribe fenfluramine, which seems to suppress the appetite by releasing serotonin, a brain chemical that inhibits the body's "feeding-reward" system but which may also make you sleepy. Drugs are generally prescribed only for patients for whom other weight-loss therapies have been unsuccessful.

▼ No small number of over-the-counter diet drugs prove to be fraudulent, yet their sales comprise a multimillion-dollar industry. One mail-order diet pill company alone collected more than $1.6 million from 30,000 customers in a single mailing, according to the National Council against Health Fraud.

▼ A review of 100 over-the-counter diet drug ingredients by an advisory panel of the Food and Drug Administration concluded that only two were possibly safe and effective.

One is phenylpropanolamine (PPA), an ingredient in over-the-counter appetite suppressants such as Acutrim and Dexatrim. Some scientific evidence suggests that it works by stimulating the part of the brain that says you're full. A person taking drugs containing PPA, advises one diet expert, should follow the instructions carefully and use only before a tempting meal that might derail the diet, rather than on a regular basis.

The other is benzocaine, the ingredient in Ayds candy. A topical anesthetic that numbs taste buds, it supposedly makes sweets less appetizing. A few studies indicate it may indeed help some people lose weight.

▼ The effectiveness of diet pills varies. According to a study from Michigan State University, 86 percent of women who used over-the-counter products that contained PPA said it was not effective over the long run, had limited or no appetite-suppressant effect, or was totally ineffective.

A Guide to Weight-Loss Surgery

Surgery as an aid to weight loss has been performed for more than 30 years. But these very serious forms of surgery aren't for everyone, says Charles Yale, M.D., professor of surgery at the University of Wisconsin Medical School. Patients considering surgery must meet certain criteria, he says. First, they should be morbidly obese, or at least 100 pounds over their ideal weight. (Weights over this level are life-threatening.) Furthermore, they must have repeatedly tried and failed to lose weight on conventional diets or with the aid of a physician. Finally, they should have no serious medical or psychiatric problems that can complicate surgery.

Type of Surgery	Procedure	Effectiveness	Possible Complications
Intestinal bypass	In this oldest form of weight-loss surgery, a section of the small intestine is closed off so that food bypasses it. The calories are not totally absorbed by the body. An estimated 150,000 people have had this surgery.	Produced excellent loss, says one expert, in a group of patients operated on between 1972 and 1976, but the procedure has serious complications and has been largely abandoned.	Cirrhosis of the liver, malnutrition with serious vitamin and mineral deficiencies, kidney stones, arthritis. As many as 74,000 patients have developed life-threatening complications, 44,000 have liver malfunctions, and 31,000 have recurring kidney stones.
Stomach stapling	This is actually a group of different procedures—including gastric bypass and gastroplasty—in which a tiny artificial stomach is created out of a portion of the original stomach, often through the use of a staple gun. These operations cause weight loss by limiting food intake. No more than a few mouthfuls can be eaten without vomiting. An estimated 300,000 people may have had this surgery.	Five years after gastric bypass, the average patient has lost almost one-third of his or her original weight, one surgeon reports. Fewer than 15% of the operations are failures, he says. In a review of 6,000 cases, however, another surgeon found that more than 50% of patients failed to lose even 15% of their initial weight. One study showed that 75% of surviving patients regained all weight lost.	Infections at site of surgery, cancer, anemia, lung collapse, osteoporosis, kidney and urinary infections, liver and gallbladder diseases.
Gastric balloon	A cylindrical plastic balloon is placed in the stomach within a plastic tube. The balloon is then inflated and the tube removed. The balloon automatically seals closed and is left to	One study reported that 97 of 100 patients reported decreased appetite. The average weight reduction was 40 pounds after 6 months and 76 pounds after 10 months. In another	Gastric ulcers, gastric erosions, partial gastric obstruction. In one study 9% of the balloons deflated spontaneously, and in one patient a deflated balloon passed into the

Type of Surgery	Procedure	Effectiveness	Possible Complications
	float freely in the stomach. More than 20,000 balloons have been inserted.	study, however, no significant difference was reported between amount of weight lost with the balloon or without it.	intestine and obstructed the bowel.
Jaw wiring	The patient's teeth are fastened together to limit the intake of most nonliquid foods.	May be helpful in the short-term for patients who are not good at dieting. However, in many cases, weight lost is regained once the wires are removed unless the person continues a low-calorie diet.	Shifts in tooth position, gum disease, promotion of tooth decay, and danger of inhaling sputum or other substances into the lungs.
Liposuction	In this popular form of plastic surgery, (more than 99,000 liposuctions were performed in the United States in 1986 alone), deposits of excess fat are dislodged with a metal straw inserted beneath the skin. A suction machine then vacuums up the fat. Liposuction differs from other diet surgeries because ideally it is performed on people of normal weight or those who are only minimally overweight. Candidates are disproportionately heavy in certain areas, such as the thighs or hips.	Because only 1 or 2 pounds of fat are removed per procedure per site, body weight is not appreciably affected. Those fat cells that are removed are permanently gone, though fat cells remaining can increase in size if the person gains weight.	Permanent discoloration of the skin, dents, temporary bruising, swelling and numbness in the treated area, blood clots, infections, and shock.

Weight Loss Doesn't Buy Love

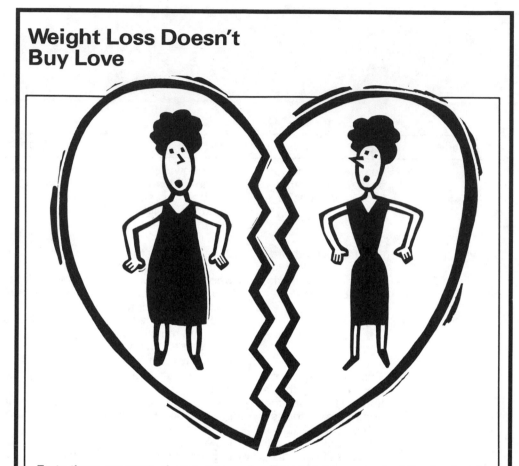

Forty-three percent of one group of patients were motivated to have weight-loss surgery out of a desire to become more attractive to their partner or spouse.

Five out of six of those did so because they feared that their obesity threatened the continuation of their marriage.

Following weight loss, nearly all the patients felt more attractive and interested in sex. However, the interest was frequently not reciprocated.

Twenty-one percent of the husbands of female patients became impotent and an additional 35 percent reported a "cooling of interest."

Thirty-six percent of the spouses, both male and female, had extramarital affairs following their spouses' weight loss.

Seventeen to 21 percent of patients become divorced or separated within the first two years after the surgery.

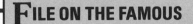

FILE ON THE FAMOUS

Too-Thin Stars
of the Silver Screen

Ultrathin movie stars and models are constantly paraded before us as the epitome of attractive femininity. But the walking-clothes-hanger look is not a healthy goal. Singer Karen Carpenter took obsession with thinness to extremes, descending into anorexia nervosa and dying in 1983 at age 33.

The more things change, the more they stay the same. The fat/thin obsession is not a new one. As long as 60 years ago physical culturist Bernarr Macfadden was warning against "The Menace of Skinny Movie Stars" in his health magazine *Physical Culture*. "Where are the strong, free-limbed goddesses to whom the old Greeks so wisely paid homage?" the magazine lamented in a September 1930 article. Replaced by the scrawny likes of 5-foot, 5-inch, 115-pound Mary Astor, 16 pounds underweight according to the magazine's calculations—as were Joan Crawford and Janet Gaynor. Apparently Mary Nolan was out to drive Macfadden mad: She weighed 23 pounds less than she should have for her 5-foot, 6-inch frame. Greta Garbo was 5 feet, 7 inches and should have tipped the scales at 139 pounds, 14 pounds more than her working weight.

Macfadden blamed the requirements of Hollywood contracts for the skinny binge. "No good can come of it" for actors or for the majority of young women who aren't actors but aspire to look like them, the magazine warned.

"Our womanhood . . . are ruining their health with ill-advised, get-thin-quick diets," the article thundered. "The craze for the boyish form is indeed far-reaching. Like an evil octopus it reaches out its tentacles and survives on the natural beauty and health it consumes."

One actress who fought with the studios over her weight, Nita Naldi, was quoted as saying, "I have hips and I have breasts where God meant a woman to have them." The article held her up as an example of "sturdy health and super-womanhood." In contrast to Jeanne Eagels, who had a "frail physique and underweight conditon" and "suffered a complete breakdown and premature death."

Naldi had to move to a less-finicky Europe to continue her career. And 60 years later, too many American women still consider themselves fat failures if they aren't as thin as the models men drool over in commercials.

Food Choices:
The Fat and the Lean

Help yourself and your figure by developing an awareness of the fat content of some common foods.

High-Fat Foods

For effective weight loss, steer clear of these and other foods with a high percentage of their calories coming from fat.

Low-Fat Foods

Make foods from this list part of your low-fat weight-loss plan.

Food	Percentage of Calories from Fat
Oil	100.0
Butter	99.1
Mayonnaise	98.3
Margarine	98.2
Creamy dressing	88.8
Cream, light	87.9
Cream cheese	87.8
Sour cream	85.2
Frankfurter, beef	82.2
Pepperoni	80.8
Avocado	79.5
Walnuts	79.0
Liverwurst	78.5
Bacon, broiled or fried	77.5
Almonds	75.9
Pork, blade roll, cured	73.7
Cheese, cheddar	72.5
Peanuts, roasted, salted	71.3

Food	Percentage of Calories from Fat
Apple cider	trace
Raisins, seedless	1.3
Acorn squash	1.5
Peach, fresh	1.8
Bread, Italian	2.0
Grapefruit	2.7
Macaroni, cooked	3.1
Kidney beans, cooked	3.5
Milk, skim	4.5
Turkey breast	4.9
Tuna, canned in water	5.6
Apricots, fresh	6.7
English muffin	7.3
Nectarine	7.7
Watermelon	11.3
Oatmeal	13.9
Lobster, broiled	14.2
Saltines	20.8

More than 1 million people participate in weight-loss groups each week, but fewer than 20 percent stay in programs long enough to lose an appreciable amount of weight.

What Makes a Food "Light"?

The designation of a food or beverage as "light" or "lite" can mean several things.

▼ Light meat or poultry must have 25 percent fewer calories than regular versions.

▼ Other types of food have to have 33 percent fewer calories in their light versions.

▼ Light beer typically has 20 percent fewer calories than the producer's regular brew.

To make matters more confusing, in some cases "light" or "lite" means the product is light in color or weight, such as "lite pears," though not necessarily low in calories.

A Long List of Lights

No fewer than 454 new food and beverage products labeled "low," "light," or "natural" (another inexact term) were introduced during the first six months of 1987 alone.

Foods and beverages marketed in light versions at a typical grocery store include, but are not limited to:

American cheese, apple juice, bacon, baked apple rolls, beefsteak burritos, beer, black cherry soda, borscht, breakfast cereal, breakfast ham, broccoli and cheese baked potato, brown rice pilaf, canned peaches, canned pears, canned green beans, cheesecake, cheese cannelloni, cheese enchiladas, cheese pizza, chicken cacciatore, chicken à la king, chicken fettucini, chili, chocolate candy, chocolate chip cookies, chocolate milk, chocolate mousse, corn chips, corn oil, cottage cheese, cream of mushroom soup, crispbread, custard, dill pickles, dips, dried fruit, fish fillets, French bread pizza, fruit cocktail, fruit juice bars, gefilte fish, gelatin desserts, grape jelly, gravy, gum, ham, hard candy, hot chocolate, hog dogs, ice cream, instant breakfast, Italian bread, ketchup, lemon cake, linguine with clam sauce, lunch meat, margarine, matzohs, mayonnaise, milk, milk shakes, mints, orange juice, Oriental beef with vegetables and rice, pasta primavera, pancake mix, peanut butter, peanut butter cups, popcorn, pork and beans, potato bread, potato chips, pudding, raspberry jam, ricotta cheese, roasted peanuts, rye bread, salad dressings, Salisbury steak, sardines, sausage, scalloped potatoes and ham, seltzer water, sesame sticks, sherbet, sliced turkey breast in mushroom sauce, soup stocks, spaghetti sauce, stuffed cabbage with meat, swiss cheese, syrup, tuna, turkey divan, vanilla wafers, veal marsala, vegetable juice, wheat bread, whipped topping, white sauce, wine, yogurt, and zucchini lasagna. And, yes—dog food.

Fast (and Fattening) Foods

You're probably best off limiting fast-food forays if you're aiming to lose weight, because calorie and fat content run high.

Foods	Calories	Percentage of Calories as Fat
Breakfast		
Roy Rogers Pancake Platter w/sausage	608	43
Burger King Croissan'wich w/sausage	538	69
McDonald's Biscuit w/sausage and egg	529	60
Burger King Great Danish	500	65
Burger King French Toast Sticks	499	52
Roy Rogers Pancake Platter w/syrup, butter	452	30
Roy Rogers Breakfast Crescent w/sausage	449	58
Roy Rogers Breakfast Crescent w/bacon	431	61
McDonald's Hotcakes w/butter and syrup	413	20
Roy Rogers Breakfast Crescent	401	61
McDonald's Apple Danish	389	39
McDonald's Sausage McMuffin	372	51
Wendy's Breakfast Sandwich	370	46
Burger King Croissan'wich	304	56
McDonald's Egg McMuffin	293	34
Wendy's Omelet w/eggs, ham, cheese, and mushrooms	250	61
Roy Rogers Apple Danish	249	40
Chicken		
Burger King Specialty Chicken Sandwich	688	52
Wendy's Chicken Club	509	47
Arby's Chicken Breast Sandwich	509	51
Arby's Turkey Deluxe	375	38
Roy Rogers Chicken Breast	324	50
McDonald's Chicken McNuggets	288	50
Roy Rogers Chicken Thigh	282	60
Burger King Chicken Tenders	204	44
Roy Rogers Chicken Wing	142	57
Roy Rogers Chicken Leg	117	46
Fish		
Arby's Fish Filet Sandwich	580	48
Burger King Whaler Sandwich	488	49
McDonald's Filet-O-Fish	442	52
Hamburgers/cheeseburgers		
Burger King Whopper w/cheese	711	54

Foods	Calories	Percentage of Calories as Fat
McDonald's McDLT	674	56
Burger King Whopper	628	51
Roy Rogers RR-Bar Burger	611	57
McDonald's Big Mac	562	51
McDonald's Quarter Pounder w/Cheese	517	50
Burger King Bacon Double Cheeseburger	510	54
Roy Rogers Hamburger	456	55
McDonald's Quarter Pounder	414	43
Wendy's Hamburger, multigrain bun	350	43
Wendy's Hamburger, white bun	350	41
Burger King Whopper Jr.	322	47
McDonald's Cheeseburger	308	37
Burger King Hamburger	275	39
McDonald's Hamburger	257	31

Salads

Foods	Calories	Percentage of Calories as Fat
Taco Bell Taco Salad w/dressing	1,167	66
Taco Bell Taco Light Platter	1,062	49
Taco Bell Seafood Salad, no dressing	648	56
Taco Bell Taco Salad, no shell	524	32
Wendy's Taco Salad w/taco sauce	440	38
McDonald's Chef's Salad	231	50
McDonald's Chicken Salad Oriental	141	19
McDonald's Garden Salad	112	48

Roast beef

Foods	Calories	Percentage of Calories as Fat
Arby's Bac n' Cheddar Deluxe Roast Beef	526	61
Arby's Super Roast Beef	501	39
Arby's King Roast Beef	467	36
Roy Rogers Roast Beef w/cheese, large	467	38
Arby's Beef n' Cheddar	455	51
Roy Rogers Roast Beef w/cheese, regular	424	40
Roy Rogers Roast Beef, large	360	27
Arby's Regular Roast Beef	353	35
Roy Rogers Roast Beef, regular	317	28
Arby's Junior Roast Beef	218	33

A Whale of an Appetite

A typical blue whale, the largest animal in the world, eats up to 5,000 pounds of krill (a type of shrimp) each day—or 1,825,000 pounds a year. On land, this would be equivalent in weight to an annual order of 1,310,841 Arby's Fish Fillet Sandwiches, 1,943,190 McDonald's Filets-O-Fish, and 1,787,541 Wendy's Fish Fillets—buns, lettuce, and tartar sauce included.

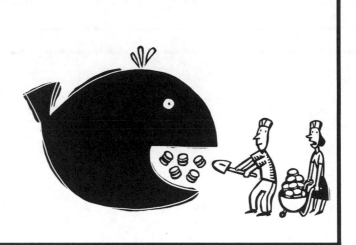

Is THAT A FACT?

Obese people are psychologically unstable.

Several studies have shown that emotional disturbance is no more common among the obese than among normal-weighted persons. In fact, some studies have suggested that the obese actually exhibit less psychopathology than the nonobese.

Overweight is glandular.

Experts estimate that no more than 5 percent of obesity problems are attributable to glandular, chromosomal, or metabolic dysfunctions.

Your stomach shrinks while you diet.

Your stomach doesn't get smaller or larger, says one expert, but is like a crumpled paper bag that can change shape to accommodate more food. When you eat less, you feel full faster because your stomach is still in the crumpled-up state.

Exercise increases an overweight person's appetite.

Several studies have found that exercise does not make you hungrier. One study of overweight women, for instance, found that they continued to consume the same amount of calories no matter how sedentary or active they were, though of course they *burned* more calories when they were active.

Exercising in a plastic suit accelerates weight loss.

The suit makes you sweat so you lose water weight, but you regain it the instant you drink or eat after your exercise session. Plastic sweatsuits can be dangerous, by the way. The danger of heatstroke, especially in hot weather, is very real.

Still Sweet on Sugar

Artificial sweeteners were supposed to serve as low-calorie substitutes for sugar, but they haven't put a dent in America's craving for the real thing. Per capita consumption of the substitutes in 1988 was more than three times what it was in 1975, yet the average American still managed to consume 15.6 more pounds of caloric sweeteners than he did in 1975. Actually, Americans do eat less refined sugar than they used to, but they compensate with more corn sugar sweeteners, which have become common ingredients in canned fruits, jellies, candy, and baked goods.

Consumption per Person (lb.)	Year					
	1975	1978	1980	1983	1985	1988
Sugar, refined	89.2	91.4	83.6	71.1	63.3	62.8
Corn sweeteners	27.5	33.7	40.2	52.2	66.5	69.5
Honey	1.0	1.1	0.8	0.9	1.0	1.0
Syrups	0.4	0.4	0.4	0.4	0.4	0.4
Total caloric sweeteners	118.1	126.6	125.1	124.6	131.2	133.7
Saccharin*	6.1	6.9	7.7	9.5	6.0	6.0
Aspartame*	0.0	0.0	0.0	3.5	12.0	14.0
Total low-calorie sweeteners*	6.1	6.9	7.7	13.0	18.0	20.0
Total of all sweeteners	124.2	133.5	132.8	137.6	149.2	153.7

*Sugar sweetness equivalent, based on saccharin being ounce for ounce 300 times as sweet as sugar and aspartame 200 times as sweet.

Ninety-five percent of all people who lose weight regain it within a year.

The Best Exercises for a Woman's Five Worst Fat Zones

As a woman loses weight, certain key trouble spots—especially the upper arms and breasts—may remain flabby. Other spots tend to be diet-resistant, particularly the abdomen, hips, thighs, and buttocks. In both cases, toning exercises can make all the difference, tightening flaccid tissue, strengthening your muscles, and improving your posture.

Upper Arms

Dumbbell curl. Tone and define your biceps (the large muscle at the front of your upper arm) without enlarging them.

Stand erect and hold a dumbbell (5 pounds or less) in each hand, your arms at your sides with palms facing forward. Slowly bend your arms at the elbows and bring the weights up until they touch your chest. Repeat ten times.

Dumbbell extension. This tones the triceps (the large muscle on the back of the upper arm), reducing flab.

Lie on your back on the floor. With a dumbbell (5 pounds or less) in each hand, raise your straightened arms directly overhead to a position perpendicular to your body. Then slowly lower the weights toward your chest, bending your elbows. You can work both arms simultaneously or one at a time. Repeat ten times.

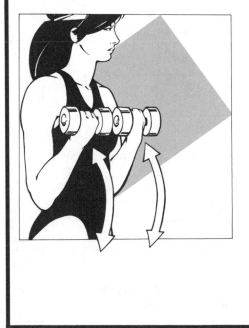

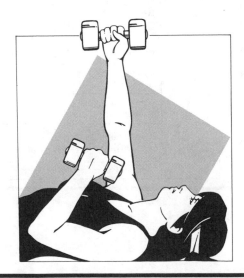

Chest

Dumbbell fly. This is an excellent toning exercise for the pectorals, the muscles underlying your breasts.

Lie on your back on the floor and hold a dumbbell (5 pounds or less) in each hand. Hold the dumbbells directly over your chest with your arms straight, palms facing each other. Then, keeping your arms straight, slowly lower the weights to the floor on each side of you so your body forms a cross. Now, bring the weights to the upright position again. Repeat 10 times, gradually working up to 20 repetitions.

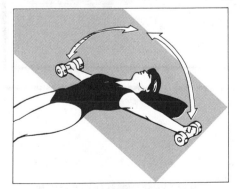

Abdomen

Crunch sit-up. This exercise helps flatten your stomach by firming the underlying abdominal muscles.

Lie on the floor with your knees bent. Don't anchor your feet. Cross your arms on your chest, tighten your abdomen, and slowly raise your upper body halfway until your shoulder blades clear the floor. Hold for five counts, release. Repeat 15 times or until your muscles tire.

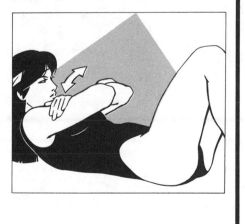

(continued)

The Best Exercises for a Woman's Five Worst Fat Zones – *Continued*

Hips and Thighs

Hydrants. This exercise strengthens the muscles along the side of your hips and minimizes fatty deposits there.

Get down on your hands and knees. Your hands should be positioned directly under your shoulders; your knees should be hip width apart. Lift your right knee to the side at about shoulder height, straighten your leg, bend your knee again, and return to starting position. Repeat 10 to 15 times. Switch to the left leg for another 10 to 15 reps.

Buttocks

Hydrant variation. These strengthen the gluteus maximus muscles that extend from your hips across your buttocks to the back of your thighs.

Repeat the hydrant position described above. With your right leg extended to the rear, lift to hip level, then return leg to floor. Repeat 10 to 15 times with each leg.

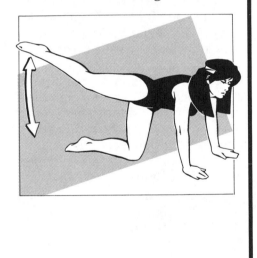

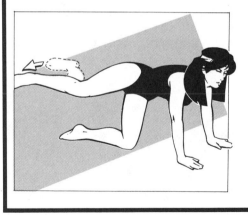

In a study of over 6,000 men, those who watched 3 hours of TV a day were twice as likely to be obese as those who watched less than 1 hour.

Workouts That Burn Off Weight

A regular program of exercise —at least 30 minutes a day three times a week—helps you lose weight faster and more consistently than if you're only cutting back on food calories. But be aware that the more pounds you lose the more efficient your body becomes, and hence the fewer calories you burn during a workout. So you need to exercise more to keep losing weight. The chart shows a number of exercises and their calorie-burning potential, depending on your weight. For best results, strive for an exercise program that burns about 300 calories or more per session.

Exercise	Calories Burned per Hour		
	110 lb.	154 lb.	198 lb.
Martial arts	620	790	960
Racquetball (2 people)	610	775	945
Basketball (full-court game)	585	750	910
Skiing—cross country (5 mph)	550	700	850
downhill	465	595	720
Running—8 min. mile	550	700	850
12 min. mile	515	655	795
Swimming—crawl, 45 yards/min.	540	690	835
crawl, 30 yards/min.	330	420	510
Stationary bicycle—15 mph	515	655	795
Aerobic dancing—intense	515	655	795
moderate	350	445	540
Walking—5 mph	435	555	675
3 mph	235	300	365
2 mph	145	185	225
Calisthenics—intense	435	555	675
moderate	350	445	540
Scuba diving	355	450	550
Hiking—20 lb. pack, 4 mph	355	450	550
20 lb. pack, 2 mph	235	300	365
Tennis—singles, recreational	335	425	520
doubles, recreational	235	300	365
Ice skating	275	350	425
Roller skating	275	350	425

Your Ideal Calorie Intake

Use this chart to calculate how many calories you should eat each day to maintain your ideal weight.

To lose weight, of course, you would need to eat fewer calories.

If You Are ...	And Want to Keep Your Weight at ...	Multiply by ...	For Your Total Daily Calorie Limit
Very inactive (don't exercise)	———————	× 13 =	———————
Mildly inactive (exercise once in a while)	———————	× 14 =	———————
Reasonably active (exercise once or twice a week, walk a fair amount, and put physical energy into the job)	———————	× 15 =	———————
Very active (do aerobic workouts 3–4 hours a week and have a somewhat physically demanding job)	———————	× 17 =	———————
Superactive (training for a marathon or working on a loading dock)	———————	× 21 =	———————

Example: You're reasonably active —you work out two or three times a week and do some walking each day on your job—and want to maintain your weight at 130 pounds. Multiplying 130 by 15 you find your total daily limit of 1950 calories.

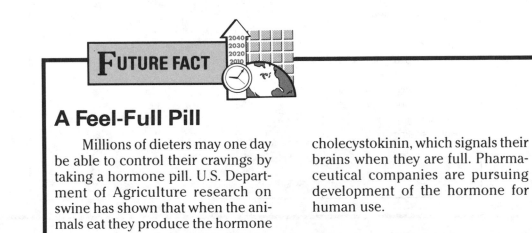

FUTURE FACT

A Feel-Full Pill

Millions of dieters may one day be able to control their cravings by taking a hormone pill. U.S. Department of Agriculture research on swine has shown that when the animals eat they produce the hormone cholecystokinin, which signals their brains when they are full. Pharmaceutical companies are pursuing development of the hormone for human use.

SOURCES

Accidents

Page 2
"Who Dies in Accidents" adapted from *Accident Facts,* National Safety Council, 1988.

Page 2
"Leading Causes of Death" adapted from *Accident Facts,* National Safety Council, 1988.

Page 3
"Men Are at Greater Risk" adapted from *Accident Facts,* National Safety Council, 1988.

Page 4
"Where It Hurts" adapted from *Accident Facts,* National Safety Council, 1988.

Page 5
"Every 4 Seconds" adapted from *Accident Facts,* National Safety Council, 1988.

Page 5
"The Most Dangerous Months" adapted from *Accident Facts,* National Safety Council, 1988.

Page 6
"The Most Dangerous States" adapted from *Accident Facts,* National Safety Council, 1988.

Page 7
"High Risks on the Highway" adapted from *Accident Facts,* National Safety Council, 1988.

Page 8
"Best and Worst Drivers" adapted from *Accident Facts,* National Safety Council, 1988.

Page 9
"How Not to Drive" adapted from *Accident Facts,* National Safety Council, 1988.

Page 9
"High-Risk Holidays" adapted from *Accident Facts,* National Safety Council, 1988.

Page 10
"Accidents at Home" adapted from *Accident Facts,* National Safety Council, 1988.

Page 11
"Is Nothing Safe?" adapted from *Product Summary Report,* U.S. Consumer Product Safety Commission, 1988.

Page 12
"The Dangers of Child's Play" adapted from *Product Summary Report,* U.S. Consumer Product Safety Commission, 1988.

Page 13
"Rating the Workplace" adapted from *News* (Washington, D.C.: U.S. Department of Labor, December 1988).

Page 14
"When Tornadoes Are Most Likely to Strike" adapted from *News* (Washington, D.C.: U.S. Department of Labor, December 1988).

Aging

Page 16
"An Aging Nation" adapted from *Aging America: Trends and Projections* (Washington, D.C.: U.S. Senate Special Committee on Aging, 1988).

Page 17
"Men: Outnumbered and Outlived" adapted from *Aging America: Trends and Projections* (Washington, D.C.: U.S. Senate Special Committee on Aging, 1988).

Page 18
"The Ailments That Come with Age" adapted from *Answers about the Aging Woman* (Washington, D.C.: U.S. Department of Health and Human Services).

Page 18
"Lapse in Lung Power" adapted from *Normal Human Aging,* Nathan W. Shock, et al. (Washington, D.C.: U.S. Department of Health and Human Services, November 1984).

Page 23
"Limitations of the Aged" adapted from *Statistical Abstract of the United States* (Washington, D.C.: U.S. Department of Commerce, 1988).

Page 24
"Where People Fall" adapted from "Fall Injuries among the Elderly: Community-Based Surveillance," *Journal of the American Geriatrics Society,* vol. 36, no. 11, November 1988.

Page 25
"Who Takes Care of the Elderly" adapted from *Aging America: Trends and Projections* (Washington, D.C.: U.S. Senate Special Committee on Aging, 1988).

Page 27
"Slower to React" adapted from *Normal Human Aging,* Nathan W. Shock, et al. (Washington, D.C.: U.S. Department of Health and Human Services, November 1984).

AIDS

Page 31
"AIDS across the Nation" adapted from *HIV/AIDS Surveillance* (Atlanta: Centers for Disease Control, November 1989).

Page 32
"AIDS Rates around the World" adapted from *Update: AIDS Cases Reported to Surveillance, Forecasting, and Impact Assessment Unit,* World Health Organization, October 1, 1989.

Page 34
"The AIDS Iceberg" adapted from *Report of the Surgeon General's Workshop on Children with HIV Infection and Their Families* (Washington, D.C.: U.S. Department of Health and Human Services, 1987).

Page 35
"AIDS Incidence Rising in the New Decade" adapted from *Global AIDS into the 1990s,* V International Conference on AIDS (Montreal: World Health Organization, June 4, 1989).

Page 36
"The Symptoms of Infection" adapted from "Characterization of the Acute Clinical Illness Associated with Human Immuno-deficiency Virus Infection," *Archives of Internal Medicine,* vol. 148, April 1988.

Page 37
"What's Your Risk of HIV Infection?" adapted from "Preventing the Heterosexual Spread of AIDS," *Journal of the American Medical Association,* vol. 259, no. 16, April 22–29, 1988.

Alcohol

Page 39
"Most Drinks Pack the Same Punch" adapted from *Family Medical Guide* (New York: American Medical Association, 1987).

Page 41
"What to Expect from That Next Drink" adapted from *Family Medical Guide* (New York: American Medical Association, 1987).

Page 42
"Worldwide Alcohol Use" data provided by Fred Stinson, Ph.D., affiliated with the National Institute of Alcohol Abuse and Alcoholism, telephone interview, November 28, 1989.

Page 43
"Where Americans Drink the Most . . . and Least" adapted from *Quick Facts,* National Institute of Alcohol Abuse and Alcoholism, 1989.

Page 44
"How Alcohol Harms Society" adapted from Donatelle, et al., *Access to Health* (Englewood Cliffs, N.J.: Prentice Hall, 1988; and from *Disease Prevention/Health Promotion: The Facts,* U.S. Department of Health and Human Services (Palo Alto, Calif.: Bull Publishing Company, 1988).

Allergies and Asthma

Page 46
"Who's Allergic to What" adapted from *News and Notes,* vol. 86, no. 3 (Milwaukee, Wis.: The American Academy of Allergy and Immunology, Winter 1986).

Page 47
"An Insect Sting Can Be Fatal" adapted from *Insect Allergy* (Washington, D.C.: U.S. Department of Health and Human Services, 1981).

Page 51
"A Bath for Your Stuffy Nose" adapted from "Effects of Inhaled Humidified Warm Air on Nasal Patency and Nasal Symptoms in Allergic Rhinitis," *Annals of Allergy,* vol. 60, no. 3, March 1988.

Page 53
"Asthma Deaths on the Upswing" adapted from "Mortality from Asthma, 1979–1984," *Journal of Allergy and Clinical Immunology,* vol. 82, no. 5, part 1, November 1988.

Page 54
"What Triggers Asthma" adapted from *Understanding Asthma,* National Jewish Center for Immunology and Respiratory Medicine, 1985.

Angina
Page 56
"Who Has Angina?" adapted from *Current Estimates from the National Health Interview Survey, United States 1987* (Hyattsville, Md.: U.S. Department of Health and Human Services, September 1988).

Page 56
"When Angina Is Most Likely to Strike" from "Frequency of ST-Segment Depression Produced by Mental Stress in Stable Angina Pectoris from Coronary Artery Disease," *American Journal of Cardiology,* vol. 61, no. 15, June 1, 1988.

Page 57
"Where Do They Live?" from *Current Estimates from the National Health Interview Survey, United States 1987* (Hyattsville, Md.: U.S. Department of Health and Human Services, September 1988).

Page 58
"The Hostile Heart" adapted from "Hostility as a Risk Factor for Mortality and Ischemic Heart Disease in Men," *Psychosomatic Medicine,* vol. 50, no. 4, July–August 1988.

Page 60
"Can Aspirin Block a Heart Attack?" from "Aspirin, Heparin, or Both to Treat Acute Unstable Angina," *The New England Journal of Medicine,* vol. 319, no. 17, October 27, 1988.

Page 61
"High-Tech Treatments Are on the Rise" from *1989 Heart Facts* (Dallas, Tex.: American Heart Association).

Page 62
"How Safe Is Coronary Bypass Surgery?" from "Changing Controversies in Surgery for Angina," *British Journal of Hospital Medicine,* vol. 39, no. 1, January 1988.

Page 62
"How Safe Is Balloon Surgery?" from "Percutaneous Transluminal Coronary Angioplasty in 1985–1986 and 1977–1981," *The New England Journal of Medicine,* vol. 318, no. 5, February 4, 1988.

Page 63
"Fish Oil Prevents Repeat Treatment" from "Reduction in the Rate of Early Restenosis after Coronary Angioplasty by a Diet Supplemented with n-3 Fatty Acids," *The New England Journal of Medicine,* vol. 319, no. 12, September 22, 1988.

Arthritis
Page 65
"The Major Types of Arthritis" adapted from "Living with Arthritis," *Newsweek,* March 20, 1989.

Page 66
"The Price We Pay for Arthritis" adapted from *The Upjohn Arthritis Report,* Ansaid Tablets/Arthritis Survey (Kalamazoo, Mich.: The Upjohn Co., 1986).

Page 67
"Where Osteoarthritis Strikes" adapted from *Understanding Arthritis* (New York: Arthritis Foundation, 1984).

Page 68
"Where Rheumatoid Arthritis Strikes" adapted from *Understanding Arthritis* (New York: Arthritis Foundation, 1984).

Page 72
"The Most Popular Pain Relief Remedies" adapted from *The Upjohn Arthritis Report,* Ansaid Tablets/Arthritis Survey (Kalamazoo, Mich.: The Upjohn Co., 1986); and from *Getting Maximum Good from Arthritis Drugs,"* vol. 40, no. 10, October 1988.

Back Problems
Page 75
"Where You Live Affects Your Back" adapted from *Vital and Health Statistics, Current Estimates from the National Health Interview Survey, 1988* (Hyattsville, Md.: National Center for Health Statistics, October 1989).

Page 77
"The Pressures of Everyday Life" adapted from *The Fit Back* (Alexandria, Va.: Time-Life Books, 1988).

Page 78
"Who Gets a Sprained Back?" adapted from *The Frequency of Occurrence, Impact, and Cost of Selected Musculoskeletal Conditions in the United States* (Chicago: American Academy of Orthopedic Surgeons, 1984).

Page 79
"Getting Back to Work" adapted from "A Prospective Two-Year Study of Functional Restoration in Industrial Low Back Injury," *Journal of the American Medical Association,* vol. 258, no. 13, October 2, 1987.

Page 80
"What You're Most Likely to Be Doing When You Sprain Your Back" adapted from *Back Injuries Associated with Lifting* (Washington, D.C.: U.S. Department of Labor, August 1982).

Page 82
"Back Pain Relief—Who's Got the Knack?" adapted from *Backache Relief,* Klein and Sobel (New York: Times Books, a division of Random House, 1985).

Page 83
"Fit Backs Don't Get Hurt" adapted from *The Fit Back* (Alexandria, Va.: Time-Life Books, 1988).

Body Cycles
Page 88
"A Headache for All Seasons" adapted from "Seasonal and Meteorological Factors in Primary Headaches," *Headache,* vol. 28, no. 2, March 1988.

Page 89
"When Should You Get a Tooth Filled?" adapted from *The Timing of Biological Clocks,* Arthur T. Winfree (New York: Scientific American Books, Inc., 1987).

Page 89
"A Year in the Life of Vitamin D" adapted from "Vitamin D Status of the Elderly in Relation to Age and Exposure to Sunlight," *Human Nutrition: Clinical Nutrition,* vol. 38C, no. 2, March 1984.

Page 90
"Do You Really Have a Fever?" adapted from *The Timing of Biological Clocks,* Arthur T. Winfree (New York: Scientific American Books, Inc., 1987).

Page 90
"The Most Dangerous Drink of the Night" adapted from *The Rhythms of Life,* Edward S. Ayensu, et al. (New York: Crown Publishers, Inc., 1982).

Page 91
"Where People Are Sad" adapted from "From Diet to Jobs, to Sex, How Seasons Affect Mood and Behavior," *Washington Post,* February 28, 1989.

Page 92
"When Hearts Beat Fastest" adapted from *The Rhythms of Life,* Edward S. Ayensu, et al. (New York: Crown Publishers, Inc., 1982).

Page 92
"Some Mornings Can Kill You" adapted from "Circadian Variation in the Frequency of Sudden Cardiac Death," *Circulation,* vol. 75, no. 1, January 1987.

Page 93
"The Highs and Lows of Cholesterol" adapted from "Seasonal Cholesterol Cycles: The Lipid Research Clinic's Coronary Primary Prevention Trial Placebo Group," *Circulation,* vol. 76, no. 6, December 1987.

Bone Health
Page 95
"Who Gets Osteoporosis?" adapted from *Osteoporosis* (Bethesda, Md.: National Institute of Arthritis and Musculoskeletal and Skin Diseases, May 1986).

Page 96
"Which Bones Break Most Often" adapted from "Osteoporosis: A Decade's Findings in Prevention, Diagnosis, and Treatment," *The Female Patient,* vol. 11, September 1986.

Page 99
"Where Were You When You Broke Your Hip?" adapted from *The Frequency of Occurrence, Impact, and Cost of Selected Musculoskeletal Conditions in the United States* (Chicago: American Academy of Orthopaedic Surgeons, 1984).

Page 101
"How Exercise Can Mineralize Your Bones" adapted from "Weight-Bearing Exercise Training and Lumbar Bone Mineral Content in Postmenopausal Women," *Annals of Internal Medicine,* vol. 108, no. 6, June 1988.

Page 102
"Where to Find Calcium" adapted from *Nutritive Value of Foods* (Washington, D.C.: U.S. Department of Agriculture, 1985).

Page 104
"Calcium Intake: The Ideal versus the Reality" adapted from "Osteoporosis: A Decade's Findings in Prevention, Diagnosis, and Treatment," *The Female Patient*, vol. 11, September 1986.

Page 106
"Where We Get Our Calcium" adapted from *Introductory Nutrition*, Helen A. Guthrie (St. Louis: C.V. Mosby Co., 1986).

Caffeine and Coffee
Page 108
"How Much Coffee Do You Drink?" from "United States of America, Coffee Drinking Study, Winter 1988," (London, England: International Coffee Organization, 1988).

Page 109
"Young People Have Kicked the Habit" from "United States of America, Coffee Drinking Study, Winter 1988" (London, England: International Coffee Organization, 1988).

Page 109
"Who Drinks the Most Coffee?" from "Green Coffee Statistics" (Washington, D.C.: USDA/ Foreign Agricultural Service, 1989; and from Glenn D. Considine, *Foods and Food Production Encyclopedia* (New York: Van Nostrand Reinhold Company, Inc., 1982).

Page 110
"England Is Losing Her Thirst for Tea" adapted from "Britain's Thirst for Tea Wanes," *New York Times*, September 21, 1987.

Page 110
"How Much Caffeine Is Okay?" adapted from "Dictionary of Healing Techniques & Remedies," *Prevention*, vol. 41, no. 3, March 1989.

Page 113
"A Protective Role against Asthma" adapted from "Dictionary of Healing Techniques & Remedies," *Prevention*, vol. 41, no. 3, March 1989.

Cancer
Page 116
"What Causes Cancer?" adapted from *Understanding Cancer*, Mark Renneker, M.D. (Palo Alto, Calif.: Bull Publishing Co., 1988).

Page 117
"It Matters Where You Live" adapted from *Cancer Facts and Figures—1989* (Atlanta: American Cancer Society, 1989).

Page 118
"Worldwide Cancer Rates—The Best and the Worst" adapted from *Cancer Rates and Risks* (Washington, D.C.: U.S. Department of Health and Human Services, April 1985).

Page 120
"Who's at Risk" adapted from *Cancer Facts and Figures—1989* (Atlanta: American Cancer Society, 1989).

Page 121
"Smoker's Roulette" adapted from *Cecil Textbook of Medicine*, James Wyngaarden, ed. (Philadelphia: W. B. Saunders Co., 1988).

Page 124
"What the Experts Recommend" adapted from *Understanding Cancer*, Mark Renneker, M.D. (Palo Alto, Calif.: Bull Publishing Co., 1988).

Page 125
"50 Cancer-Fighting Foods" from "Eat to Beat Cancer," *Prevention*, vol. 41, no. 2, February 1989.

Page 129
"Cancer Treatment Options" adapted from *Cancer Facts and Figures—1989* (Atlanta: American Cancer Society, 1989).

Page 130
"Advanced Treatments Not Fully Utilized" adapted from *Cancer Treatment 1975–1985* (Gaithersburg, Md.: U.S. General Accounting Office, January, 1988).

Cholesterol
Page 132
"How High Is Too High?" adapted from *So You Have High Blood Cholesterol* (Washington, D.C.: National Institutes of Health, September 1987).

Page 133
"Global Highs and Lows" adapted from Art Ulene, *Count Out Cholesterol* (Los Angeles: Feeling Fine Programs, Inc., 1989).

Page 133
"Women 'Win' in the End" from *So You Have High Blood Cholesterol* (Washington, D.C.: National Institutes of Health, September 1987).

Page 134
"A Healthy Ratio" adapted from "All about Your Cholesterol Numbers," *Prevention*, vol. 41, no. 3, March 1989.

Page 135
"High Cholesterol Kills" adapted from "Is Relationship between Serum Cholesterol and Risk of Premature Death from Coronary Heart Disease Continuous and Graded?" *Journal of the American Medical Association*, vol. 256, no. 20, November 28, 1986.

Page 136
"Are You at Risk?" adapted from "An Approach to the Management of Hyperlipoproteinemia," *Journal of the American Medical Association*, vol. 255, no. 4, January 24–31, 1986.

Page 136
"The Framingham Study: How HDL Protects" adapted from "Incidence of Coronary Heart Disease and Lipoprotein Cholesterol Levels," *Journal of the American Medical Association*, vol. 256, no. 20, November 28, 1986.

Page 137
"Can Heart Disease Be Stopped?" adapted from "Diet, Lipoproteins, and the Progression of Coronary Atherosclerosis," *The New England Journal of Medicine*, vol. 312, no. 13, March 28, 1985.

Page 139
"Which Diet Lowers Cholesterol the Most?" adapted from "Plasma Lipids and Lipoprotein Cholesterol Concentrations in People with Different Diets in Britain," *British Medical Journal*, vol. 295, no. 6,594, August 8, 1987.

Page 139
"How Much Saturated Fat Is Too Much?" from *Good Fat, Bad Fat: How to Lower Your Blood Cholesterol in Adults*, Griffin & Castelli (Tucson, Ariz.: Fisher Books, 1989).

Page 140
"How Much Saturated Fat and Cholesterol Are You Eating?" from *Eating to Lower Your High Blood Cholesterol* (Washington, D.C.: National Institutes of Health, September 1987).

Page 143
"Which Fat Should You Reach for First?" adapted from "Nutrition, Cholesterol, and Heart Disease Part III: How Diet Affects Blood Cholesterol Levels," *Nutrition Forum*, vol. 6, no. 3, May–June 1989.

Page 144
"Take a 'CSI' Tally" adapted from *The New American Diet System*, Sonja L. Connor, M.S., R.D., and William E. Connor, M.D. (New York: Simon and Schuster, 1991).

Page 147
"How Long Does It Take to Lower Cholesterol?" from *So You Have High Blood Cholesterol* (Washington, D.C.: National Institutes of Health, September 1987).

Page 147
"Drugs That Drop Cholesterol" adapted from "Lipid Disorders: Diet and Drug Therapy," *Modern Medicine*, vol. 56, no. 9, September 1988; and "New Guidelines for the Evaluation and Treatment of Hypercholesterolemia," *Modern Medicine*, vol. 56, no. 12, December 1988.

Page 148
"The Stress Effect" adapted from "Serum Cholesterol and Thyroxine in Young Women during Mental Stress," *Experimental and Clinical Endocrinology*, vol. 83, no. 3, 1984.

Page 149
"Divers Have Their Ups and Downs" adapted from "Serum Uric Acid and Cholesterol Variability," *Journal of the American Medical Association*, vol. 206, no. 13, December 23–30, 1968.

Death
Page 151
"The Ten Leading Causes of Death" from *Health, United States, 1988* (Hyattsville, Md.: U.S. Department of Health and Human Services, March 1989).

Page 152
"When Four Killers Reach Their Peak"
adapted from *Accident Facts* (Chicago:
National Safety Council, 1988).

Page 153
"The Decline of Heart Disease" from *Health,
United States, 1988* (Hyattsville, Md.: U.S.
Department of Health and Human Services,
March 1989).

Page 154
"Where and When Lightning Kills" infor-
mation provided by Paul Hudspeth, National
Climatic Data Center, telephone interview,
November 20, 1989.

Page 155
"What Are Your Odds of Being Murdered?"
information provided by Bruce Taylor,
Ph.D., U.S. Bureau of Justice Statistics,
telephone interview, November 28, 1989.

Page 156
"What Are Your Chances of Dying This
Year?" from *Almanac of the American
People,* by Tom and Nancy Biracree. Copy-
right © 1988 by Tom and Nancy Biracree.
Reprinted with the permission of Facts on
File, Inc., New York.

Page 157
"Where People Live the Longest" from *U.S.
Decennial State Life Tables* (Hyattsville,
Md.: National Center for Health Statistics).

Page 158
"How Many of Your Classmates Are Left?"
from *Vital Statistics of the United States,
1986,* Life Tables, vol. II, section 6
(Hyattsville, Md.: U.S. Department of Health
and Human Services, October 1988).

Page 158
"Where People Die" adapted from "A
Survey of the Last Days of Life: Overview
and Initial Results," (Washington, D.C.:
Social Statistics Section Proceedings of the
American Statistical Association, 1987).

Page 159
"File on the Famous: They Did So Much in
So Little Time" from *The New Encyclopae-
dia Britannica, Micropaedia* (Chicago: Ency-
clopaedia Britannica, Inc., 1977); and from
Information Please Almanac 1989 (Boston:
Houghton Mifflin Company, 1989).

Dental Problems

Page 161
"Dental Emergencies: What to Do" information provided by Phil Weinstraub, American Dental Association, telephone interview,
November 20, 1989.

Page 161
"Cavities are Commonplace" adapted from
Oral Health of United States Adults (National
Institute of Dental Research, 1987).

Page 162
"Dental Fillings—What's Right for You?"
adapted from "Dental Fillings," *Prevention,*
vol. 40, no. 8, August 1988.

Page 163
"Children Are Getting Fewer Cavities"
adapted from *Caries Prevalence in U.S.
Schoolchildren 1986–1987* (Washington,
D.C.: Department of Health and Human
Services, 1988).

Page 164
"Are People Really Afraid of Dentists?"
adapted from "The Prevalence and Practice Management Consequences of Dental
Fear in a Major U.S. City," *Journal of the
American Dental Association,* vol. 116, May
1988.

Page 165
"How Long Since Your Last Dental Visit?"
adapted from *Oral Health of U.S. Adults*
(National Institute of Dental Research,
1987).

Page 166
"How Many Teeth Are Left?" adapted from
Oral Health of U.S. Adults (National Insti-
tute of Dental Research, 1987).

Page 167
"When Teeth Meet the Acid Test" from
"Beautiful Teeth: A Practical-Tip Update,"
Prevention, vol. 36, no. 4, April 1984.

Diabetes

Page 171
"Where is Diabetes Most Common?" adapted
from *Current Estimates from the National
Health Interview Survey, United States 1987*
(Hyattsville, Md.: U.S. Department of Health
and Human Services, 1988).

Page 172
"Diabetes Is on the Rise" adapted from
"The Demographics of Diabetes," *Ameri-
can Demographics,* April 1987.

Page 173
"How to Recognize Diabetic Emergencies"
reprinted with permission from *A Word to
Teachers and School Staff.* Copyright ©
1986 American Diabetes Association.

Page 174
"A Higher Rate of Hospitalization" from
*Direct and Indirect Costs of Diabetes in the
United States in 1987.* Copyright © 1988
American Diabetes Association. Reprinted
with permission.

Page 175
"Eye Disease—A Likely Complication"
adapted from "Diabetic Retinopathy," *Postgraduate Medicine,* vol. 81, no. 6, May 1,
1987.

Page 176
"Diet Recommendations Have Changed"
adapted from *Diabetes Forecast,* October
1989.

Page 177
"Life Expectancy for Diabetics" adapted
from *Diabetes in America* (Alexandria, Va.:
National Diabetes Data Group of National
Institutes of Health, 1985).

Digestive Problems

Page 179
"Chronic Problems for Many" adapted
from *Disease Prevention/Health Promotion:
The Facts* (Washington, D.C.: U.S. Department of Health and Human Services,
1988).

Page 179
"Who's at Greatest Risk?" adapted from
*Disease Prevention/Health Promotion: The
Facts* (Washington, D.C.: U.S. Department
of Health and Human Services, 1988).

Page 180
"Off-the-Shelf Digestive Aids" adapted from
The Complete Book of Better Digestion,
Michael Oppenheim, M.D. (Emmaus, Pa.:
Rodale Press, 1990).

Page 181
"A Guide to Digestive Diseases" adapted
from *Listen to Your Body,* Michaud, et al.
(Emmaus, Pa.: Rodale Press, 1988).

Page 183
"Where Gas Comes From" from "Management of Irritable Bowel Syndrome," *Modern Medicine,* vol. 57, no. 5, May 1989.

Page 184
"Choosing the Right Firefighter" adapted
from "Why You Must Counsel Your Antacid
Patient," *U.S. Pharmacist,* vol. 13, no. 4,
April 1988.

Page 188
"Understanding Ulcers" adapted from *The
Complete Book of Better Digestion,* Michael
Oppenheim, M.D. (Emmaus, Pa.: Rodale
Press, 1990); and from *The American
Medical Association Family Medical Guide*
(New York: Random House, 1987).

Environment and Health

Page 193
"Pollution: Our Most Pressing Problem?"
adapted from "The Environment," *Gallup
Report,* no. 285, June 1989.

Page 193
"The 20 Areas with the Worst Smog"
adapted from "Health and Fitness," *The
Walking Magazine,* July–August 1989.

Page 194
"Toxic Emissions: The Top Ten States"
adapted from "Is Breathing Hazardous to
Your Health?" *Newsweek,* April 3, 1989.

Page 195
"Carbon Monoxide—An Indoor Problem,
Too" adapted from "Air Quality in the
Home," *EPRI Journal,* March 1982, as
appeared in *Healthy Living in an Unhealthy
World,* Calabrese and Dorsey (New York:
Simon and Schuster, 1984).

Page 196
"Where Air Pollutants Come From" adapted
from "Indoor and Outdoor Pollutants and
the Upper Respiratory Tracts," *Journal of
Allergy and Clinical Immunology,* vol. 81,
no. 5, May 1988.

Page 197
"Now Your Oven's Clean, but . . ." adapted from "Air Quality in the Home," *EPRI Journal,* March 1982, as appeared in *Healthy Living in an Unhealthy World,* Calabrese and Dorsey (New York: Simon and Schuster, 1984).

Page 198
"What's Going Up in Smoke?" adapted from *Healthy Living in an Unhealthy World,* Calabrese and Dorsey (New York: Simon and Schuster, 1984).

Page 199
"Are Neighbors of Nuclear Plants at Risk?" adapted from *Cancer Mortality Changes around Nuclear Facilities in Connecticut,* Dr. E. J. Sternglass, testimony at the Congressional Seminar on Low-Level Radiation, February 10, 1978, Washington, D.C., as appeared in *Radiation Alert: A Consumer's Guide to Radiation,* David I. Poch (Canada: Doubleday Canada Ltd., 1985).

Page 200
"Where Radon Risk Is Greatest" adapted from *Executive Fitness,* vol. 20, no. 2, February 1989.

Page 201
"Other People's Smoke Can Pollute Your Lungs" adapted from *Indoor Air Quality and Human Health,* Isaac Turiel (Stanford, Calif.: Stanford University Press, 1985).

Page 202
"Water: What's Safe to Drink" adapted from *Rodale's Practical Homeowner,* January 1987.

Page 203
"What We're Doing to Make the Environment Healthier" adapted from *Gallup Report,* no. 285, June 1989.

Fitness
Page 205
"The Best Fitness Activities" adapted from *The Athlete Within: A Personal Guide to Total Fitness* by Harvey B. Simon, M.D., and Steven R. Levisohn, M.D. Copyright © 1987 by Charter Oak Trust and Harvey B. Simon Family Trust. By permission of Little, Brown and Company.

Page 206
"Where You'll Find the Fit" adapted from *Prevention Index 1988,* (Emmaus, Pa.: Rodale Press, 1988).

Page 207
"The More Degrees, the More Activities" adapted from "Where's the Boom?" *American Demographics,* vol. 9, no. 3, March 3, 1987.

Page 209
"Active People Live Longer" adapted from "More Good News for Walkers," *Walker's World Newsletter,* vol. 1, no. 1, Summer 1986.

Page 210
"Train at the Rate That's Right for Your Heart" adapted from *Running for a Healthy Heart* (Dallas, Tex.: American Heart Association, 1988).

Page 211
"How Hot Is Too Hot?" adapted from "Too Hot to Exercise," *Muscle and Fitness,* vol. 48, no. 10, October 1987.

Page 212
"How Fit Are Kids Today?" adapted from "The National Children and Youth Fitness Study II," *Journal of Physical Education, Recreation, and Dance,* November–December 1987.

Page 212
"Fitness for Mr. Fix-It" from "Heart Disease Prevention for Nonexercisers," *Body Bulletin,* July 1988.

Page 213
"Walking on the Job: Who Does the Most?" adapted from "Healthy Occupations: Work to Walk," *American Health Magazine,* vol. 7, no. 1, January–February 1988.

Page 214
"Steroids–A Dangerous Trap for Young Athletes" adapted from "Estimated Prevalence of Anabolic Steroid Use among Male High School Seniors," *Journal of the American Medical Association,* vol. 260, no. 23, December 16, 1988.

Page 215
"The Sports with the Most Injuries" adapted from "Athletic Injuries: Comparison by Age, Sports, and Gender," *American Journal of Sports Medicine,* vol. 14, no. 3, May–June 1986.

Food and Health
Page 217
"What Concerns Shoppers Most" adapted from *Trends: Consumer Attitudes and the Supermarket* (Washington, D.C.: Food Marketing Institute, 1988).

Page 218
"Fixing Food Differently" adapted from *Trends: Consumer Attitudes and the Supermarket* (Washington, D.C.: Food Marketing Institute, 1988).

Page 219
"The Fat Finder" adapted from "The Fat-Fighter's Bible" parts 1–4, *Prevention,* vol. 41, nos. 5–8, May–August 1989.

Page 228
"Who Eats the Most Fish?" adapted from *Food Consumption, Prices, and Expenditures, 1966–1987* (Washington, D.C.: U.S. Department of Agriculture, January 1989).

Page 230
"The Omega-3 Fish Oil Finder" adapted from *Composition of Foods: Finfish and Shellfish Products* (Washington, D.C.: U.S. Department of Agriculture, September 1987.)

Page 232
"The Fiber Finder" adapted from "100 Top Fiber Foods," *Prevention,* vol. 41, no. 11, November 1989.

Page 234
"More Vegetables, Less Lung Cancer" adapted from "Vegetable Consumption and Lung Cancer Risk: A Population-Based Case-Control Study in Hawaii," *Journal of the National Cancer Institute,* vol. 81, no. 15, August 2, 1989.

Page 236
"The 100 Healthiest Foods" adapted from "Best Diet and Healing Foods," *Prevention,* vol. 41, no. 9, September 1989.

Page 240
"Dumpty Takes Plunge" adapted from *Food Consumption, Prices, and Expenditures, 1966–1987; Food Consumption, Prices, and Expenditures, 1963–1983;* and *U.S. Food Consumption, 1906–1963* (Washington, D.C.: U.S. Department of Agriculture, 1989, 1984, 1964).

Page 241
"Trends in Healthy Eating" adapted from *Food Consumption, Prices, and Expenditures, 1966–1987* (Washington, D.C.: U.S. Department of Agriculture, January 1989).

Page 242
"Our Favorite Salad Fixings" adapted from *The Packer Focus: Fresh Trends 1989* (Lincolnshire, Ill.: Vance Publishing Corp., 1989).

Page 243
"Heads above Iceberg: The Best Leafy Greens" adapted from "Heads above Iceberg: Better Alternatives," *Quick and Healthy Cooking,* Summer 1987; and *Composition of Foods: Vegetables and Vegetable Products* (Washington, D.C.: U.S. Department of Agriculture, August 1984).

Page 244
"Food, Guilt, and Self-Indulgence" adapted from *Fish & Fitness* (Cleveland, Ohio: North Atlantic Seafood Association, 1988); and "Alert '88: Key Trends & Predictions," *Research Alert,* vol. 5, no. 15, January 8, 1988.

Page 245
"When Do People Eat Fresh Fruit?" adapted from *The Packer Focus: Fresh Trends 1987* (Lincolnshire, Ill.: Vance Publishing Corp., 1986); and "Fruit: Something Good That's Not Illegal, Immoral, or Fattening," *FDA Consumer,* May 1988.

Page 245
"Comparing Diets: Soviets and Americans" adapted from "Comparing Soviet and U.S. Food Supplies," *National Food Review,* vol. 11, no. 1, January 3, 1988.

Page 246
"America's Favorite Ethnic Cuisines" adapted from "You Are Where You Eat," *American Demographics,* July 1987. Used with permission.

Foot Problems

Page 248
"Why Your Tootsies Are Tired Tonight" adapted from *Ten Steps to Comfort,* Charles S. Smith (Dayton, Va.: CSS Publications, Inc., 1986).
Page 249
"The Top Five Foot Complaints" information provided by Debra Ponczek, Porter/Novelli for Scholl, Inc., telephone interview, August 31, 1989.
Page 249
"Pronation vs. Supination: Which Side Are You On?" adapted from "Running Injuries," *Clinical Symposia,* vol. 32, no. 4, 1980. Additional information supplied by Neal Kramer, M.D., Bethlehem, Pa., interview, September 21 & 25, 1989.
Page 253
"A Quick and Easy Foot Massage" adapted from *Executive Fitness,* vol. 15, no. 11, May 26, 1984.

Gender Differences

Page 257
"Women Have More Chronic Illness" adapted from "A Life-and-Death . . ." *American Demographics,* vol. 10, no. 7, July 1988.
Page 258
"Different Ways of Dying" adapted from "Sex-Related Differences in Health and Illness," *Psychology of Women Quarterly,* vol. 12, 1988.
Page 259
"Life Expectancy at Birth: Girls Have the Edge" adapted from "Life Expectancy Remains at Record Level," *Statistical Bulletin,* vol. 70, no. 3, July–September 1989.
Page 260
"How Many Years Are Still Ahead?" adapted from "Life Expectancy Remains at Record Level," *Statistical Bulletin,* vol. 70, no. 3, July–September 1989.
Page 262
"Answering Nature's Call" adapted from "Rest Area Usage Design Criteria Update," Washington State Department of Transportation, January 1989.
Page 263
"The Creativity Connection" adapted from *The Opposite Sex,* Anne Campbell (Topsfield, Mass.: Salem House Publishers, 1989).
Page 264
"Who's in the Office (and Who Isn't)" adapted from "Loss of Workdays for Medical Reasons among Metropolitan's Employees in 1982–1983," *Statistical Bulletin.* vol. 66, no. 1, 1985.
Page 265
"Gender at the Gym" adapted from "Survival of the Fittest" *American Demographics,* May 1989.

Headaches

Page 267
"How Long Do Headaches Last?" adapted from "An Epidemiologic Study of Headache among Adolescents and Young Adults," *Journal of the American Medical Association,* vol. 261, no. 15, April 21, 1989.
Page 268
"Frequency of Headaches" adapted from "An Epidemiologic Study of Headache among Adolescents and Young Adults," *Journal of the American Medical Association,* vol. 261, no. 15, April 21, 1989.
Page 268
"The Top Ten Headache Triggers" adapted from *The Nuprin Pain Report,* Humphrey Taylor, et al., September 1985.
Page 269
"A Guide to Common Headaches" adapted from "The Complete Headache Chart" (Chicago: National Headache Foundation).
Page 272
"Pain Patterns in Headaches" adapted from *Migraine and Other Headaches,* James W. Lance, M.D. (New York: Charles Scribner's Sons, 1986).
Page 273
"Foods That Bring Pain" adapted from *Help for Headaches,* Joel R. Saper, M.D., F.A.C.P. (New York: Warner Books, 1987).
Page 274
"Treatment Success Rates" adapted from "Clinical Characterization of Patients with Chronic Headache," *Headache,* vol. 28, no. 9, October 1988.

Health History of the World

Page 278
"Cro-Magnon Man Ate Only the Leanest Meat" adapted from "The Stone-Age Diet," *Men's Health,* vol. 2, no. 7, July 1986.
Page 279
"Stone-Age Health Prescription" reprinted from "The Stone-Age Diet," *Men's Health,* vol. 2, no. 7, July 1986.
Page 281
"Pox, Plague, and Famine: A Grim Scorecard" from *Encyclopedia of Medical History,* Roderick E. McGrew (New York: McGraw-Hill Publishing, 1985); and *The Timetables of Science,* Hellemans and Bunch (New York: Simon and Schuster, 1988); and *The 1989 Information Please Almanac* (Boston: Houghton Mifflin Company, 1988).
Page 283
"Microbe Hunting" adapted from *A Short History of Medicine,* Erwin H. Ackerknecht, M.D. (New York: The Ronald Press Company, 1968); and *The Timetables of Science,* Hellemans and Bunch (New York: Simon and Schuster, 1988).

Hearing

Page 286
"Hearing Problems Increase with Age" adapted from *Vital & Health Statistics* (Hyattsville, Md.: U.S. Department of Health and Human Services, 1988).
Page 287
"How Loud Is That Sound?" adapted from "Noise-Induced Hearing Loss: The Family Physician's Role," *American Family Physician,* vol. 36, no. 6, December 1987; and *The American Medical Association Family Medical Guide,* Kunz and Finkel, eds. (New York: Random House, 1987); and "The Ear," *Better Health and Living,* vol. 3, no. 6, December 1987; and "Your Life Is Too Loud If . . ." *Body Bulletin,* March 1987; and *The Guinness Book of World Records,* Donald McFarlan, ed. (New York: Sterling Publishing Company, Inc., 1988).
Page 288
"Noise Exposure: Safe Limits" adapted from "Noise-Induced Hearing Loss: The Family Physician's Role," *American Family Physician,* vol. 36, no. 6, December 1987.
Page 289
"Comparing Ear Protectors" adapted from *Noise, Ears & Hearing Protection* (Washington, D.C.: American Academy of Otolaryngology—Head and Neck Surgery, Inc., 1985); and "Hearing Protection Guide Directs Users to Manufacturers/Devices by Category," *Occupational Health & Safety,* vol. 57, May 1988.
Page 290
"Why It's Hard to Sleep in a Hospital" adapted from "The Effects of Progressive Muscular Relaxation on Subjectively Reported Disturbance Due to Hospital Noise," *Behavioral Medicine,* vol. 14, no. 1, Spring 1988.
Page 292
"How Sign Language Works" adapted from *Signing/Signed English: A Basic Guide,* Bornstein and Saulnie (New York: Crown Publishers, 1986).
Page 294
"A Guide to Hearing Aids" adapted from "Who's Who in Hearing Aids," *Body Bulletin,* March 1987; and *Hearing Aids: What Are They?* (Washington, D.C.: National Information Center on Deafness, 1987); and information supplied by Bill Mahon, *The Hearing Journal,* telephone interview, December 15, 1989.

Herbs

Page 296
"Herbs That Heal" adapted from *The New Honest Herbal,* Varro E. Tyler (Philadelphia: George F. Stickley Company, 1987). Additional information supplied by Varro E. Tyler, Ph.D., Purdue University, telephone interview, December 1989.

Page 299
"Instead of Salt" adapted from *Cooking with the Healthful Herbs,* Jean Rogers (Emmaus, Pa.: Rodale Press, 1983).
Page 299
"Seven Ancient Immune Helpers" adapted from "Immunomodulating Agents of Plant Origin, 1: Preliminary Screening," *Journal of Ethnopharmacology,* vol. 18, 1986.
Page 301
"Land of 1,000 Healing Herbs" adapted from "Important Chinese Herbal Remedies," *Clinical Therapeutics,* vol. 9, no. 4, 1987.
Page 302
"New Drugs, Old Ingredients" adapted from *Pharmacognosy,* Tyler, Brady, and Robbers (Philadelphia: Lea & Febiger, 1988).
Page 303
"Toxic Tea" adapted from "Toxic Effects of Herbal Teas," *Archives of Environmental Health,* vol. 42, no. 2, May–June 1987.

High Blood Pressure
Page 305
"Defining the 'High' in High Blood Pressure" adapted from *The 1988 Report of the Joint National Committee on Detection, Evaluation, and Treatment of High Blood Pressure* (Bethesda, Md.: National Institutes of Health, May 1988).
Page 306
"Who Has High Blood Pressure?" adapted from "Hypertension and Other Cardiovascular Risk Factors: Focus on Minority Population," *Hypertension Highlights,* vol. 8, no. 1, Spring 1987; and from *Disease Prevention/Health Promotion: The Facts,* U.S. Department of Health and Human Services (Palo Alto, Calif.: Bull Publishing Company, 1988).
Page 307
"What Do People Know about Hypertension?" adapted from *Disease Prevention/Health Promotion: The Facts,* U.S. Department of Health and Human Services (Palo Alto, Calif.: Bull Publishing Company, 1988).
Page 308
"The Geography of High Blood Pressure" adapted from *Current Estimates from the National Health Interview Survey, United States, 1987* (Hyattsville, Md.: U.S. Department of Health and Human Services, September 1988).
Page 310
"The Risks Rise with Pressure" from *High Blood Pressure,* Shulman, Saunders, and Hall (New York: Macmillan Publishing Co., 1987).
Page 311
"A Guide to Home Blood Pressure Monitors" adapted from *Buying and Caring for Home Blood Pressure Equipment* (Dallas, Tex.: American Heart Association).

Page 313
"Where You'll Find the Sodium" from Agriculture Handbook Nos. 8-1, 8-7, 8-8, 8-10, 8-11, 8-12, 8-13, 8-15, 8-16 (Washington, D.C.: U.S. Department of Agriculture); and from *Bowes & Church's Food Values of Portions Commonly Used,* 14th edition, Pennington and Church (Philadelphia: J. B. Lippincott Co., 1985.)
Page 316
"As Obesity Goes, So Goes Hypertension" adapted from "Obesity and Hypertension: Long-Term Effects of Weight Reduction on Blood Pressure," *International Journal of Obesity,* September 1985.
Page 317
"The Hypertension Pharmacy" adapted from "Outsmarting the 'Silent Killer,'" *Prevention,* vol. 41, no. 10, October 1989.

The Human Body
Page 320
"A Full Range of Possible Sizes" adapted from *The Guinness Book of World Records,* Donald McFarlan, ed. (New York: Sterling Publishing Co., Inc., 1989).
Page 321
"The Body You've Always Wanted" adapted from "Survey Finds Desired Body Type Changing," *Executive Fitness,* vol. 19, no. 11, November 1988.
Page 321
"The Major Organs Ranked by Weight" adapted from *Atlas of the Body and Mind* (Chicago: Rand McNally and Company, 1976).
Page 322
"Some Surprising Surface Areas" adapted from *Atlas of the Body and Mind* (Chicago: Rand McNally and Company, 1976).
Page 323
"Body Temperature: The Extremes" adapted from the *Guinness Book of World Records,* Donald McFarlan, ed. (New York: Sterling Publishing Co., Inc., 1989).
Page 323
"If You Can't Stand the Heat . . ." adapted from the *Guinness Book of World Records,* Donald McFarlan, ed. (New York: Sterling Publishing Co., Inc., 1989).
Page 329
"Baby's a Half-Pint, But Not for Long" adapted from *Atlas of the Body and Mind* (Chicago: Rand McNally and Company, 1976).
Page 338
"Water In Equals Water Out" adapted from *Introductory Nutrition,* Helen A. Guthrie, Ph.D., D.Sc., R.D. (St. Louis: Times Mirror/ Mosby College Publishing, 1989).
Page 343
"Bad News Travels Fast" adapted from *Human Physiology and Mechanisms of Disease,* Arthur C. Guyton, M.D. (Philadelphia: W.B. Saunders Co., 1987).

Page 345
"A Nail's Pace" adapted from *Principles of Anatomy and Physiology,* Tortora and Anagnostakos (New York: Harper & Row Publishers, Inc., 1984).

Infections
Page 350
"Is It a Cold or the Flu?" adapted from *Harrison's Principles of Internal Medicine,* Eugene Braunwald, et al. (New York: McGraw-Hill Book Company, 1987).
Page 352
"The Negative Impact of Infections" adapted from *Disease Prevention/Health Promotion: The Facts,* U.S. Department of Health and Human Services (Palo Alto, Calif.: Bull Publishing Company, 1987).
Page 354
"Day Care: A High Infection Rate" adapted from "Frequency and Severity of Infections in Day Care," *The Journal of Pediatrics,* vol. 112, no. 4, April 1988.
Page 355
"A Guide to Childhood Immunizations" adapted from "Recommended Schedule for Active Immunization of Normal Infants and Children," *Morbidity and Mortality Weekly Report,* April 7, 1989.
Page 356
"Putting the Chill on Food-Borne Infections" adapted from "Food Poisoning and Traveller's Diarrhea," *Nutrition and Health,* vol. 9, no. 2, 1987.
Page 358
"Immunizations—Protection for Adults, Too" adapted from *Cecil Textbook of Medicine,* Wyngaarden and Smith, et al. (Philadelphia: W. B. Saunders Co., 1988).

Medical Care
Page 361
"How Did You Select Your Current Doctor?" adapted from "I Love My Doctor But . . .," *Prevention,* vol. 41, no. 8, August 1989.
Page 362
"How Long Since Your Last Contact?" adapted from *Health, United States, 1988* (Washington, D.C.: U.S. Department of Health and Human Services, March 1989).
Page 363
"Hey, Doc, Tell Me More About . . ." adapted from "I Love My Doctor But . . .," *Prevention,* vol. 41, no. 8, August 1989.
Page 364
"How Much Time Is Spent with Each Patient?" adapted from "National Study of Medical and Surgical Specialties," University of Southern California, *Washington Post,* April 4, 1989.

Page 365
"What Doctors Do That Their Patients Dislike" adapted from "I Love My Doctor But . . .," *Prevention*, vol. 41, no. 8, August 1989.

Page 366
"How Doctors Rate Each Other" adapted from "How Physicians Size Each Other Up," *Medical Economics*, vol. 64, no. 14, July 13, 1987.

Page 367
"The Number of Physicians Continues to Rise" adapted from *Health, United States, 1988* (Washington, D.C.: U.S. Department of Health and Human Services, March 1989).

Page 368
"Where in the World Are the Doctors?" adapted from *World Development Report 1989* (Washington, D.C.: International World Bank, 1989).

Page 375
"Hospital Stays Are Getting Shorter" adapted from *Health, United States, 1988* (Washington, D.C.: U.S. Department of Health and Human Services, March 1989).

Page 377
"The Most Common Hospital Infections" adapted from "Nosocomial Infection Surveillance, 1984," *Centers for Disease Control Surveillance Summaries*, vol. 35, no. 155.

Page 378
"Nursing Home Population Soars" adapted from *Health, United States, 1988* (Washington, D.C.: U.S. Department of Health and Human Services, March 1989).

Page 379
"The Most Frequently Performed Operations" adapted from *Socio-Economic Factbook for Surgery 1989*, American College of Surgeons, 1989.

Page 379
"More Women Are Becoming Surgeons" adapted from *Socio-Economic Factbook for Surgery 1989* (American College of Surgeons, 1989).

Page 380
"Who Undergoes Surgery?" adapted from "1987 Summary: National Hospital Discharge Survey," *Advancedata*, U.S. Department of Health and Human Services, September 9, 1988.

Page 381
"How Surgical Risk Can Vary" adapted from "Investigation of the Relationship between Volume and Mortality for Surgical Procedures Performed in New York State Hospitals," *Journal of the American Medical Association*, vol. 262, no. 4, July 28, 1989.

Page 381
"Transplant Trends" adapted from *Socio-Economic Factbook for Surgery 1989* (American College of Surgeons, 1989).

Page 382
"The Most Important Health Care Issues" adapted from *Rights and Responsibilities: A National Survey of Healthcare Opinions* (Lexington, Ky.: The American Board of Family Practice).

Page 383
"Health Care Coverage—Where the Gaps Are" adapted from *Health, United States, 1989* (Washington, D.C.: U.S. Department of Health and Human Services, March 1989).

Page 384
"What the United States Spends for Health" adapted from *Health Care Financing Review*, U.S. Department of Health and Human Services, vol. 7, no. 1, Fall 1985; and vol. 10, no. 2, Winter 1988.

Medical Oddities

Page 396
"Making the Most of Multiple Births" adapted from "Multiple Births: An Upward Trend in the United States," *Statistical Bulletin*, January–March 1988.

Page 399
"Wasp-Waisted Women" adapted from *ABC's of the Human Body*, Reader's Digest (Pleasantville, N.Y.: Reader's Digest Association, 1987).

Medications

Page 401
"The Ten Most Prescribed Drugs" information provided by Tina Pugliese, American Pharmaceutical Association, telephone interview, January 10, 1990.

Page 402
"How Drugs Enter the Body" adapted from *Guide to Prescriptions and Over-the-Counter Drugs* (New York: American Medical Association, 1988).

Page 403
"Decoding Your Prescription" adapted from *Guide to Prescription and Over-the-Counter Drugs* (New York: American Medical Association, 1988).

Page 404
"Eight Items That Belong in Every Medicine Cabinet" adapted from "10 Essential Healers and Helpers," *Prevention*, vol. 40, no. 7, July 1988.

Page 406
"Drugs That Contain Alcohol" adapted from *Physicians' Desk Reference* (Oradell, N.J.: Medical Economics Company, 1989).

Page 407
"Side Effects of Common Prescription Drugs" adapted from *Physicians' Desk Reference* (Oradell, N.J.: Medical Economics Company, 1989).

Page 410
"How Beta-Blockers Work" adapted from *Guide to Prescription and Over-the-Counter Drugs* (New York: American Medical Association, 1988).

Page 411
"Choosing an Antihistamine" adapted from *Guide to Prescription and Over-the-Counter Drugs* (New York: American Medical Association, 1988).

Page 411
"Taken as Prescribed?" adapted from "How Often Is Medication Prescribed?" *Journal of the American Medical Association*, vol. 261, no. 22, June 9, 1989.

Page 412
"First-Aid Products Compared" adapted from "Comparison of Topical Antibiotic Ointments, a Wound Protectant, and Antiseptics for the Treatment of Human Blister Wounds Contaminated with Staphylococcus aureus," *The Journal of Family Practice*, vol. 24, no. 6, 1987.

Page 413
"Finding the Right Antibiotic for the Job" adapted from *The American Medical Association Guide to Prescription and Over-the-Counter Drugs* edited by Charles B. Clayman, M.D. Copyright © 1988 by Random House, Inc. Reprinted by permission.

Page 415
"Generics versus Brand Names" information provided by Ron Stocker, Walter's Pharmacy, Allentown, Pa., telephone interview, December 28, 1989.

Mental Illness

Page 417
"The Risks: In the Course of a Month" adapted from "One-Month Prevalence of Mental Disorders in the United States," *Archives of General Psychiatry*, vol. 45, November 1988.

Page 417
"The Risks: In the Course of a Lifetime" adapted from "One-Month Prevalence of Mental Disorders in the United States," *Archives of General Psychiatry*, vol. 45, November 1988.

Page 418
"The Major Mental Illnesses" adapted from *Anxiety Disorders*, American Psychiatric Association, 1988; and *Schizophrenia*, American Psychiatric Association, 1988.

Page 421
"On the Couch, by the Hour" data compiled from information supplied by Sue Heffner, American Psychiatric Association, telephone interview, December 20, 1989.

Page 423
"Where Are the Seriously Mentally Ill?" adapted from "What Is Serious Mental Illness," *Public Citizen*.

Mind/Body Interactions

Page 425
"Where the Body Is Targeted by Stress" adapted from "Take the AMA Stress Test," *Prevention*, vol. 38, no. 7, July 1986.

Page 426
"How the Skin Mirrors Emotion" adapted from "Emotional Aspects of Cutaneous Disease," *Dermatology in General Medicine,* ed. by T. B. Fitzpatrick, et. al (New York: McGraw-Hill, 1979).

Page 427
"Stress Hits Home with Baby Boomers" adapted from *National Center for Health Statistics-Advancedata* no. 126 (Hyattsville, Md.: U.S. Department of Health and Human Services, September 19, 1986).

Page 429
"The Cancer Personality" adapted from "Personality Predicts Early Death," *Brain/Mind Bulletin,* vol. 14, no. 6, March 1989.

Page 430
"Saved by Their Fighting Spirit" data from *Good Relationships Are Good Medicine,* Barbara Powell, Ph.D (Emmaus, Pa.: Rodale Press, 1987).

Page 431
"Optimists Are Healthier" from "Minding Your Health," *Prevention,* vol. 40, no. 5, May 1988.

Page 432
"Hypnotherapy and Kids" data from "Hypnotherapy in Children," *Post Graduate Medicine,* vol. 79, no. 4, March 1986.

Page 433
"The Healing Power of Pets" adapted from *The Kal Kan Report: Pets on Prescription* (Vernon, Calif.: Kal Kan Foods, Inc., August 12, 1986).

Page 435
"Meditators Have a Health Advantage" adapted from "Medical Care and the Transcendental Meditation Program," *Psychosomatic Medicine,* vol. 49, no. 3, September–October 1987.

Page 436
"Marriage Is Good for Your Health" adapted from "Marriage May Promote Health," *Medical World News,* December 26, 1988.

Moods
Page 439
"What Makes Us Angry or Impatient?" adapted from *Almanac of the American People,* Biracree and Biracree (New York: Facts on File, Inc., 1988).

Page 440
"What Do We Daydream About?" adapted from "Green Colors Daydreams," *USA Today,* July 1, 1989.

Page 441
"The Foods That Shape Our Moods" adapted from *Maximum Brainpower,* the editors of *Prevention* Magazine Health Books (Emmaus, Pa.: Rodale Press, 1989).

Page 442
"Anxiety—What Causes It?" adapted from *Shyness,* Jones, Check, and Briggs (New York: Plenum Publishing Corp., 1986).

Page 443
"In the Mood for Murder" adapted from "Temperature and Aggression: Ubiquitous Effects of Heat on Occurrence of Human Violence," *Psychological Bulletin,* vol. 106, no. 1, 1989.

Page 444
"How Health Habits Affect Mood" adapted from "Personal Health Habits and Symptoms of Depression at the Community Level," *Preventive Medicine,* vol. 17, no. 2, 1988.

Pain
Page 447
"How Pains Compare" adapted from *Conquering Pain,* Sampson Lipton (New York: Arco Publishing, 1984).

Page 447
"Fewer Aches As We Age" adapted from *The Nuprin Pain Report* (New York: Louis Harris and Associates, Inc. for Bristol-Myers Products, 1985).

Page 448
"Lost Workdays Due to Pain" adapted from *The Nuprin Pain Report* (New York: Louis Harris and Associates, Inc., for Bristol-Myers Products, 1985).

Page 449
"How Sufferers Rate Their Aches" reprinted from *The Nuprin Pain Report* (New York: Louis Harris and Associates, Inc. for Bristol-Myers Products, 1985). Used with permission.

Page 450
"Who's Tough Enough to Stand the Pain?" adapted from "Acute-Pain Tolerance among Athletes," *Canadian Journal of Sport Sciences,* vol. 12, no. 4, December 1987.

Page 452
"Who Treats Pain?" adapted from *The Nuprin Pain Report* (New York: Louis Harris and Associates, Inc. for Bristol-Myers Products, 1985).

Pet Health
Page 455
"When Your Pet Needs Its 'Shots' " adapted from *The Pet First-Aid Book,* Hill, Myers, and Hawkins (New York: McGraw-Hill Book Company, 1986).

Page 456
"When Your Pet Can Make You Sick" adapted from "Healthy Tips for Close People/Pet Encounters," *Prevention,* vol. 40, no. 4, April 1988.

Page 457
"How Male and Female Dogs Differ" adapted from *The Perfect Puppy,* Hart and Hart (Oxford, England: W. H. Freeman and Company, 1988).

Page 458
"If Your Dog Were Human, How Old Would It Be?" from *The Pet First-Aid Book,* Hill, Myers, and Hawkins (New York: McGraw-Hill Book Company, 1986).

Page 459
"Where Rabies Strikes" from *Rabies Surveillance 1986* (Atlanta: U.S. Department of Health and Human Services, 1987).

Page 460
"Rating the Dog Breeds for Personality" adapted from *The Perfect Puppy,* Hart and Hart (Oxford, England: W. H. Freeman and Company, 1988).

Page 461
"Walking the Dog—How Far?" adapted from *The Dog Care Manual,* David Alderton (London: Quarto Publishing Ltd., 1986).

Page 462
"When Cats Get Their Dander Up" adapted from "When the Fur Flies," *Rodale's Allergy Relief,* July 1986.

Page 462
"Animal Facts of Life" adapted from *The Pet First-Aid Book,* Hill, Myers, and Hawkins (New York: McGraw-Hill Book Company, 1986).

Page 463
"Selecting a Pet Bird" adapted from *The Bird Care Book,* Sheldon L. Gerstenfeld, V.M.D. (Reading, Mass.: Addison-Wesley Publishing Company, 1981).

Sex
Page 465
"Marital Sex—How Often?" adapted from *American Couples: Money, Work, Sex,* Blumstein and Schwartz (New York: William Morrow & Co., 1983).

Page 466
"Why Couples Argue" from *Bruskin Report* (New Brunswick, N.J.: R. H. Bruskin Associates).

Page 467
"Happy . . . and Not Interested" adapted from "Some Facts (and Figures) of Life," *Men's Health,* Fall 1987.

Page 468
"About as Satisfying as a Good Book" from *Roper Report 86-4* (New York: Roper Organization, March 1986).

Page 469
"When Sex Is Wrong: Some Opinions" adapted from *General Social Survey—1988,* National Opinion Research Center, 1988; and from *Unchurched Americans: 10 Years Later* (Princeton, N.J.: Gallup Organization, 1988).

Page 470
"Sexual Activity of Teen-Age Girls" from *A Report to the Utah Board of Education on a Federal Family Life Project* (Provo, Utah: Brigham Young University, 1985).

Page 471
"Contraception Methods" adapted from *Understanding U.S. Fertility* (Washington, D.C.: National Center for Health Statistics, December 1984).

Page 473
"Syphilis, Gonorrhea Trends" adapted from *Health, United States, 1988* (Hyattsville, Md.: U.S. Department of Health and Human Services, March 1989).

Skin Problems
Page 477
"Hives: Things That Go Bump in Your Life" adapted from *Urticaria-hives,* American Academy of Dermatology, 1987.

Page 477
"Burns: A Matter of Degree" adapted from *Guard Your Child against Burns,* National Burn Victim Foundation.

Page 478
"Cosmetic Reactions" adapted from "Cosmetic Allergies," *FDA Consumer,* vol. 20, no. 9, November 1986.

Page 479
"An Antiaging Cream That Really Helps" adapted from "Caution Advised in Use of New Antiaging Creams," *Men's Health,* June 1988.

Page 480
"Moles That May Be Dangerous" adapted from *Common Sense about Moles,* American Academy of Dermatology, 1988.

Page 480
"How to Pick the Right Sunscreen" adapted from "Skin Sense," *Children,* Summer 1987.

Page 481
"Reversing the Skin's Signs of Aging" adapted from *The Face Book,* American Academy of Facial and Reconstructive Surgery (Washington, D.C.: Acropolis Books Ltd., 1988).

Page 482
"Should I Have Cosmetic Surgery?" adapted from *The Face Book,* American Academy of Facial and Reconstructive Surgery (Washington, D.C.: Acropolis Books Ltd., 1988).

Sleep
Page 485
"The Patterns of Sleep" adapted from *Secrets of Sleep,* Alexander Borbely (New York: Basic Book Publishers, 1986).

Page 486
"How Long We Sleep" adapted from *Secrets of Sleep,* Alexander Borbely (New York: Basic Book Publishers, 1986).

Page 487
"Neither a Long Nor a Short Sleeper Be" adapted from *Secrets of Sleep,* Alexander Borbely (New York: Basic Book Publishers, 1986).

Page 488
"The 25-Hour Day" adapted from *Secrets of Sleep,* Alexander Borbely (New York: Basic Book Publishers, 1986).

Page 489
"The Sleep/Dream Cycle" adapted from *The Sleep Instinct,* Ray Meddis (London: Routledge Kegan Paul, Ltd., 1977).

Page 490
"The Four Biggest Sleep Complaints" adapted from *Sleep the Gentle Tyrant,* Wilse B. Webb (Englewood Cliffs, N.J.: Prentice Hall, 1975).

Page 491
"What We Dream About" adapted from *Secrets of Sleep,* Alexander Borbely (New York: Basic Book Publishers, 1986).

Page 492
"How Sleeping Pills Affect Sleep Quality" adapted from *Get a Better Night's Sleep,* Oswald and Adam (New York: Arco Publishing, 1983).

Page 493
"Age Brings Less Sleep, Fewer Dreams" adapted from *The Brain,* Richard Restak (New York: Bantam Books, 1984).

Page 494
"Sleep Positions: What They Mean" adapted from *Bruce Jenner's Better Health and Living,* vol. 1, no. 1, August 1988.

Strokes
Page 497
"Stroke Deaths on the Decline" adapted from *1989 Heart Facts,* American Heart Association, 1989.

Page 498
"Where Stroke Deaths Strike" adapted from *Health, United States, 1988* (Washington, D.C.: U.S. Department of Health and Human Services, 1988).

Page 499
"Stroke Risk-An Ethnic Mix" adapted from *Disease Prevention/Health Promotion: The Facts,* U.S. Department of Health and Human Services (Palo Alto, Calif.: Bull Publishing Company, 1988).

Page 500
"Strokes around the Globe" adapted from "WHO World Health Statistics," *Public Health Reports: Journal of the U.S. Public Health Service,* vol. 101, no. 3, May–June 1986.

Page 501
"The Damage Diagrammed" adapted from *Strokes: A Guide for the Family,* American Heart Association, 1981; and from *Stroke: Why Do They Behave That Way?* American Heart Association, 1974.

Page 502
"Strokes and Smokes" adapted from "Cigarette Smoking as a Risk Factor for Stroke," *Journal of the American Medical Association,* vol. 259, no. 7, February 19, 1988.

Page 503
"Excess Alcohol, Excess Risk" adapted from "Stroke and Alcohol Consumption," *The New England Journal of Medicine,* vol. 315, no. 17, October 23, 1986.

Page 504
"De-Stroke Your Diet" adapted from *Composition of Foods,* Agriculture Handbook Nos. 8-1, 8-9, 8-11, 8-12, 8-15, 8-16 (Washington, D.C.: U.S. Department of Agriculture, 1976, 1982, 1984, 1984, 1986, 1987).

Travel
Page 506
"Where the Risk of Digestive Upset Is Greatest" adapted from "Update on Traveler's Diarrhea," *Postgraduate Medicine,* vol. 84, no. 1, July 1988.

Page 506
"Can Traveler's Diarrhea Be Prevented?" adapted from "Prevention of Travelers' Diarrhea by the Tablet Formulation of Bismuth Subsalicylate," *Journal of the American Medical Association,* vol. 257, no. 10, March 13, 1987.

Page 507
"The Dos and Don'ts of Drinking the Water" adapted from *Everyday Health Tips,* Debora Tkac, et al. (Emmaus, Pa.: Rodale Press, 1988).

Page 508
"What You Don't Want to Bring Back From Vacation" from *Health Information for International Travel, 1988* (Washington, D.C.: U.S. Department of Health and Human Services, May 1988).

Page 509
"Think First, Eat Second" adapted from *Traveling Well,* W. Scott Harkonen, M.D. (New York: Dodd, Mead & Company, 1984); and *The Safe Food Book* (Washington, D.C.: U.S. Department of Agriculture, 1984).

Page 511
"Off the Beaten Path: Where Lyme Disease Lurks" adapted from "Lyme Disease," *MMWR,* vol. 38, no. 39, October 5, 1989.

Page 512
"Medical Emergencies Can Keep You Grounded" from "Frequency and Types of Medical Emergencies among Commercial Air Travelers," *Journal of American Medical Association,* vol. 261, no. 9, March 3, 1989.

Page 513
"Fear of Flying Soars to New Heights" from "Criticism of Flight Safety Remains High, But Concern Eases Slightly Since '87," (Princeton, N.J.: Gallup Organization, 1989).

Page 514
"Sickness in Space" adapted from *Everyday Health Tips,* Debora Tkac, et al. (Emmaus, Pa.: Rodale Press, 1988).

Page 515
"Hop on the Bus, Gus" adapted from *Accident Facts* (Chicago: National Safety Council, 1988).

Vision Problems
Page 518
"A Guide to Common Vision Problems" adapted from *Vision and Lifestyle News Backgrounder* (St. Louis, Mo.: American Optometric Association).

Page 519
"Are Nearsighted People Smarter?" adapted from "Intelligence, Education, and Myopia in Males," *Archives of Ophthalmology,* vol. 105, no. 11, November 1987.

Page 520
"Contact Lenses Compared" adapted from "Patient Health Guide," *Journal of American Optometric Association,* vol. 88, no. 8, August 1988; and "Contact Lenses: What to Consider," *Consumer Reports,* June 1989.

Page 522
"How Cataract Surgery Helps" adapted from "Impact of Cataract Surgery with Lens Implantation on Vision and Physical Function in Elderly Patients," *Journal of the American Medical Association,* vol. 257, no. 8, February 27, 1987.

Page 523
"Eye Injuries Are Part of the Game" adapted from *1988 Sports and Recreational Eye Injuries,* National Society to Prevent Blindness, 1989.

Page 524
"The Next Century Will Be a Blur for Many" adapted from "The Dimension of the Problem of Eye Disease among the Elderly," *Ophthalmology,* vol. 94, no. 9, September 1987.

Vitamins and Minerals

Page 526
"Your Recommended Dietary Allowance" adapted from *Recommended Dietary Allowances* (Washington, D.C.: National Research Council, 1989).

Page 530
"Some Additional Nutrients: Safe and Adequate Amounts" adapted from *Recommended Dietary Allowances* (Washington, D.C.: National Research Council, 1989).

Page 532
"Get Your Vitamins and Minerals Here" adapted from *Composition of Foods,* Agriculture Handbook Nos. 8-1, 8-4, 8-5, 8-7 through 8-17 (Washington, D.C.: U.S. Department of Agriculture, 1976, 1979, 1980, 1982–1984, 1986, 1987, 1989); and from *Bowes and Church's Food Values of Portions Commonly Used,* Pennington and Church (Philadelphia: J. B. Lippincott Company, 1985).

Page 535
"How Vitamins Are Lost" adapted from *Food Chemistry,* Owen R. Fennema (New York: Marcel Dekker, Inc., 1985).

Page 536
"Microwave versus Conventional Cooking" adapted from "Vitamin Losses with Microwave Cooking," *Food Sciences and Nutrition,* vol. 42F, no. 3, February 1989.

Page 539
"The Most Common Deficiencies" adapted from "Problem Nutrients in the United States," *Food Technology,* September 1981, as appeared in *Understanding Vitamins and Minerals* (Emmaus, Pa.: Rodale Press, 1984).

Page 539
"Why Do You Take Vitamins?" adapted from *The Gallup Study of Vitamin Use in the United States,* Survey VI, Volume I (Princeton, N.J.: Gallup Organization, December 1982) as appeared in *Vitamin Issues,* vol. 3, no. 2 (Nutley, N.J.: Vitamin Nutrition Information Service, Hoffmann-La Roche, Inc.).

Page 541
"Signs of Deficiency" adapted from *The Complete Book of Vitamins and Minerals for Health* (Emmaus, Pa.: Rodale Press, 1988); and from *Cecil Textbook of Medicine,* Wyngaarden and Smith, et al. (Philadelphia: W. B. Saunders Company, 1988).

Page 542
"A Link between Sunshine, Vitamin D, and Cancer?" adapted from *The Calcium Connection,* Garland and Garland (New York: A Fireside Book, Simon & Schuster, Inc., 1989).

Page 544
"Five Cancer-Fighting Factors" adapted from "Best Bets against Cancer," *Prevention,* vol. 40, no. 10, October 1988.

Weight Loss

Page 548
"How the States Rank in Weight Control" from *Health across America: Prevention Practices in Major States and Cities, Summary Report,* Louis Harris and Associates, Inc. (Emmaus, Pa.: Rodale Press, 1988).

Page 549
"The Ideal Fertility Weight" adapted from "Body Weight Control Practice as a Cause of Infertility," *Clinical Obstetrics and Gynecology,* vol. 28, no. 3, September 1985.

Page 550
"The Dieting Years" from *Calorie Control Council News* (Atlanta: Calorie Control Council, 1989); and Keith Keeney, Calorie Control Council, telephone interview, January 10, 1990.

Page 554
"A Guide to Weight Loss Surgery" compiled from "Surgery for Morbid Obesity," *Postgraduate Medicine,* vol. 83, no. 6, May 1, 1988; and "Gastric Balloons to Treat Obesity" *Postgraduate Medicine,* vol. 83, no. 6, May 1, 1988; and "Report on Weight-Loss Surgery" (Bellerose, N.Y.: National Association to Aid Fat Americans, Inc., 1986); and "Jaw Wiring: Its Role in the Treatment of Obesity" (London: J. S. Garrow); and *Rating the Diets,* Theodore Berland and the editors of Consumer Guide (Skokie, Ill.: The New American Library, Inc., 1979); and "Liposuction: Quick Fix for Fat Pads, But No Substitute for Diet, Exercise," *Environmental Nutrition,* vol. 10, no. 9, September 1987.

Page 556
"Weight Loss Doesn't Buy Love" from "Report on Weight-Loss Surgery" (Bellerose, N.Y.: National Association to Aid Fat Americans, Inc., 1986).

Page 558
"Food Choices: The Fat and the Lean" from *High Energy Living,* the editors of *Prevention* Magazine (Emmaus, Pa.: Rodale Press, 1986).

Page 560
"Fast (and Fattening) Foods" from "Fast Food Fats," *Lose Weight Naturally Newsletter,* vol. 2, no. 12, December 1988.

Page 563
"Still Sweet on Sugar" from *Sugar and Sweetener, Situation and Outlook Yearbook* (Washington, D.C.: U.S. Department of Agriculture, June 1988).

Page 567
"Workouts That Burn Off Weight" adapted from *Maximum Personal Energy,* Charles T. Kuntzleman (Emmaus, Pa.: Rodale Press, 1981).

Page 568
"Your Ideal Calorie Intake" from "A Trick to Tote Up Calories," *Lose Weight Naturally Newsletter,* vol. 1, no. 6, October 1987.

INDEX